Breastfeeding and Mothering in Antiquity and Early Byzantium

This volume offers the first comparative, interdisciplinary, and intercultural examination of the lactating woman – biological mother and othermother – in antiquity and early Byzantium. Adopting methodologies and knowledge deriving from a variety of disciplines, the volume's contributors investigate the close interrelationship between a woman and her lactating breasts, as well as the social, ideological, theological, and medical meanings and uses of motherhood, childbirth, and breastfeeding, along with their visual and literary representations.

Breastfeeding and the work of mothering are explored through the study of a great variety of sources, mainly works of Greek-speaking cultures, written and visual, anonymous and eponymous, which were mostly produced between the first and seventh century AD. Due to their multiple interdisciplinary dimensions, ancient and early Byzantine lactating women are approached through three interconnected thematic strands having a twofold focus: society and ideology, medicine and practice, and art and literature.

By developing the model of the lactating woman, the volume offers a new analytical framework for understanding a significant part of the still unwritten cultural history of the period. At the same time, the volume significantly contributes to the emerging fields of breast and motherhood studies. The new and significant knowledge generated in the fields of ancient and Byzantine studies may also prove useful for cultural historians in general and other disciplines, such as literary studies, art history, history of medicine, philosophy, theology, sociology, anthropology, and gender studies.

Stavroula Constantinou is the founder and director of the Centre for Medieval Arts & Rituals at the University of Cyprus (UCY). She is also the initiator and editor-in-chief of the peer-reviewed and diamond open access journal *Eventum: A Journal of Medieval Arts and Rituals* (first issue in November 2023). Currently, she coordinates the major EU-Horizon 2020 project *Network for Medieval Arts & Rituals* (grant agreement nr 951875) and a couple of other projects on mothering and storytelling. Her research focuses on Byzantine narratives, gender, ritual, performance, emotions, and the body. She is the author of the forthcoming book *Interactive Embodiment: Approaching Byzantine Bodies* (2024).

Aspasia Skouroumouni-Stavrinou is a postdoctoral researcher at the Centre for Medieval Arts & Rituals at UCY. Her research focuses on ancient Greek drama (with an emphasis on performance, space, gender, and reception), ancient Greek religion, ancient and early Byzantine motherhood, and family culture.

Breastfeeding and Mothering in Antiquity and Early Byzantium

Edited by
**Stavroula Constantinou and
Aspasia Skouroumouni-Stavrinou**

Routledge
Taylor & Francis Group

LONDON AND NEW YORK

First published 2024
by Routledge
4 Park Square, Milton Park, Abingdon, Oxon OX14 4RN

and by Routledge
605 Third Avenue, New York, NY 10158

Routledge is an imprint of the Taylor & Francis Group, an informa business

Funded by European Regional Development Fund and the Republic of Cyprus through the Foundation of Research and Innovation.

British Library Cataloguing-in-Publication Data
A catalogue record for this book is available from the British Library.

Library of Congress Cataloging-in-Publication Data
Names: Constantinou, Stavroula, editor. | Skouroumouni-Stavrinou, Aspasia, 1972– editor.
Title: Breastfeeding and mothering in antiquity and early Byzantium / edited by Stavroula Constantinou and Aspasia Skouroumouni-Stavrinou.
Description: Abingdon, Oxon ; New York, NY : Routledge, 2024. | Series: Routledge research in Byzantine studies | Includes bibliographical references. | Identifiers: LCCN 2023026093 (print) | LCCN 2023026094 (ebook) | ISBN 9781032208756 (hardback) | ISBN 9781032208763 (paperback) | ISBN 9781003265658 (ebook)
Subjects: LCSH: Breastfeeding—Byzantine Empire. | Motherhood—Byzantine Empire.
Classification: LCC RJ216 .B7285 2024 (print) | LCC RJ216 (ebook) | DDC 649/.3309495—dc23/eng/20230911
LC record available at https://lccn.loc.gov/2023026093
LC ebook record available at https://lccn.loc.gov/2023026094

ISBN: 978-1-032-20875-6 (hbk)
ISBN: 978-1-032-20876-3 (pbk)
ISBN: 978-1-003-26565-8 (ebk)

DOI: 10.4324/9781003265658

Typeset in Times New Roman
by codeMantra

This book is dedicated to our children
Andreas Roderich, Konstantinos, Eleni, Michail, and Marina

Contents

Figures and Tables

Figures

Tables

Preface

Breastfeeding and Mothering in Antiquity and Early Byzantium is an interdisciplinary and wide-ranging edited collection dealing with aspects of breastfeeding and mothering from antiquity to early Byzantium, focusing mainly on the period from the first to the seventh century of our common era. The study of ancient and early Byzantine breastfeeding and mothering is based on a large variety of sources: textual and visual, eponymous and anonymous, profane and religious. These sources have been approached via pioneering interdisciplinary and combinatory methods from both young and established scholars with well-grounded knowledge in different disciplines: philology, literary studies, history of ideas, history of medicine, art history, archaeology, theology, and gender and performance studies. We hope that the fresh readings that the volume provides will initiate more studies that will further illuminate not only the surveyed sources but also the importance and characteristics of the variegated and often elusive phenomena (in both senses of the word) of premodern, and consequently also of modern breastfeeding and motherhood.

This volume's contents constitute part of the results of a Cyprus-based interdisciplinary research project entitled "Lactating Breasts: Motherhood and Breastfeeding in Antiquity and Byzantium" (MotherBreast 2018–2023; https://www.ucy.ac.cy/motherbreast/), which brought into collaboration cultural historians of diverse expertise with medical practitioners dedicated to the breastfeeding cause. MotherBreast was co-financed by the European Regional Development Fund and the Republic of Cyprus through the Research and Innovation Foundation (project EXCELLENCE/1216/0020), as well as by the University of Cyprus. The project was developed while the editors were also implementing the project "Network for Medieval Arts and Rituals" (NetMAR), which has received funding from the European Union's Horizon 2020 research and innovation programme under grant agreement nr 951875. The opinions expressed in this volume reflect only the authors' views and in no way reflect the European Commission's opinions. The European Commission is not responsible for any use that may be made of the information it contains.

Most of the volume's chapters were developed from papers delivered during three of the MotherBreast project's major scholarly events: an international workshop (8–9 October 2020) entitled "Lactating Breasts: Motherhood and Breastfeeding in Antiquity and Byzantium"; a series of sessions with the general title "Breast

Rules: Motherhood and Breastfeeding in the Middle Ages" which were convened by the editors at Leeds International Medieval Congress (2020 and 2021); and finally, an international conference held in Cyprus (5–7 November 2021) entitled "Motherhood and Breastfeeding in Antiquity and Byzantium." Even though these events took a hybrid or online form due to the COVID-19 pandemic, they proved fruitful for allowing the contributors to develop their ideas and reach the results that have made this publication possible.

The editors wish to express their special thanks to all volume contributors for their insightful chapters and their keen response to and support of this project. We would also like to warmly thank the members of the MotherBreast team – Dionysios Stathakopoulos, Laurence Totelin, and Petros Bouras-Vallianatos – who reviewed and provided valuable advice and comments on different sections of the volume. Our fervent thanks go also to Jane Burkowski for her admirable editorial work, and to Michael Greenwood at Routledge for his expert help, as well as to the volume's anonymous reviewers for their constructive comments. We would also like to express our sincere thanks to our institution, the University of Cyprus (UCY), and its Centre for Medieval Arts and Rituals (CeMAR) for supporting the project's implementation and for hosting most of its events. What is more, we wish to express once again our genuine gratitude to the Cyprus Foundation of Research and Innovation and UCY, which made the MotherBreast project possible.

Finally, this volume, as our dedication discloses, is offered as a special token of gratitude to our own children. We thank Andreas Roderich, Konstantinos, Eleni, Michail, and Marina for providing us with the unique opportunity to actively practice mothering and breastfeeding: an experience which has ultimately been both our initial and our continuous source of inspiration for taking up and completing this work.

Stavroula Constantinou and Aspasia Skouroumouni-Stavrinou
Nicosia, March 2023

Note to the Reader

As far as Greek names and terms are concerned, we have generally followed the spelling in the *Oxford Classical Dictionary* (*OCD*) for ancient names and terms and the *Oxford Dictionary of Byzantium* (*ODB*) for the Byzantine ones. A Greek term is in most cases given first along with its English translation within parentheses. When repeated, the Greek term is transliterated.

For Galenic titles (English titles and abbreviations), we have followed the most recent systematic translation of Galenic titles by Singer (Singer, P.N. ed. 2013. *Galen: Psychological Writings*. Translated by V. Nutton, D. Davies, and P.N. Singer. Cambridge: Cambridge University Press). Accordingly, for Hippocratic texts we have followed the titles and abbreviations in Craik, E. 2015. *The "Hippocratic" Corpus: Content and Context*. Abingdon: Routledge. For other works, we have not followed absolute rules. Apart from well-established variants in Latin, English titles and abbreviations for primary sources have been adopted. A title is given in full at the first occurrence in each chapter and thereafter it is rendered in abbreviated form, if and where it reoccurs within the chapter, in which case the abbreviated form is always indicated in parenthesis at the first occurrence of the title within the chapter. Abbreviations of author names and titles feature also in the Index.

Regarding medical sources in particular, besides the numbering of the traditional division into books and/or sections where applicable, a reference to the edition (volume in Roman numerals, page and line/s in Arabic numerals) is also added, e.g. Sor. *Gyn.* 2.21.2.7–10 (CMG 4, 69.15–18), ed. Ilberg 1927.

The short list of abbreviations below refers to general sources used throughout the volume. Journal titles are given in full.

Athens, Nat. Lib.   Athens, National Library (Ethnike Bibliotheke).
BGU   *Berliner Griechische Urkunden* (Ägyptische Urkunden aus den Kgl. Museen zu Berlin).
LIMC   *Lexicon Iconographicum Mythologiae Classicae* (*LIMC*; 1981–1999 and 2009) and the *Thesaurus cultus et rituum antiquorum* (*ThesCRA*; 2004–2014), 2022 © *LIMC* Basel and DHLab, https://weblimc.org/.

LSJ	*Liddell–Scott–Jones Greek–English Lexicon*, Perseus Digital Library–Tufts University, online version 2011, http://stephanus.tlg.uci.edu/lsj.
OCD	*The Oxford Classical Dictionary*, 4th ed., Oxford Reference, online version 2012.
ODB	*The Oxford Dictionary of Byzantium*, 3 vols, ed. A.P. Kažhdan, Oxford Reference, online version 2005.
OLD	*The Oxford Latin Dictionary*, 2nd ed., ed. P.G.W. Glare, Oxford: Oxford University Press, 2012.
TLG	*Thesaurus linguae Graecae Digital Library*, ed. M.C. Pantelia. University of California, Irvine, http://www.tlg.uci.edu.

Notes on Editors and Contributors

Andria Andreou is a postdoctoral researcher at CeMAR of UCY (Cyprus). Her research focuses on Byzantine short narrative forms, gender, death, desire, and dreams. She is currently co-editing *Storyworlds in Collections: Toward a Theory of the Ancient and Byzantine Tale* (2023) with Stavroula Constantinou.

Petros Bouras-Vallianatos is an Associate Professor in History of Science at the University of Athens (Greece). He works on medicine and pharmacology. He has recently published *Innovation in Byzantine Medicine: The Writings of John Zacharias Aktouarios* (2020) and *Exploring Greek Manuscripts in the Library at Wellcome Collection in London* (2021).

Stavroula Constantinou is the founder and director of CeMAR at UCY (Cyprus). Currently, she coordinates the major EU-Horizon 2020 NetMAR project. Her research focuses on Byzantine narratives, gender, ritual, performance, emotions, and the body. She is the author of the forthcoming book *Interactive Embodiment: Approaching Byzantine Bodies* (2024).

Barbara Crostini is a Senior Lecturer in Church History, Art History, and Cultural Studies at the Newman Institute, Uppsala, and an Adjunct Lecturer in Greek at the University of Uppsala (Sweden). Her publications question the relation between material culture and theology, stressing continuity between Late Antiquity and Byzantium.

Maria Parani is an Associate Professor in Byzantine and Post Byzantine Art and Archaeology at UCY (Cyprus). Her research interests comprise daily life and material culture in Byzantium and the exploration of alternative sources for their study, such as written texts and artistic representations, to supplement archaeological data.

Tim Parkin is the Tatoulis Classics Chair of the University of Melbourne (Australia). His publications include *Old Age in the Roman World* (2003), *Roman Social History* (2007), and *The Oxford Handbook of Childhood in the Classical*

World (2014). He is currently working on ancient sexual health and Roman domestic violence.

Aspasia Skouroumouni-Stavrinou is a postdoctoral researcher at CeMAR of UCY (Cyprus). Her research focuses on ancient Greek drama (with emphasis on performance, space, gender, and reception), ancient Greek religion, ancient and early Byzantine motherhood, and family culture.

Dionysios Stathakopoulos is Assistant Professor of Byzantine History at UCY (Cyprus). He has taught at King's College London (UK), the Central European University (Hungary), and the University of Vienna (Austria). His latest book is *A Short History of the Byzantine Empire* (2014).

Laurence Totelin is Professor of Ancient History at Cardiff University (UK). She is a historian of Greek and Roman science, technology, and medicine, with a focus on the history of gynaecology, botany, and pharmacology. Her most recent publication is *Bodily Fluids in Antiquity* (2021), co-edited with Mark Bradley and Victoria Leonard.

1 The Lactating Woman

Breastfeeding and Mothering in Antiquity and Early Byzantium*

Stavroula Constantinou
and Aspasia Skouroumouni-Stavrinou

Introduction

> A creature from another planet visiting the Earth might ask, "If women are
> the ones that keep the human race going, why do they get the rough deal?"
> We need to answer that question, environmentally, economically, politically.
> And we can. There are so many huge and complex problems to tackle, but
> breastfeeding is one of the simpler ones. (Palmer 2009³, 362)

In a succinct and graphic way, Gabrielle Palmer captures a key paradox of human societies, both past and present: the problematic, yet fully integrated into our daily lives, depreciation of breastfeeding and women's essential mothering work in general. Even though Palmer's exhortation to take seriously breastfeeding and mothering by dealing with their significant environmental, economic, and political aspects was first expressed in the previous century, and more precisely in the late 1980s,[1] it is now, in the third decade of the second millennium – when we are most affected by global warming, pandemic diseases, and a global food crisis – that this exhortation becomes more urgent than ever.[2] And, as Palmer emphatically points out, "breastfeeding is one of the simpler" problems that we have to deal with.

* The research for this chapter was co-funded by the European Regional Development Fund and the Republic of Cyprus through the Foundation of Research and Innovation (Project: EXCEL-LENCE/1216/0020), as well as by the University of Cyprus within the framework of an internal research project. Some of the ideas that inform the article's arguments were developed within the framework of the project "Network for Medieval Arts and Rituals" (NetMAR), which received funding from the European Union's Horizon 2020 research and innovation programme under grant agreement nr 951875. The opinions expressed in this document reflect only the authors' views, and in no way reflect the European Commission's opinions. The European Commission is not responsible for any use that may be made of the information it contains.

1 The first edition of Palmer's book entitled *The Politics of Breastfeeding: When Breasts Are Bad for Business* came out in 1988.
2 According to the EU's Copernicus Climate Change Service (C3S), 2021 was the world's warmest year on record, while levels of planet-warming carbon dioxide and methane in the atmosphere hit new highs in this year (https://climate.copernicus.eu/c3s-european-state-climate-2021-shows-year-contrasts-europe; accessed 15 March 2023). The coronavirus disease 2019 (COVID-19), which is still in progress, has had unmatched effects on the health of millions of people, spread uncertainty in

DOI: 10.4324/9781003265658-1

If sustainable development is an imperative and the most vital concern in our era, the milky breast is an amulet we need to hold on to. Breastmilk is a natural, free, and renewable source of nutrition, which is environmentally harmless, as it is produced and delivered to the consumer at the right temperature without causing pollution, needless packing, or waste. Breastfeeding improves the survival, health, and development of children. It benefits mothers and mother–child relationships while at the same time contributing to human capital development. For these essential reasons, laws, policies, and actions protecting, promoting, and supporting breastfeeding should have a priority in the agendas of politicians, policy makers, educators, and managers in all sectors. There is thus an imperative need for political and other initiatives that will encourage and allow (working) mothers to breastfeed.

If the establishment of a breastfeeding-friendly culture requires initiatives from various sectors and individuals holding key positions in society, research has a significant role to play in this process: for example, research in the humanities that helps to complement, contextualize, and make more accessible purely biomedical, technical, and other similar accounts of what it means to breastfeed is particularly relevant and needed. An awareness of and reflection on the ideology and medical contexts surrounding, for instance, premodern – in this case ancient and early Byzantine (1st–7th c. AD) – ecological practices concerning childbirth, breastfeeding, and mothering could prove extremely useful for the promotion of breastfeeding in contemporary societies. Knowledge of the past will not just deepen cultural awareness but will also inform political, social, and public health decision-making for the present and the future.

In the last few decades, ancient and medieval mothering has started to receive increasing scholarly attention.[3] Within this context, the figure of the (wet) nurse has also surfaced in multiple studies.[4] What is more, in the context of studies on mothers and (wet) nurses, the ancient and Byzantine female breast and the practice of breastfeeding have appeared as a side interest. These studies are mainly concerned with the breast's medical history[5]; the depiction of the breast in classical art and Byzantine iconography (focussing primarily on icons of the Virgin

---

society and economy, and affected daily life, global economy, travel, and trade (https://www.un.org/en/coronavirus; accessed 15 March 2023). Since May 2022, an outbreak of monkeypox has been causing further socio-economic problems (https://www.who.int/health-topics/monkeypox; accessed 15 March 2023). Due to the ongoing Russian war in Ukraine, food prices have increasingly risen, causing a global crisis pushing millions of people into life-threatening poverty (https://www.worldbank.org/en/topic/agriculture/brief/food-security-update; accessed 15 March 2023).

3   For studies on motherhood, see e.g. Petersen and Salzman-Mitchell 2012; Leyser and Smith 2011; Augoustakis 2010; Parsons and Wheeler 1996; Demand 1994; Dixon 1988 (for antiquity), and Töpfer 2020; Beth Rose 2017, 1–71; Bleek 2017; Woodacre and Fleiner 2016, 2015; Leyser and Smith 2011; Hatlie 2009; Dockray-Miller 2000; Skinner 1997; Parsons and Wheeler 1996; Mulder-Bakker 1995; Atkinson 1991 (for the Middle Ages).

4   See e.g. Pedrucci 2020a, 2020b, 2019c; Parca 2017; Tawfik 1997; Abou Aly 1996; Bradley 1994a, 1991, 1986, 1980 (for antiquity), and Sperling 2013; Giladi 1999 (for the Middle Ages).

5   See e.g. Lawrence 2021; Pedrucci 2020c; Laskaris 2008; Holman 1997; Aboul 1998.

Galaktotrophousa – the one who nurtures with milk);[6] its literary (chiefly archaic and classical) enunciations;[7] the connotations of breast and milk as literal and metaphorical entities in mythical Greco-Roman tales of transgressive or divine breastfeeding[8] and in religious literature (theological treatises, homiletics, and hagiography);[9] and the bioarchaeology of breastfeeding and weaning practices.[10]

Conducive to the "breastfeeding turn" in scholarship on premodern societies, a small number of invariably non-English-language monographs and edited volumes dedicated to the ancient history of breastfeeding appeared in the previous decade.[11] Giulia Pedrucci authored and edited some of the first studies focussing on ancient Greek breastfeeding. Her 2013 monograph *L'allattamento nella Grecia di epoca arcaica e classica* examines breastfeeding and mothering in archaic and classical Greece, concentrating on the theory of the *hematogenesis* of human milk, the differentiated understandings of human and divine motherhood, and male stances on the nursing mother.[12]

Pedrucci's *Maternità e allattamenti nel mondo greco e romano* (2018) investigates the intersection of religious and motherhood studies to reveal aspects of breastfeeding and mothering in Greco-Roman antiquity.[13] The religious perspective remains dominant also in her subsequent multilingual edited volume *Breastfeeding(s) and Religions* (2019), which discusses how discourses and images from different religious traditions (Greco-Roman, Christian, Jewish, Hindu,

---

6 See e.g. Räuchle 2022; Bolman 2015, 2004; Zellmann-Rohrer 2019; Coccagna 2014; Meyer 2012 and 2009, 80–94, 105–114; Gkegkes et al. 2007; Stafford 2005; Williamson 1998; Bonfante 1997; Cohen 1997; Langener 1996; Gourevitch 1992.

7 See e.g. Marshall 2017; Salzman-Mitchell 2012; Hanson 2003; Newbold 2000; O' Neill 1998; De Forest 1993; Gerber 1978.

8 See e.g. Pedrucci 2019a, 2019b, 2017, 2016; Mulder 2017.

9 See e.g. Constantinou 2023a, 2023b, 2023c, 2015; Totelin 2021; D-Vasilescu 2018; Dova 2017; Penniman 2017; LaValle 2015; Engelbrecht 1999; Corrington 1989.

10 See e.g. Centlivres Challet 2017; Bourbou 2016; Bourbou et al. 2013. See also publications coming out of two recent major Swiss projects on ancient and medieval infancy ("Lactation in History: A Cross-cultural Research on Suckling Practice, Representations of Breastfeeding and Politics of Maternity in a European Context"; "To Be a Child in Roman Aventicum/Avenches (1st–3rd c. AD): Evidence on Health, Disease and Feeding Practices from Bioarchaeology"): Bourbou and Dasen 2018; Bourbou 2017.

11 Previous works that take into consideration antiquity up to the Middle Ages invariably provide a very general analysis which is not representative of premodern realities. See e.g. Yalom 1997 (discussing only in passing – within the context of her general chapters on the "sacred" and the "medical" breast – ancient Greek and Western medieval evidence related to breastfeeding); Fildes 1988 and 1986 (devoting a few pages to the breastfeeding and weaning practices of the whole period from antiquity to the Middle Ages). Ancient or medieval symbolic and practical uses of human milk have been briefly treated also within the context of overviews of premodern societies in edited collections or monographs examining the diachronic history of milk from ancient to modern times (see e.g. Rzeźnicka and Kokoszko 2020; Kokoszko et al. 2018; Anagnostakis and Pellettieri 2016; Velten 2010; Walker 2000).

12 Pedrucci 2013a. The second section, relating to Sicily, has also been published as a separate monograph (*L'isola delle madri*, Pedrucci 2013b).

13 Pedrucci 2018.

and Islamic), have described and influenced the practice of breastfeeding.[14] Finally, *Visiones sobre la lactancia en la Antigüedad*, an edited collection by Reboreda Morillo, which was published in the same year (2019b),[15] opens up the spectrum to deal with religious and non-religious aspects of breastfeeding and weaning practices with an important emphasis on themes and motifs related to divine breastfeeding in the ancient Near East, Egypt, Greece, and Rome.

The present volume, which examines breastfeeding and mothering in antiquity and early Byzantium from a variety of perspectives and approaches, aims to contribute significantly to the newly emerging fields of breast and motherhood studies by developing the lactating woman as a new critical category for approaching premodern mothering practices alongside their familial, social, ideological, legal, religious, philosophical, didactic, medical, artistic, and literary uses. The lactating woman – blood mother and othermother – is approached here through the notions of "gender," "body," and "performance," which are inextricably related, since each is defined through the others. These three concepts constitute cultural constructs determining social identities and behaviours.

The notion of "gender" was introduced by feminism that makes a distinction between sex, connoting the biological differences between men and women, and gender, designating the meanings of these differences in culture.[16] As for the notion of "performance," it comes from another discipline, performance studies, and it includes both Butler's concept of "performativity" and a "broad spectrum of human actions ranging from ritual, play, sports, popular entertainments, the performing arts and everyday performances to the enactment of professional, race, and class roles, and on to healing."[17] In our approach, performativity is mainly used to talk about the lactating woman's construction as a gendered social role, while performance is employed to refer to practices, rituals, and healings related to childbirth, breastfeeding, and mothering.

The construction of the lactating woman as a gendered social role is first and foremost imputed by language. For example, the ancient Greek word "θῆλυς" (*thēlus*; female),[18] according to its etymology, correlates the category of woman with the nursing quality of the breast, its ability to produce milk and be suckled. The modern Greek words "θηλυκός" (*thēlukos*; female), "θηλή" (*thēlē*; nipple), and "θηλάζω" (*thēlazō*; to breastfeed, nurse, or suckle) also derive from the same root. The identification of woman with nursing in the Greek language reveals a certain belief system in which breastfeeding is treated as her most essential activity. On the one hand, it is not surprising that motherhood and breastfeeding are at the very centre of the conception of womanhood, given how premodern societies were characterized by both ecological practices and strong patterns of family structures.

14 Pedrucci 2019d.
15 Reboreda Morillo 2019b.
16 De Beauvoir 1949; Ortner and Whitehead 1981.
17 Schechner 2002, 2.
18 Translations, unless otherwise indicated, are our own.

This word choice, on the other hand, is highly indicative of the patriarchal character of societal attitudes towards the lactating woman. In Greek culture from antiquity to the present, processes of the female body, such as milk production and breastfeeding, have been presented through language as ways of confining women to the private-sphere role of the mother/nursing figure as determined through the long-established institution of motherhood.[19]

Due to their multiple interdisciplinary dimensions, ancient and early Byzantine lactating women and mothering are in this volume approached through three interconnected thematic strands, each having a twofold focus: society and ideology, medicine and practice, and art and literature. The society and ideology strand concerns the types, identities, and roles of the lactating woman, in association with her social, legal, and religious treatment, as well as in relation with the network of her familial, kinship, and other interpersonal relationships. The relationships between blood mothers, othermothers, and their nurslings, as well as the anxieties surrounding wet nursing, along with breastfeeding's function as a means of female empowerment and networking, are also relevant. All in all, the general ideology (social, political, and religious) that surrounds and defines the lactating woman, her types, and her imposed roles are relevant to this strand. In short, this first strand attempts to comprehend the lactating woman's social performativity in association with the ideological consciousness of the examined cultures.

The strand of medicine and practice involves ancient and early Byzantine ideas about the biology of breastfeeding, including the origin of breastmilk and the bodily substances and organs involved, along with their characteristics; related practices, such as diet and exercise; breast diseases, such as mastitis and breast engorgement, and their treatment; lactation cessation; the composition, qualities, benefits, and medical uses of milk; and finally milk theories and debates, along with their literary dimensions. Most of these aspects are examined against the background of ancient medical pluralism, involving three interconnecting sectors of healthcare: the popular, the professional, and the religious/magical. Mostly, the popular sector is the one activated first, and it determines an individual's engagement with the other two sectors. While being non-professional and non-specialist, the popular sector first recognizes and defines any medical problems or ill health. This sector includes all the healing options that people freely make use of without recourse to medical professionals and religious or magical healers. The professional sector includes physicians and those who either support (wet nurses) or complement their work (midwives).[20] Finally, the religious/magical sector consists of priests, living saints, magicians, healing shrines, objects (icons, relics, amulets, and phylacteries), and words (prayers, exorcisms, and spells).[21]

19 For the perennial institution of motherhood, which establishes and defines women's social role as mothers and nurturers, see Rich 1995.
20 See Bacalexi 2005.
21 Nutton 2013, 1992; Oberhelman 2013; Chirban 2010, 1991; Lloyd 2003, 1983, 1979; Bennett 2000, 279–291; Miller 1997; French 1986; Vikan 1984, 65–86.

The last strand (art and literature) concentrates on the artistic and literary conceptions and representations of the lactating woman and her mothering within the context of the relevant social, ideological, philosophical, religious, and medical discourses which lie at the centre of the previous two strands. In this case, the focus is on the cultural logic of the works, visual and literary, which use the lactating woman and mothering as thematizing structures. The cultural logic of the discussed works refers, on the one hand, to the social and cultural space they occupy both as products of the ancient and early Byzantine worlds and as agents at work in these very worlds. On the other hand, this cultural logic also denotes the examined works' artistic and literary character, which requires interpretation according to relevant artistic and literary theories. The visual and literary analysis attempted here concerns chiefly the typology, rhetoric, symbolisms, visual and narrative meanings, and functions of the lactating woman and the mother.

The three thematic strands (society and ideology, medicine and practice, and art and literature) structure not only the subsequent discussion but also the remaining chapters of the volume, which fall into three parts named after the strands. Of course, not all issues that are relevant to each strand can be sufficiently discussed within the framework of a collected volume such as this one. The volume's chapters focus on a selection of those issues, inviting further studies for their better understanding. Concerning the following analysis in particular, we pursue some significant issues pertaining to each strand that are mostly exemplified through an examination of the *Passion of Perpetua and Felicity* (*PPF*), a literary account of the imprisonment and martyrdom of two lactating mothers (Perpetua and Felicity) and their male fellow prisoners, who were martyred together in Roman Carthage on 7 March AD 203.[22] In addition

---

22 The *PPF* has come down to us in a Latin and a Greek version (for the debates concerning the priority of either version, see e.g. Cobb 2021, 8–10; Shaw 2020; Gold 2018, 13–20; Heffernan 2012, 60–99). The Latin version, which is now considered the oldest one, is also preserved in two short *Acta – Acta* A and *Acta* B – the latter being a bit shorter than the former (for the *Acta*, see Cobb 2021, 67–93; Cotter-Lynch 2016, 43–62; Kitzler 2015; Guazzelli 2009). Two very brief Greek parallels of the *Acta* can be found in the *Synaxarion of Constantinople* (10th c. AD) and the *Menologion of Basil II* (11th c. AD). For the second of February, the *Synaxarion* includes an extremely short entry (around 11 printed lines) on Perpetua and her fellow martyrs (Day 2.2, ed. Delehaye (1902) 1984). Basil's *Menologion* has an entry of approximately double the size – around 20 printed lines (*Patrologia Graeca* (*PG*) 117, 292, ed. Migne 1857–1866). The titles of these two short Greek entries follow the later title appearing first on the single known manuscript preserving the Greek *PPF*, which mentions Perpetua first and then her male fellow martyrs. In all three cases, Felicity's name is given last. Our analysis is based on the Greek *PPF* (*BHG* 1482, ed. and trans. Cobb 2021, 46–65, that reprints the edition of Van Beek 1936), which probably dates to the early sixth century AD, and not the late third century AD as has been previously thought (Shaw 2020, 342). In a more recent publication Stephanie Cobb, by contrast, dates the Greek *PPF* to around AD 260 (Cobb 2021, 44), thus following the date suggested by previous scholars (see e.g. Bremmer and Formisano 2012b, 4). This earlier dating, however, does not sound as convincing as that of the early sixth century AD that has been suggested by Brent Shaw (Shaw 2020). The Greek *PPF* appears to be a translation of

to the analysis of the *PPF*, the chapter's arguments are supported by the use of relevant passages from other earlier, contemporary, and later sources.

In both its Latin and Greek versions, the *PPF* includes three maternal figures belonging to different social classes: a noble nursing mother (Perpetua);[23] a pregnant slave giving birth in prison (Felicity); and a woman of low social status – probably a free woman or a freedwoman (the anonymous Christian mother who adopts Felicity's newborn baby after her violent death).[24] As already pointed out, the first two mothers – Perpetua and Felicity – play a central role in this composite text, which consists of three parts: an editor's framing text (*PPF* 1–2, 14–21), including Felicity's story (*PPF* 2.1, 15, 18, 20.1–6); Perpetua's prison diary (*PPF* 3–10); and the visionary account of the Christian prisoners' spiritual father and fellow martyr Saturos (*PPF* 11–13).

A significant part of Perpetua's diary presents her worldly and otherworldly experiences as a lactating woman and nursing mother in prison. As for Felicity, her story as an imprisoned pregnant woman who longs to give birth so that she can die as a martyr with her Christian fellow prisoners constitutes the largest part of the editor's text. The maternal milk leaking from Felicity's breasts while she is taken

---

a Latin text closer to the third-century original, which is now lost (Bremmer and Formisano 2012b, 4). The Latin version that has come down to us is discussed in Chapter 5 of this volume.

23 Based mostly on the facts that Perpetua did not hire a wet nurse as was the norm in elite Roman families of her times and that her father was not treated by Roman officials as a member of the aristocracy, some scholars have argued that Perpetua must have belonged to a lower social strand (e.g. Cooper 2011). However, the (Greek) text clearly states that she "was nobly born and lavishly reared" ("ἦν γεννηθεῖσα εὐγενῶς καὶ τραφεῖσα πολυτελῶς," *PPF* 2.1; trans. Cobb 2021, 47), just as it plainly declares that Felicity was a slave (*PPF* 2.1). As the following discussion will indicate, there were elite Roman and Byzantine women who undertook the breastfeeding of their own babies. Furthermore, as Hanne Sigismund-Nielsen rightly points out, "we cannot tell whether young mothers in the area around Carthage usually nursed their infants in pre-Christian times. The fact that Perpetua does so and that it is not commented as extraordinary could point in the direction of a local habit" (Sigismund-Nielsen 2012, 108). Finally, even if Perpetua did not come from the highest stratum of Roman society, her social class seems to be higher than that of the other two mothers in the *PPF* (Felicity and the surrogate mother of the former's daughter). The three women's different social statuses are important for our purposes, as they determine their differentiated treatments as lactating mothers.

24 According to Roman law, Felicity's child was a slave that belonged to her master. Yet, due to her Christianity and imminent execution, Felicity's master, who is not mentioned in the text, may have lost his interest in having her offspring, whose father also remains unknown (it has been suggested that the father might be Revocatos, Felicity's fellow slave, but again there is no such clear indication in the *PPF*; see e.g. Van Henten 2012, 127–128; Ronsse 2006, 303; Habermehl 2004, 209; Bradley 2003, 171; Schöllgen 1985, 248–249; Poirier 1970, 306–309). The *PPF* does not reveal either the name or the social class of the Christian woman adopting Felicity's newborn daughter. We could, however, assume that she may have been a free woman of low social status or a freedwoman, since a slave or an elite woman would not have the liberty to raise a slave child as her own ("one of the sisters … brought her up herself as a daughter"; "μία τῶν ἀδελφῶν … εἰς θυγατέρα ἀνέθρεψεν αὐτῇ," *PPF* 15.6; trans. Cobb 2021, 59). For slavery in the Roman Empire, see Glancy 2006; Joshel and Murnaghan 1998; Bradley 1994b, 1987; For freedwomen, see Perry 2014.

with the other martyrs to the arena further reinforces the emphasis that the *PPF* places on lactation and maternity. All in all, the *PPF* is a unique text paying attention to mothering and to different experiences of lactation, as well as to lactation cessation.[25] Furthermore, the *PPF* is the earliest and the only work in our corpus featuring a lactating woman's own voice and experience. Of course, we have no way of proving whether Perpetua was the actual author of the *PPF*'s autobiographical narrative.[26] Yet, even if what appears as the holy woman's diary is not the work of a historical woman called Perpetua, it reflects the experiences and agonies of an imprisoned lactating mother.[27]

As the premodern text *par excellence* of the lactating woman, the *PPF* is eminently suitable for bringing to the fore her typology, socio-ideology, and medical and literary treatments.[28] As the following analysis will show, the *PPF* reflects various earlier and contemporary discourses and ideologies – moralist, philosophical, theological, medical, and rhetorical – around the lactating woman and mothering. As well as influencing the production of hagiographical and other literary texts,[29] the stories of Perpetua and Felicity inspired the creation of visual works, such as the two martyrs' mosaic in the Archiepiscopal Chapel in Ravenna and that of the Basilica Eufrasiana in Poreč.[30] However, none of the late antique and early medieval works in question presents the two holy women as (lactating) mothers, and consequently, their visual representations are not of interest here. The fact that both Perpetua and Felicity are represented as virgins and not as mothers in late antique and later religious art might be related to contemporary theologians' and hagiographers' tendency to conceptualize female martyrdom and holiness in virginal terms.[31]

---

25 See also Chapter 5.
26 Questions about the text's authorship and authenticity have been widely debated, with most scholars accepting that Perpetua either dictated her prison experiences to a scribe or wrote them down on her own (see e.g. Cobb 2021, 6–8; Gold 2018, 13–17; Bremmer and Formisano 2012b, 5–6). In a very recent article, Ellen Muehlberger has once again brought back the discussion of the work's authenticity, suggesting that "Perpetua's words align with a tradition of late ancient writers ventriloquizing women renowned and honoured, but for whom no words had been previously recorded" (Muehlberger 2022, 313). Yet again, there is no way of proving that Perpetua was not the author of the prison diary attributed to her by the anonymous redactor of the *PPF*.
27 For testimonies of contemporary imprisoned mothers echoing Perpetua's anxieties, see Scheffler 2002, 175–220.
28 The examination of the *PPF*'s rewritings in later, mostly Latin and Western vernacular, texts that provide new understandings of the lactating woman is beyond the scope of this chapter. For some of these rewritings, see Cobb 2021, 97–259.
29 In Thomas Heffernan's words, the *PPF* was the "primal document in the development of the conventions which were to shape female sacred biography for a millennium," offering "medieval female sacred biography exquisite models for the portrayal of female heroism along with the complex philosophical matrix from which these biographies of saintly women were to be cast" (Heffernan 1988, 186, 230).
30 For the late antique visual works representing Perpetua and Felicity, see Cobb 2021, 337–358.
31 See Weitbrecht 2012; Atkinson 1991, 144; cf. Heffernan 1988, 231–299. For Perpetua's treatment as a virgin by Augustine, for example, see Sigismund-Nielsen 2012, 116–117.

Even though lactation and maternity are so central in the *PPF*, a text that has attracted immense scholarly attention,[32] apart from relatively few exceptions,[33] scholars tend to ignore these essential elements of the text. In her appraisal of the *PPF*, Danuta Shanzer, for example, describes it as an

> extraordinary and moving text [that] preserves at its heart the first preserved autobiographical account written by an ancient woman. No other single text can convey as vivid an impression of the impact of an imperial persecution upon the individual, from arrest, to courtroom, to prison, to execution in the amphitheatre. This text too provides wonderful material on the dreams of the martyrs and their expectations and fears of death and the afterlife. It also raises fundamental issues of language and communication.[34]

Shanzer's list of the work's characteristics and merits fails to mention its most important element: (lactating) maternity, which sets the story going both in Perpetua's diary and the account of Felicity.[35] In fact, (lactating) maternity is the reason why the *PPF* is such an "extraordinary and moving text": two imprisoned women who are sentenced to public suffering and death have to come to terms with the physicality of their maternal bodies and the fate of their orphaned babies. Without realizing it, most scholars have fallen into the trap of late antique and medieval ideologies concerning female holiness that identifies it with virginity.

Interestingly, this very fact is brought to the fore by one of the text's most eloquent readers, Marina Werner, who remarks: "I have been mistaken … I have been including Saints Perpetua and Felicity among the ranks of the Virgin Martyrs. … But the error I have been making is revealing."[36] By ignoring or forgetting the two holy women's maternity, scholars not only provide incomplete readings of the *PPF* but also promote Christian ideology concerning the virginal status of female saints. But let us now see how approaching the *PPF* through the concept of the lactating

---

32 The scholarship on the Latin *PPF* goes back to the seventeenth century AD (Holstenius 1664: first edition of the text). It was, however, in the last decades of the nineteenth century AD (see e.g. Pillet 1885) and particularly after 1889 when the Greek *PPF* was discovered in the Convent of the Holy Sepulchre in Jerusalem (first edition in 1890 by Harris and Gifford) that scholars started showing increasing interest in the *PPF*. Some studies of the last two decades are provided here: Cobb 2022, 2021, 2019; Muehlberger 2022; Klein 2020; Shaw 2020; Gold 2018; Dova 2017; Rea 2016; Cardoso 2015; Constantinou 2015, 300–304; Gonzalez 2014; Solevåg 2013, 199–248; Bremmer and Formisano 2012a; Heffernan 2012; Hunink 2012; Cooper 2011; Dunn 2010; Farina 2009; Kraemer 2008; Perkins 2007; Butler 2006; Ronsse 2006; Hérnandez Lobato 2005; Bremmer 2004, 2003, 2002, 2000; Castelli 2004, 85–92; Habermehl 2004; Osiek 2002; Kraemer and Lander 2000.

33 It is mostly after Judith Perkins' seminal article "The Rhetoric of the Maternal Body in the Passio of Perpetua" (2007) that scholars have started paying attention to the central role of maternity in the *PPF*. These studies include Cobb 2022, 15–21; Totelin 2021, 247–250; Dova 2017; Parkhouse 2017; Cotter-Lynch 2016; Solevåg 2013, 199–248; Van Henten 2012; Weitbrecht 2012; Moss 2010; Burrus 2008; Perkins 2007.

34 Shanzer 2009, 934.

35 See below, under "Art and Literature."

36 Warner 2012, 356.

woman provides not only a better understanding of the text and its literariness, but also illuminates a variety of late antique, and even later, ideologies surrounding breastfeeding and mothering.

Society and Ideology

Even though archaeological evidence suggests that alternative sources for infant feeding were sought already in antiquity,[37] the lactating woman's services were in high demand in premodern societies, as human milk was the safest nutrition for the newborn.[38] In Pliny the Elder's (AD 23/24–79) words, "mother's milk" was "the most useful thing" (*"[Lac] utilissimum … maternum*, *Natural History* 28.123, ed. and trans. Rackham 1938, 86, 87). In addition to her milk, infants also needed the lactating woman's soothing and loving care, a reality voiced by Perpetua's father when he tells her that her son "cannot live" without her ("ζῆν οὐ δύναται," *PPF* 5.3; trans. with a modification Cobb 2021, 51). The lactating woman was thus indispensable and extremely desired in the examined societies.

As our multifarious sources allow us to discern, there existed at least four types of lactating women in antiquity and Byzantium: biological nursing mothers, voluntary nurses, compelled nurses, and mercenary wet nurses. These lactating women fulfilled the vital need for babies' nurturing – even for those that were exposed or abandoned[39] – thus enabling the continuation of family traditions and the increase of slavery forces.[40] The engagement of each type of lactating woman, as will be further discussed below, was determined by a number of factors – physical, practical, medical, economic, familial, social, and ideological.

In the examined sources, a considerable number of terms can be detected designating one, two, or all types of lactating women. For the blood mother, the terms *mētēr* ("μήτηρ"; mother), *tiktousa, tekousa* ("τίκτουσα," "τεκοῦσα"; the one giving birth), *teknotrophos, teknotrophoūsa, paidotrophos*, and *paidotrophoūsa* ("τεκνοτρόφος," "τεκνοτροφοῦσα," "παιδοτρόφος," "παιδοτροφοῦσα"; child-nourisher) are employed. It is not always clear, however, whether these terms refer

37 Throughout the Roman Empire, clay and glass feeding bottles and breast pumps dating from the first to the fifth century AD have been found in children's tombs, domestic contexts, and pottery workshops. See e.g. Bécares Rodríguez 2019; Centlivres Challet 2017, 899 and 2016; Bourbou 2016; Bourbou et al. 2013; Gourevitch 1990. The use of animal milk directly suckled from the animal's udder is also another possibility which is documented in mythical stories; see e.g. Centlivres Challet 2017, 901. For animals as wet nurses in myth, see Pedrucci 2019a, 2016.
38 See e.g. Matthews Grieco 1991; Hill et al. 1987.
39 For child exposure and abandonment, see e.g. Evans Grubbs 2013a, 2011, 2010, and 2009a; Miller 2003, 141–175; Corbier 2001; Boswell 1988, 51–265; Patlagean 1977, 116, 363.
40 Through children a family's name was continued and patrimony was transmitted. Married couples wished to conceive children, whom they were supposed to look after. Children, on the other hand, were expected to honour their parents and take care of them in their old age. See e.g. Vuolanto 2013; Congourdeau 2009; Evans Grubbs 2009b; Bradley 1994a; Saller 1994, 105–114, 161–203; Rawson 1991. Slave-owning families acquired more slaves through their female slaves' children. For slave-breeding, see Scheidel 1997; Bradley 1987, 47–80 and 1986; Treggiari 1979, 188.

also to the breastfeeding mother.[41] While one of the most common terms signifying the lactating woman – *trophos* ("τροφός") – sometimes refers to the biological (nursing) mother,[42] it mainly concerns the surrogate mother, who provides her services either for free or against payment.

Trophos can also mean the dry nurse, and often we are not sure whether the author means a wet nurse, a dry nurse, or both. Some other frequently used terms for the surrogate nursing woman include the nouns *titthē* ("τίτθη," "τιτθή"), *titthēnē* ("τιτθήνη"), *tithēnē* ("τιθηνή"), and *tithēnos* ("τιθηνός"). The term *tithēnos*, like *trophos*, is at times subject to ambiguity, signifying a wet nurse, a dry nurse, or both.[43] The words *tittheutria* ("τιτθευτρία"), *thēlō* ("θηλώ"), *thēlamōn* ("θηλαμών"), *thēlastria* ("θηλάστρια"), and *visastria* ("βυζάστρια"), which mean exclusively the wet nurse, voluntary, compelled, or mercenary, are much less commonly used.[44] The term *ammas* or *amma* ("ἀμμάς," "ἀμμά"), which might mean either the nurse, both wet and dry, or the biological mother, is also less frequently used and is mostly found in Byzantine sources.[45]

The fact that the terms assigned to breastfeeding women do not always allow a distinction between nursing and non-nursing biological mother, blood mother and othermother, voluntary, compelled, and mercenary wet nurse, or wet and dry nurse constitutes a first indication of the difficulties we encounter in our attempt to understand ancient and Byzantine approaches to the lactating woman and her roles. A sociolinguistic study dedicated to the various ancient and Byzantine Greek terms that are

41 In his etymological lexicon, the fifth-century grammarian Orion of Thebes, for example, defines "mother" as "the one whose breasts create the food for the gestating foetus" ("Μήτηρ ἡ μαστεύουσα τὰ πρὸς τροφὴν τοῖς κυηθεῖσιν," letter m, p. 101.11, ed. Sturz 1820).
42 For example, the *Lexikon* of Hesychios (5th/6th c. AD) defines *trophos* as "mother" (τ 1518, ed. Schmidt 1861–1862). Some early Byzantine authors, such as Anastasios of Sinai (7th c. AD), refer to the lactating mother by using the term *trophos*: "Τελείαν γυναῖκα λέγει, τουτέστι πρᾶγμα τέλειον, οἰκοδέσποιναν, μητέρα, τροφὸν καὶ γεννήτριαν καὶ κτήτορα τέκνων πολλῶν" (Anastasios of Sinai, *Hexaemeron* 10.4–6, eds Baggarly and Kühn 2007). For uncertainties about the exact meaning of the Latin term *nutrix* (wet or dry nurse), with wet nursing being the primary meaning of the term (as the analogue to the Greek *tithē*), see Dasen 2010, 700–701; Bradley 1991, 30, n. 2 and 1986, 222, n. 6; Beaucamp 1982, 550. For similar ambiguities in the Egyptian terminology concerning wet nurses (*ménat* used for wet nurses, mothers, priestesses, or mother goddesses), see Spieser 2012, 21, 35.
43 See e.g. how Ptolemy the Grammarian (2nd c. BC/2nd c. AD) differentiates between *titthē* and *tithēnē* or *trophos*: "There is a difference between *titthē* and *trophos* or *tithēnos*, for *titthē* is the one who offers the breast, whereas *trophos* or *tithēnos* is the one who takes care of the child after weaning" ("τιτθὴ καὶ τροφὸς καὶ τιθηνὸς διαφέρει· τιτθὴ μὲν γάρ ἐστιν ἡ μαστὸν παρεχομένη· τροφὸς δὲ καὶ τιθηνὸς ἡ τὴν ἄλλην ἐπιμέλειαν ποιουμένη τοῦ παιδὸς καὶ μετὰ τὸν ἀπογαλακτισμόν," *On Differences of Terms* 394.18–21, ed. Heylbut 1887).
44 See e.g. the meaning of the words in ancient lexica: "breastfeeder: nurse, wet nurse" ("θηλώ· τροφός, τήθη," Hesychios, *Lexikon* 499, ed. Latte 1953–1966); "breastfeeder: the wet nurse" ("θηλαμών· ἡ τροφός," Philoxenos *fr.* 100, ed. Theodoridis 1976); "breastfeeder: the one who feeds infants through her nipple" ("θηλάστριαν· τῶν παίδων τὴν τροφὸν διὰ τὴν θηλήν," *Moeris* 21, ed. Hansen 1998).
45 See e.g. "*Amma*: the nurse … and the mother" ("Ἀμμάς· ἡ τροφὸς … καὶ ἡ μήτηρ," Hesychios, *Lexikon* 3692 Latte); "*Amma* means the mother" ("Ἀμμά,᾽ ὅπερ ἑρμηνεύεται μήτηρ"; *Life and Passion of Mamas* (5th/7th c. AD) 5.3, ed. Berger 2002).

employed in different sources to refer to this form of mothering could yield interesting results about the socio-ideological position and treatment of nursing biological mothers and voluntary, compelled, and mercenary othermothers in different periods and traditions. Since the examined texts rarely specify whether a wet nurse is voluntary, compelled, or mercenary, it is very difficult, if not impossible, to explore the social implications of wet nursing as an act of generosity, a forced labour, and a profession. Thus, our discussion of the lactating woman's socio-ideology is structured around the binary of blood mother and othermother. Of course, when available, different nuances of the wet nurse's situation are also taken into consideration.

Nursing Blood Mothers

Whereas mothers breastfeeding their own children rarely appear in Greco-Roman sources,[46] they are frequently mentioned in early Byzantine texts. In one of the poetic epitaphs for his mother Nonna, for example, Gregory the Theologian (ca. AD 330–389) highlights his strong bond with his mother, which he presents as the result of his nursing at her breast. He was deeply thankful for this maternal nursing, showing his gratitude in the relatively great number of poems he wrote for his mother: "The mother's blood was burning with love for her two sons, but mainly for [me] whom she breastfed. It is for this reason, mother, that I have paid you back with so many epigrams" ("τὸ δ' ἔζεεν αἷμα τεκούσης | ἀμφοτέροις ἐπὶ παισί, μάλιστα δὲ θρέμματι θηλῆς· | τοὔνεκα καὶ σὲ τόσοις ἐπιγράμμασι, μῆτερ, ἔτισα," *Anthologia Graeca* 8.30.4–6, ed. Beckby 1965–1968).[47] For Gregory, maternal breastfeeding did not only establish a fervent mother–son bond – one that for unexplained reasons his brother was not fortunate enough to experience – but it was also a powerful sign of the mother's love for her offspring. As further discussed below, the idea that breastfeeding indicated maternal love was promoted by the Roman and Byzantine institutions of motherhood.

Nursing biological mothers feature most frequently in late antique and Byzantine hagiography, which apart from being an important literary genre is a rich source on early Christian and Byzantine social life.[48] Concerning the nursing mothers of early hagiography in particular,[49] these, as is the case with those appearing

---

46 Some of the few references to nursing mothers in the Greco-Roman world include the three breast-feeding mothers documented in the Italian inscriptions catalogued by Bradley 1991, Plutarch's (AD 46–120) wife nursing their son Chaeron (Plut. *Consolation to His Wife* 609e, ed. Sieveking (1929) 1972), and, as already mentioned, Perpetua in the *PPF*. Musonius Rufus' exhortation to Roman mothers to breastfeed their own children, for instance, suggests that surrogate breastfeeding was a common practice in Imperial Rome (Muson. *Discourses* (*Disc.*) 3.50, ed. Lutz 1947). For Musonius Rufus, see below and Chapter 2.

47 For mother–child bonding in the Church Fathers, see Burnett 2009.

48 See e.g. Patlagean 1987 and 1981, 106–126.

49 For breastfeeding mothers in middle Byzantine hagiography, see Ariantzi 2012, 82–91. As for late hagiographical texts mentioning breastfeeding mothers, see, for example: Nikephoros Xanthopoulos' (14th c. AD) *Life of Euphrosyne the Younger* (37; ed. *Acta Sanctorum* Nov. III. 1910, 861–877), where the saint heals mothers having difficulties with breastfeeding; Makarios Makres' (AD

in later Byzantine hagiographical texts, include holy mothers,[50] the saintly protagonists' mothers and wives (if the saint is a married man), whose names are not always provided,[51] and new mothers, mostly anonymous, seeking saintly assistance for breastfeeding or for their infants' rearing and health.[52] The nursing biological mothers depicted in hagiographical sources belong to both the upper and lower social classes – while there is no mention of breastfeeding mothers who are slaves. Possibly the reason for the absence of nursing slave mothers from the examined hagiography is that these mothers were separated from their babies, which were abandoned, sold, or given away to be breastfed and raised by surrogate mothers.[53]

In general, most nursing biological mothers in our sources are women of a lower social status. Most probably, these sources reflect another social reality, as poor mothers, in contrast to elite mothers, did not have the means to hire wet nurses. Elite women, on the other hand, were often expected to employ wet nurses, as breastfeeding was considered humble work reserved for slave and poor women. The latter resorted to wet nursing to sustain themselves and their families, while masters sold their female slaves' milk for their own profit. In short, prevalent social ideas about the servile character of breastfeeding, as well as the tiring nature and pains of breastfeeding, led elite mothers in both antiquity and Byzantium to refrain from nursing their own infants, which were entrusted to wet nurses.[54]

That Byzantine sources depict much more nursing blood mothers than their Greco-Roman counterparts might be related to the new ideals of motherhood which started crystallizing in the early Roman Empire. These ideals were later adopted by the first Christian authors and found their highest expression in the Church Fathers' works,

---

1383–1431) *Enkomion on Andrew of Crete* (13.240–241, ed. Argyriou 1996, 131–139), and Joseph Kalothetos' (14th c. AD) *Enkomion on Andrew of Crete* (1.11, ed. Tsames 1980, 435–451). In the latter two texts, Andrew's motherly breastfeeding is highlighted.

50 To the example of Perpetua we could add, for instance, saints Sophia (mother of saints Pistis, Elpis, and Agape; *Passion of Pistis, Elpis, Agape, and Sophia* (*PPEAS*; 7th/11th c. AD) 8.16, ed. Halkin 1973), Ioulitta (*Enkomion on Kirikos and Ioulitta* 3.7–8, ed. Halkin 1987–1989), and Martha (mother of Saint Symeon Stylites the Younger; *Life of Symeon Stylites the Younger* (*LSSY*; 6th/7th c. AD) 4.1–4, ed. Van den Ven 1962).

51 See e.g. the nameless mother of Saint Symeon the Holy Fool (Leontios of Neapolis (7th c. AD), *Life of Symeon the Holy Fool* 1700D.22, eds Festugière and Rydén 1974).

52 These include a group of mothers who cannot produce milk in the *LSSY* 138; an anonymous breast-feeding mother whose baby suffers from hernia in a story from Saint Artemios' miracle collection (*Miracles of Artemios* (7th c. AD) 11, ed. Papadopoulos-Kerameus 1909). For (breastfeeding) mothers in early Byzantine miracle collections, see Chapter 10.

53 See e.g. Bradley 1986; Joshel 1986. In contrast to the much-studied Roman female slavery (see e.g. Perry 2014; Harper 2011, 70–83, 108–112; Keith 2011; Rodger 2007; Glancy 2006; Bradley 1994b, 34–59 and 1978; Günther 1987), female slavery in Byzantium is understudied. Some studies on Byzantine slavery include Penna 2022; Rio 2017, 136–141; Prinzig 2014 and 2010; Evans Grubbs 2013b; Rotman 2000, 2004; Köpstein 1993, 1976, 1966; Hadjinicolaou-Marava 1950.

54 See Chapter 2; Constantinou and Skouroumouni-Stavrinou 2024. See also Parca 2017; Talbot 2017, 241 and 1997, 125; Bretin-Chabrol 2015; Dasen 2012a, 2012b, 2010; Salzman-Mitchell 2012; Spieser 2012; Pitarakis 2009, 211–212; Ray 2004; Corbier 2001; Schulze 1998; Karydas 1998; Holman 1997; Abou Aly 1996; Bradley 1994a, 1991, 1986, and 1980; Dixon 1988, 141–167; Rühfel 1988; Joshel 1986; Hermann 1959.

which,[55] in turn, exercised great influence on later Byzantine moralists, theologians, and hagiographers.[56] A number of studies have shown how, after becoming the first Roman emperor, Augustus (27 BC–AD 14) promoted new familial ideals,[57] which "remained relatively stable" until early Byzantium.[58] Treating marriage and childrearing as the sources of the new empire's well-being and power, the new regime sought to control family life and particularly children's nourishment and education. As John David Penniman has convincingly shown, a new discourse, which permeated different genres including medical and moral treatises, philosophy, biography, historiography, and literature, highlighted the "power of nourishment in the formation of souls."[59]

In this context, maternal milk, breastfeeding, and childrearing became focal points and essential qualities of good mothering – the kind of mothering which Gregory, as shown above, appreciated and promoted through his poetry. The Stoic philosopher Musonius Rufus, a contemporary of Augustus, described the female philosopher and thus the good woman – meaning the free and particularly the elite Roman woman – as the one who underwent the pains of childrearing, including breastfeeding: "so it is that such a woman is … strong to endure pain, prepared to nourish her children at her own breast" ("ὅθεν εἰκὸς εἶναι τὴν γυναῖκα … κακόπαθον, οἵαν ἃ μὲν ἂν τέκη τρέφειν μαστῷ τῷ ἑαυτῆς," Muson. *Disc.* 3.41–42, ed. and trans. Lutz 1947, 43).

Plutarch, another contemporary author, eulogized his own wife for showing her maternal love through breastfeeding their son: "and yet you had nursed him at your own breast and had submitted to surgery when your nipple was bruised. For such a conduct was noble, and it showed true mother love" ("καίτοι τῷ σεαυτῆς ἐκεῖνον ἐξέθρεψας μαστῷ καὶ τομῆς ἠνέσχου, τῆς θηλῆς περίθλασιν λαβούσης· γενναῖα γὰρ ταῦτα καὶ φιλόστοργα," Plut. *Consolation to His Wife* 609e; trans. De Lacy and Einarson 1959, 591). Interestingly, both Musonius and Plutarch identified good mothering not just with breastfeeding but also with painful nursing as the result of ineffective suckling, inflammation, or tiredness. What made the good mother and exemplary woman was the pain she suffered without complaint in her attempt to nurse and take care of her children. The ideal woman or woman philosopher in Musonius' words was the one who "love[d] her children more than life itself" ("τέκνα μᾶλλον ἀγαπᾶν ἢ τὸ ζῆν," Muson. *Disc.* 3.32; trans. Lutz 1947, 41).

The mother's milk, like the father's semen, was seen by medical authors, such as Galen (AD 129–ca. 216/217), moralists, such as Favorinus (ca. AD 85–155), as reported by Aulus Gellius (ca. AD 125–180), and Christian writers, such as Clement of Alexandria (ca. AD 150–215), as transformed blood.[60] Having been the

55 See Penniman 2017 and 2015.
56 For the Church Fathers' influence on later Byzantine culture, see e.g. Trovato 2023, 3–22; Lössl 2000; Moffatt 1986, 709.
57 See e.g. Milnor 2008; Severy 2003; Gardner 1998, 47–54; Galinsky 1996, 128–140; Syme 1960, 440–458.
58 Cooper 2007, 108.
59 Penniman 2017, 37.
60 Gal. *On the Function of the Parts of the Body* 14.8, 4.176.1–179.14K, ed. Kühn 1822; Aulus Gellius, *Attic Nights* 12.1.12–15, ed. Marshall 1969; Clement of Alexandria, *Paedagogus* 1.6.39.3–5, ed. Harl et al. 1960.

menses or the foetus' nourishment in the womb, maternal blood turned into milk to feed the newborn. Thus, a mother who offered her milk to her own baby "sustained a father's seminal patterning of his child and imbued her own positive traits in the hopes of shaping her child toward ideal man- or womanhood."[61] In short, (painful) breastfeeding was seen as a mother's ethical obligation to the family of her husband and to her children, who were nursed according to familial and social expectations. This ideology found one of its most eloquent expressions in late antique and Byzantine hagiography, whose mostly high-born saintly protagonists are depicted receiving milk from their mothers' breasts. Maternal breastfeeding in hagiography appears to determine the protagonists' exemplarity and future holiness. Through her milk, the Christian mother is presented as transmitting her faith and its values to her newborn babies.

In the aforementioned anonymous *Passion of Pistis, Elpis, Agape, and Sophia*, for example, Pistis – the Greek term for faith – attempts to convince her two younger sisters (Elpis (Hope) and Agape (Love)) to remain steadfast before their upcoming cruel tortures, by telling them: "we suckled milk from her [the mother's] holy breasts and she nurtured us in godly wisdom" ("γάλα ἀπὸ μαστῶν ἁγίων αὐτῆς μετειλήφαμεν, καὶ ἐπαίδευσεν ἡμᾶς τὴν ἔνθεον σοφίαν," *PPEAS* 8.16–17). Similarly, the mother, who, as the hagiographer points out, is a Roman noblewoman named Sophia (Wisdom),[62] encourages her oldest daughter, who is tortured first, with the following words: "I gave you birth, I nourished you with my own milk. I suffered pains and agonies for you" ("Ἐγώ σε ἐγέννησα, ἐγώ σε τῷ γάλακτι τῷ ἐμῷ ἀνέθρεψα, ἐγὼ πόνους καὶ ὠδῖνας ἔσχον διὰ σέ," *PPEAS* 9.1–3). Once again, (painful) breastfeeding and rearing become powerful signs of maternal love and care. Sophia expects her daughter to repay these maternal pains through the sufferings of martyrdom. Both mother (Sophia) and daughter (Pistis), and through them the hagiographer, understand maternal milk as an important means of Christian formation. Sophia's milk becomes Christian nourishment, turning its three consumers (Pistis, Elpis, and Agape) into future martyrs.

As for the importance of both paternal seed and maternal milk to character formation, it is brought up in the *PPEAS* through the words of Sophia's youngest daughter (Agape), who is presented as the wisest of the three sisters. She says to the torturer while he tries to convince her to renounce her faith:

Tyrant, do you forget that the seed of the same father created both me and the ones who have just died; that the same mother gave us birth; that we drank the same milk; that we were brought up with the same character; and that we were educated in the same holy letters?

Τύραννε, ἀγνοεῖς ὅτι ὁ αὐτός με ταῖς ἀποθανούσαις ἔσπειρεν πατὴρ καὶ ἡ αὐτὴ ἐγέννησε μήτηρ καὶ τὸ αὐτὸ ἐπίομεν γάλα καὶ τῇ αὐτῇ προαιρέσει ηὐξήθημεν καὶ τὰ αὐτὰ ἱερὰ γράμματα πεπαιδεύμεθα; (*PPEAS* 12.2–6)

---

61 Myers 2017, 79.
62 As in Perpetua's case, no husband is mentioned; see also n. 23.

Having been conceived through the same paternal seed and having shared the same maternal milk with her martyred sisters, Agape is destined, too, to become a Christian martyr.

Our Perpetua, therefore, who, like Sophia, does not entrust her baby to a wet nurse but undertakes the pains of breastfeeding, incorporates the Roman, but also Byzantine, ideals of the good mother. As Chapter 3 of this volume shows, Byzantine women, who refrained from breastfeeding their infants, were treated as bad mothers deserving eternal punishment in hell. Being a good mother, Perpetua suffers when she cannot have her nursling with her: "I was afflicted on account of my infant child" ("κατεπονούμην διὰ τὸ νήπιον τέκνον," *PPF* 3.6.9; trans. Cobb 2021, 49). Perpetua's words reveal a mother who is totally broken not because she is in prison, but because she is separated from her baby. For her, nothing is more important than the baby's welfare, to which she is wholly devoted. In Musonius' terms, Perpetua is a woman philosopher who sacrifices her own needs in lieu of those of her child. Her happiness is tightly linked with her son's well-being. Despite being imprisoned, Perpetua is pleased when her baby stays with her, because she can still be a good mother for her son.

While Perpetua embodies the ideal mother – she breastfeeds, loves, takes care of, and suffers for her nursling – she is treated by her non-Christian father and Hilarianus, the Roman officer who questions her and condemns her to death, as an evil mother that abandons and sacrifices her own child. With the baby in his hands and just before Perpetua's first public trial, the father tells her: "look at your son who is not able to live after you. ... Sacrifice having pity on the baby" ("ἴδε τὸν υἱόν σου ὃς μετὰ σὲ ζῆν οὐ δύναται. ... Ἐπίθυσον ἐλεήσασα τὸ βρέφος," *PPF* 5.3, 6.2; trans. Cobb 2021, 51). Hilarianus then adds: "spare your child's infancy" ("φεῖσαι τῆς τοῦ παιδίου νηπιότητος," *PPF* 6.3; trans. Cobb 2021, 51).[63] In contrast to Perpetua herself, her fellow Christians, and the other members of her family (her mother and brothers), the two men see her Christianity as incompatible with her maternal role. For them, a good mother and daughter should not deviate from the paternal law and the religious customs and traditions of her society. Furthermore, she should not behave in ways which would threaten her life and consequently that of her children, who depend on her.

In their attempt to convince Perpetua to abandon her religion, both father and tormentor use the same strategy: inducing guilt. By attacking her in her role as a mother – a role that is essential to her – they try to make her feel broken and thus follow their commandments to sacrifice to the Roman gods. However, their guilt mechanism proves ineffective, as it is initiated when Perpetua already feels confident about herself and her maternity. She replies: "'I do not sacrifice.' ... 'I am a Christian'" ("Οὐ θύω. ... 'Χριστιανή εἰμι,'" *PPF* 6.4; trans. Cobb 2021, 51–52).

---

63 Interestingly, modern scholars adopt a similar stance when they argue that Perpetua "gives up her infant son" (Vierow 1999, 617); see also Moss 2010 and Lefkowitz 1976. Whereas these scholars talk about Perpetua's abandonment of her child, other scholars claim that the heroine does not deny her motherhood but that she transcends it instead (e.g. Jensen 2002, 202–208).

Gathering that Perpetua's empowerment derives to a great extent from her ongoing breastfeeding and contact with her son, associated with her good maternal feelings, the father becomes more drastic and crueller. He prevents Perpetua from being the good mother she has set out to be by taking her boy away from her.

Even though the father's progressively harsher attacks intended to make Perpetua feel bad about herself as mother prove unsuccessful – evidently her boy survives, and her family takes good care of him – the *PPF* incorporates a tension between good and bad motherhood. There is an opposition between the ideal mother, who is selfless, loving, and totally devoted to her child, and the cruel mother, who leaves her son behind to die for her faith. This contestation constitutes an additional struggle of social rather than literary origin structuring the *PPF* that has not been identified by Mieke Bal or Marco Formisano, who refer to the text's internal struggles between "mundane prison and eternity, male and female, reality and dreams, autobiographical form and historical content, incomplete narrative and narrated closure."[64] In fact, the *PPF* is not original in its juxtaposition between good and bad motherhood. It continues a tradition established in Augustan Rome, whose art and literature incorporate tensions and paradoxes between good and bad mothering to regulate actual Roman mothers' behaviour.[65]

These tensions and paradoxes, however, concern free and elite Roman women such as Perpetua. In the case of Felicity, who is a slave, there is no problematization of her social role as a mother. As Anna Rebecca Solevåg rightly remarks:

> The text expresses no concern for Felicitas' separation from her baby immediately after giving birth, whereas Perpetua gets heavenly help so that she does not worry about her son or suffer inflammation from weaning. Felicitas suffers physically in childbirth, but not, as it seems, emotionally from the separation. … [T]he abrupt dismissal of the baby is better explained as revealing a disinterest in a slave's emotions. … It was common for a slave to have to give up her child.[66]

Felicity's violent death necessitates the services of a surrogate mother who could provide her newborn daughter with nourishment and affection. It is to surrogate mothering and its characteristics that we now turn.

Surrogate Mothers

Whereas high maternal mortality in the examined period generated large numbers of nurslings in need of surrogate nutrition, an equally high infant mortality made available considerable numbers of lactating women who could undertake the wet nurse's

---

64 Bal (1991) 2012; Formisano 2012, 339.
65 See Liveley 2012.
66 Solevåg 2013, 233–234.

task, either for free or against payment.[67] Surrogate breastfeeding was needed also in cases where blood mothers could not produce milk or had difficulties with nursing. Such mothers, as noted above, feature in Byzantine hagiography, yet their lactation problems are solved by divine intervention. One could assume, however, that such "miracles" were rare and that premodern women who could not breastfeed had to resort to wet nursing. Surrogate breastfeeding served other purposes, too, such as a mother's easier recovery from childbirth, resumption of sexual life,[68] and the quicker acquisition of more children. Finally, as already mentioned, aristocratic women preferred to refrain from the pains of breastfeeding and from a task that was considered unfit for their class, while slave owners would – for their own reasons and for profit – hire wet nurses to nurture the infants of their female slaves.

The families, protectors, or masters of mothers who did not want or were unable to breastfeed, as well as those of mothers who lost their lives in childbirth or through violence, like the martyr Felicity, and who could not afford a mercenary wet nurse, must have made arrangements for friendly cross-nursing. This could be provided by other female members of the biological mother's extended family, her friends, her neighbours, or her fellows from the same religious group. The anonymous mother in *PPF*, for example, who is Felicity's fellow Christian and becomes the surrogate mother of the martyr's daughter, belongs to the last category, of volunteer or non-mercenary nurses. Unfortunately, friendly cross-nursing is very rarely documented in ancient and Byzantine sources, possibly because it took place in the context of informal and personal arrangements and consequently was not subject to contracts and formalities.

An ancient example of friendly cross-nursing is detected in a literary work, Menander's *Samia* (4th c. BC; ed. Sandbach 1972), where it takes a comic twist. The play's protagonist, a concubine from Samos named Chrysis who is impregnated by Demeas and whose baby dies without the father knowing, breastfeeds the illegitimate child of Moschion, Demeas' adopted son. The baby is also nursed by its own mother Plangton, who is the daughter of Demeas' neighbour. A funny confusion is created about the identity of the baby's father as the plot develops.[69]

As far as early Byzantine sources are concerned, there are some references to friendly cross-nursing once again in hagiography. In Eustratios' *Life of Patriarch Eutychios* (*LE*, 6th–7th c. AD), there is an episode in which a woman whose milk dries up takes her nursling and goes to the saint's monastery asking for a cure. After

---

67 The frequency of premature infant death is recorded in ancient and Byzantine sources and archaeological remains. For evidence from bioarchaeology, see Bourbou et al. 2013. For overviews of other kinds of evidence, see e.g. Parkin 2013, 44–47; Papaconstantinou and Talbot 2009, 283–308; and Chapter 5 in this volume. On the demographic estimates of maternal mortality and the complexities of reading the inscriptional data, see Saller 1994, 9–43; Parkin 1992, 103–105.

68 According to medical and other authorities, breastfeeding was incompatible with sex, since it was believed that the latter destroyed the lactating woman's milk. See Chapter 2.

69 For a discussion of breastfeeding in this text, see Marshall 2017, 197–199. For some potential cases of allomaternal nursing attested in the epigraphic record, see Sparreboom 2014, 147; see also Centlivres Challet 2017, 901–902.

receiving Eutychios' prayer and holy oil, the woman's breasts start overflowing with milk. Thus, this mother who used to visit other nursing women asking for their milk is now offering her own excessive milk to other infants, relieving both her maternal body and other anxious mothers (*LE* 1681–1694, ed. Laga 1992). Albeit very few, these two cases of friendly cross-dressing and the one found in *PPF* reveal the existence of networks of friendly, individual, and supportive interactions and relationships between mothers sharing the same concerns about their maternal bodies and their infants' nurture and well-being. These female networks empowered the involved mothers, who took initiatives and immediate action to help each other.

The type of surrogate mother that is most well documented in our sources is the mercenary wet nurse of low social status, who was a free, freed, or enslaved mother, a fact suggesting that wet nursing was a usual practice in the examined period.[70] That is the reason why medical authors, such as Soranos (1st–2nd c. AD), Oribasios (fl. 4th c. AD), Paul of Aegina (fl. early 7th c. AD), and Aetios of Amida (fl. ca. AD 530–560), philosophers, such as "Myia" (3rd/2nd c. BC), and influential Church Fathers, such as John Chrysostom (AD 340/350–407), as shown in Chapter 2, gave advice on how to choose a wet nurse and how to monitor her mothering. As already indicated, the popularity of wet nursing is also manifested through philosophers', moralists', and theologians' exhortations to families to avoid hiring wet nurses and to have blood mothers breastfeed their own children instead.[71]

In the Egyptian papyri, nurslings under contract for wet nursing were primarily non-citizen foundlings or domestic slave babies.[72] Nurslings recorded in Roman epitaphs were not only elite children of senatorial or equestrian families but also slaves or freed children of intermediate status.[73] Wet nurses in Byzantine sources, chiefly hagiographical, were Christian women who were hired to breastfeed mostly elite children and orphans.[74] While medical authors of antiquity, such as Soranos, asked parents to hire Greek wet nurses so that their children could learn the best speech and culture,[75] Christian authors expected their contemporaries to employ Christian nurses so that children were from an early age introduced into the values of their faith. For this reason, the father of the future martyr Theodore, for instance, undertook to feed his baby son with wheat and barley porridge because he could not find a Christian wet nurse (*Life of Theodore 'the Recruit'* (10th c. AD), 225, ed. Sigalas 1925).

70 This is apparently the reason why most studies on premodern breastfeeding focus on the wet nurse. For ancient and Byzantine wet nurses, see most of the references provided above in n. 4.
71 For the mother/wet nurse debate, see Constantinou and Skouroumouni-Stavrinou 2024.
72 For listings and statistics, see e.g. Parca 2017, 212; Tawfik 1997, 942–943.
73 See Bradley 1986, 204–206.
74 For example, a wet nurse was hired by the rich couple Emmelia of Caesarea and Basil the Elder to breastfeed their children, including saints Macrina, Basil the Great, and Gregory of Nyssa (*Life of Macrina* (*LM*, AD 382/383), 3.1–3, ed. Maraval 1971). A wet nurse also rears the orphan Febronia, who is brought up in the nunnery of her aunt, the abbess Bryene (*Life of Febronia* (7th c. AD) 7.2–4, ed. Chiesa 1990). For orphans in Byzantium, see Miller 2003.
75 See Chapter 2.

That the employment of wet nurses was a self-evident, and even natural, under-taking for elite families in the examined period was manifested through the words of high-born authors, such as the Roman emperor Marcus Aurelius (AD 121–180) and the Cappadocian Father Basil the Great (AD 329–379). In Marcus Aurelius' autobiographical *Meditations*, we read the following:

> I travel along nature's way until I fall down and take my rest, breathing out my last into the air, from which I draw my daily breath, and falling down to that earth from which my father drew his seed, my mother her blood and my nurse her milk, from which for so many years I have taken my daily food and drink, the earth which carries my footsteps and which I have used to the full in so many ways.
>
> Πορεύομαι διὰ τῶν κατὰ φύσιν, μέχρι πεσὼν ἀναπαύσωμαι, ἐναποπνεύσας μὲν τούτῳ, ἐξ οὗ καθ᾽ ἡμέραν ἀναπνέω, πεσὼν δὲ ἐπὶ τούτῳ, ἐξ οὗ καὶ τὸ σπερμάτιον ὁ πατήρ μου συνέλεξε καὶ τὸ αἱμάτιον ἡ μήτηρ καὶ τὸ γαλάκτιον ἡ τροφός· ἐξ οὗ καθ᾽ ἡμέραν τοσούτοις ἔτεσι βόσκομαι, καὶ ἀρδεύομαι, ὃ φέρει με πατοῦντα, καὶ εἰς τοσαῦτα ἀποχρώμενον αὐτῷ. (Marc. Aur. *Med.* 5.4, ed. Farquharson (1944)1968; trans. Gill 2013, 31)

Marcus saw his life as a journey following the laws of nature. As such, it took a twofold form: "one's biological life" from the first to the final breath and "one's end as dispersal into the elements."[76] In the first part of Marcus' life journey, three people played a central role. These were Marcus' father, mother, and wet nurse, to whom he owed his very life. He was generated through his father's seed and his mother's blood, in whose womb he took his first nourishment. When he was brought to the world it was the wet nurse's milk that sustained and raised him. The fluids of father, mother, and wet nurse (seed, blood, and milk) were viewed as earthly harvests collected and housed in human bodies, whose processes and life cycle were also determined by the laws of nature. Through this understanding, the three social roles of father, mother, and wet nurse emerged as natural: they were intended by nature to create and support new lives that followed, in turn, their own natural cycles.[77] Thus, the cultural norm of delegating the nursing of high-born infants to wet nurses became a natural law.

As for Basil, he wrote in one of his letters (*Let.* 37), whose recipient remains unknown:

> But I have only one foster-brother, this man who is the son of the woman who nursed me, and I pray that the household in which I was brought up may remain at its old assessment. … I urge you with this thought to spare the family in which I was nourished. … Furthermore, there is one thing that I want

---

76 Gill 2013, 147.
77 For the compatibility of human nature with universal nature in Marcus' philosophy, see Long 2012; Hadot 1998, 35–53.

your modesty to know as beyond question the truth – that most of the slaves belong to this man as a gift from us as remuneration for our sustenance, our parents having bestowed them upon him.

σύντροφον δὲ τῆς θρεψαμένης με υἱὸν τοῦτον ἔχω ἕνα, καὶ εὔχομαι τὸν οἶκον ἐν ᾧ ἀνετράφην ἐπὶ τῆς ὁμοίας καταστάσεως διαμεῖναι. ... παρακαλῶ οὕτω φείσασθαι τῆς οἰκίας ᾗ ἐνετράφην. ... Ἐκεῖνό γε μὴν πάντων ἀληθέστατον γινώσκειν σου τὴν κοσμιότητα βούλομαι, ὅτι τῶν ἀνδραπόδων τὰ πλεῖστα παρ᾽ ἡμῶν ὑπῆρξεν αὐτῷ μισθὸς τῆς τροφῆς ἡμῶν, τῶν γονέων ἡμῶν παρασχομένων. (Bas. *Let.* 37, ed. Courtonne 1957; trans. Deferrari 1926, 193, 195)

Apart from presenting wet nursing as a usual practice for elite families, Basil's letter also reveals other realities concerning the practice and the bonds it established. Wet nurses did not always move to rich families' houses to nurture their infants. Furthermore, they brought up the foster nurslings along with their own children.[78] At least Basil's sister Macrina, the family's first-born child, was nursed at home by both a wet nurse and her mother Emmelia (*LM* 3.1–3). Yet, for a family bearing ten children, with one of them dying in infancy, it must have been more convenient and less tiring for Emmelia to have some of those children reared in wet nurses' homes.[79] A nursling's integration into the wet nurse's family, which functioned as a foster family, as suggested by Basil's letter, created various bonds and relationships. Basil was strongly attached to both the woman nursing him and her son, with whom he shared the same milk and motherly affection. This emotional attachment was everlasting: when Basil wrote this and an earlier letter (Bas. *Let.* 36) to ask support from a powerful man for his foster brother, he was in his late thirties or early forties.

In that previous letter, Basil described his foster brother as his own self ("ἀντ᾽ ἐμαυτοῦ," Bas. *Let.* 36), while in the 37th letter he wrote: "I pray that the household in which I was brought up may remain at its old assessment" ("εὔχομαι τὸν οἶκον ἐν ᾧ ἀνετράφην ἐπὶ τῆς ὁμοίας καταστάσεως διαμεῖναι," Bas. *Let.* 37; trans. Deferrari 1926, 195). Basil's gratitude for his foster family was also shared by his biological family, who offered a good number of slaves and part of its estate to the foster brother. At the time of writing the letters, Basil was also prepared to undertake the increased taxation that resulted from the foster brother's possession of slaves and lands. Both letters highlight Basil's indebtedness to his foster family that not only brought him up but also continued to support him throughout his life. All in all, Basil's letters bring to the fore the powerful bonds and relationships that were created between a wet nurse, her family, and the infant under her care, as well as those between the infant's biological family and the foster family.

---

78 Wet nursing contracts that have come down to us, however, forbid wet nurses to offer their milk to other infants apart from the one they are hired for. See Parca 2013; Bradley 1986.

79 For the members of Basil's family, see Pfister 1964.

Basil's wet nurse belonged to the category of the good wet nurse. Like the category of the good mother discussed above, that of the good wet nurse included surrogate mothers who were devoted to their nurslings, whom they treated as their own children. Bad wet nurses, by contrast, were neglectful and put the nursling's life in danger through their spoiled milk and bad habits. As Constantinou and Skouroumouni-Stavrinou have shown, the binary of the good/bad wet nurse, like that of the good/bad mother, was an essential part of the ancient and Byzantine institution of motherhood.[80] Both binaries served imperial ideologies, whether Roman or Byzantine, concerning (elite) family values and the formation of social identities. Further discussion of these two binaries, as already pointed out, is provided in the two chapters of the volume's first part, on the lactating woman's society and ideology.

Chapter 2 ("Breast Rules: The Body of the Wet Nurse in Ancient and Early Byzantine Discourses") explores some ancient and early Byzantine discourses on wet nurses, focussing mainly on texts of the broader Greek medical tradition that were produced between the second century BC and the seventh century AD. The chapter covers the examined texts' prescriptions about the characteristics of the good wet nurse and recommendations concerning her diet and way of life and work. Moreover, the early history of sociomedical attitudes towards the wet nurse and her desired profile are traced, while her ambiguous status is highlighted: she was treated as both an inferior servant and a female philosopher.

Chapter 3, on the other hand, with the title "The Breast as a Locus for Punishment," turns to blood mothers who behaved as bad mothers. Drawing on the textual and visual traditions of afterlife punishments addressed to mothers who refrained from breastfeeding their babies, the chapter shows how these traditions, which probably had an Egyptian and monastic origin, aimed at controlling women of rural communities.

Having sketched the socio-ideology and the main types of the ancient and early Byzantine lactating woman – the blood mother and the surrogate mother – we now proceed to the thematic strand on medicine and practice.

Medicine and Practice

The issues of medical concern featuring in the *PPF*, which are related to maternity and breastfeeding,[81] include the eighth-month birth, a new mother's first milk, breast inflammation, and lactation cessation, along with weaning. The first two issues are experienced by Felicity, who prematurely gives birth in prison, while Perpetua, whose child is forced into abrupt weaning, is confronted with the remaining

---

80 Constantinou and Skouroumouni-Stavrinou 2024.

81 The *PPF* includes also other instances having a medical background, such as the deathly facial gangrene of Perpetua's brother Dinokrates, discussed under "Art and Literature," and the holy woman's cervical vertebrae, which the inexperienced gladiator erroneously attacks in his attempt to decapitate her. Eventually, it is Perpetua herself who directs the gladiator's hand to her clavicle (*PPF* 7.5, 11.9).

difficulties. These maternal issues were essential in the discussed cultures, which, as already mentioned, were characterized by high infant and maternal mortality. It is, therefore, no wonder that pregnancy, childbirth, and breastfeeding complications preoccupied both medical and other authors. Their treatment and uses in ancient and Byzantine medical treatises and other works – mainly philosophical and theological – reveal cultural anxieties that in some cases survive until today.[82]

For the purposes of this part, the *PPF* is discussed in the light of medical, philosophical, and theological works that circulated both in Perpetua's times and later, until the sixth century, when the text was possibly translated into Greek. The following comparative analysis is divided into four parts, each devoted to one or two of the said maternity issues.

Eighth-Month Birth

According to the *PPF*, when Felicity was arrested, "she had **an eight-month abdomen**" ("ὀκτὼ μηνῶν ἔχουσα γαστέρα," *PPF* 15.2; emphasis added).[83] Felicity's fellow Christians prayed that she could give birth before the communal martyrdom, a development that would allow her to die with all the other imprisoned Christians. As soon as the prayer is completed, "**the pains of childbirth** seized her – **difficult as is the nature of the eighth month**. And **toiling with childbirth, she felt pain**" ("ὠδῖνες αὐτὴν συνέσχον, κατὰ τὴν τοῦ ὀγδόου μηνὸς φύσιν χαλεπαί. Καὶ κατὰ τὸν **τοκετὸν καμοῦσα ἤλγει**," *PPF* 15.5; trans. Cobb 2021, 59; emphasis added). For our purposes, the two short passages given here are remarkable in two respects. First, their language relies heavily on medical terminology. Second, the extracts reflect medical and philosophical discussions about the viability of the eight-month-old foetus and about the difficulty of the eighth-month delivery. Based on numerology and the superstition that the number eight was unlucky, these discussions went back to Hippocrates and continued until the late Byzantine period.[84]

---

82 Cf. e.g. the modern superstition about the eighth-month foetus (Reiss and Ash 1988).
83 In this case, Cobb's translation has not been adopted, because it is less exact. Cobb translates the phrase as "she was eight months pregnant" (trans. Cobb 2021, 59).
84 For the origins of these discussions and their continuation by later ancient Greek writers, see Hanson 1987. Some relevant ancient and early Byzantine discussions are mentioned below. As for middle and late Byzantine treatments, see e.g. Michael Psellos' (11th c. AD) philosophical notes ("Seven-month infants survive, but not the eight-month ones …"; "Τὰ ἑπταμηνιαῖα βρέφη ζῶσι, τὰ δ' ὀκταμηνιαῖα οὔ …," *Opuscula physica* 55.1023, ed. Duffy 1992); and John Protospatharios' (13th/14th c. AD) *Commentary on Hesiod's Work and Days* ("But many say that the seventh [day] is life-giving, since seven-month infants are more viable than those of eight months. But it is good to explain how the seven-month and the nine-month infants are viable whereas the eight-month ones are not"; "Ἀλλὰ καὶ ζωογόνος παρὰ πολλοῖς ἡ ἑβδόμη λέγεται, ὅτι τὰ βρέφη ἑπταμηνιαῖα ὄντα ζωογονεῖται μᾶλλον, ἤπερ ὀκταμηνιαῖα. Ἀλλὰ πῶς μὲν τὰ ἑπταμηνιαῖα καὶ ἐνναμηνιαῖα ζωογονεῖται, τὰ δὲ ὀκταμηνιαῖα οὐδαμῶς, καλὸν εἰπεῖν," *Comm. on Hesiod*, 450, ed. Gaisford 1823).

As a short medical treatise entitled *On the Eight-Month Infant* (*Oct.*),[85] which is attributed to Hippocrates (ca. 460–370 BC), states:

> All women have the same explanation for this: they say that in the **eighth month** it is **most strenuous to carry their abdomens**. … For it happens to these children in immediate succession that they suffer both the strain that occurs in the uterus and the one after **birth has taken place**, and therefore no eight months' child survives. … When this happens, both the **mother must strain herself more**, and the child must either die or be born with **greater difficulty**.
>
> χρέωνται δὲ πᾶσαι ἑνὶ λόγῳ περὶ τούτου· φασὶ γὰρ τοὺς **ὀγδόους τῶν μηνῶν** καὶ **χαλεπώτατα φέρειν τὰς γαστέρας**, ὀρθῶς λέγουσαι. … οὐ περιγίνεσθαι τὰ ὀκτάμηνα. συγκυρεῖ γὰρ αὐτοῖς ἐφεξῆς κακοπαθεῖν τήν τε ἐν τῇ μήτρῃ γινομένην κακοπαθείην καὶ τὴν ὅταν ὁ **τόκος γένηται**, καὶ διὰ τοῦτο τῶν ὀκταμήνων οὐδὲν περιεγένετο. … τούτου δὲ γινομένου καὶ τὴν **μητέρα ἀνάγκη πονῆσαι μᾶλλον** καὶ τὸ παιδίον ἢ ἀπολέσθαι ἢ **χαλεπώτερον ἐξελθεῖν**. (Hippoc. *Oct.* 3.8–9 and 10.44, ed. and trans. Potter 2010, 81, 95; emphasis added)

The juxtaposition of this Hippocratic passage with those from the *PPF* shows how the latter's Greek translator uses medical terminology (see the words in bold) and theory to describe Felicity's situation as realistically as possible. The Greek translator adopts the medical claims that eight-month gestation is difficult and that giving birth at this stage of pregnancy is even more difficult, as it is extremely painful. Concerning the medical author's argument that eighth-month infants are not viable – which he bases on a theory that a pregnant woman and her foetus go through some illness during the eighth month – even though it is not mentioned in the *PPF*, the redactor seems to agree with it, for it supports the text's religious message. That Felicity gives birth during this difficult month, which a later medical author, Soranos, calls in his *Gynaecology* (*Gyn.*) "burdensome" ("βαρὺν ὄντα," Sor. *Gyn.* 1.56.1.2 (CMG 4, 40.9), ed. Ilberg 1927; trans. Temkin 1956, 56),[86] and

---

85 This text has come down to us with two different titles: Chapters 1–9 have the title *On the Seven-Month Infant*, while Chapters 10–13 are entitled *On the Eight-Month Infant*. Here we follow Robert Joly, who has suggested the use of the latter title for the whole work. Joly's approach is also adopted by Paul Potter, the latest editor and English translator of the text (Potter 2010, 71–101), whose edition and translation are used here.

86 Soranos, but also Galen, along with their early Byzantine followers (e.g. Orib. *Medical Collections Incerti* (*Med. Coll. Inc.*) 22.17–19 (CMG 6.2.2, 114.5–13), ed. Raeder 1933), pay special attention to eighth-month gestation, prescribing a particular diet and exercise for the pregnant woman. We read, for example, in Soranos: "With the beginning of the eighth month which people euphemistically call 'easy,' although it is burdensome and produces malaise and other distress, she [the pregnant woman] must restrict still further the amount of food and must take exercise only in a litter or a big sedan chair, unless one desires to walk short of the point of exhaustion. And if the discomfort is greater, it will also be advisable to fast for one day so that the malaise can be dispelled by the respite"; "τοῦ δὲ ὀγδόου μηνὸς ἐνστάντος, ὃν κατ' εὐφημισμὸν λέγουσιν εἶναι 'κοῦφον' βαρὺν ὄντα καὶ δυσαρέστησιν καὶ τὴν ἄλλην κακοπάθειαν ἀποτελοῦντα, τὸ τῆς τροφῆς πλῆθος

the fact that her baby survives, "renders the result of her friends' prayers all the more miraculous."[87] Examining late antique authors' accounts of Felicity's eighth-month delivery, Cobb shows their stronger emphasis on her pain in an attempt to prevent their audiences from thinking that the woman's fellow martyrs prayed for a miscarriage.[88] In so doing, these authors appear to further endorse established medical doctrines about the difficulties and dangers of eighth-month deliveries which conveniently serve their authorial purposes.

The idea that pregnant women suffer greatly during the eighth month was also expressed by an ancient philosopher, Aristotle (384–322 BC), who like Hippocrates exercised a great influence on ancient and Byzantine authors, both medical and non-medical.[89] The early Byzantine medical author Oribasios preserves the following Aristotelian fragment:

> From the work of the philosopher Aristotle, *On the Eight-Month Infant.* Some people say that eight-month infants do not survive, but this is untrue, for they do live. And this is especially evident in Egypt, because the Egyptians bring up all their infants. … Yet even in Greece, when one observes cautiously, one sees that the same happens. It is, therefore, not true that all eight-month infants are non-viable. Yet it is true that few [eight-month infants] survive and indeed fewer than the infants of seventh months and those of more months. … Women suffer most during the fourth and the ninth month, and if they have an abortion in the fourth or the ninth month they mostly die as well. Therefore, not only do the eight-month infants die, but the mothers are also endangered when they abort.
>
> Ἐκ τῶν Ἀριστοτέλους τοῦ φιλοσόφου. Περὶ ὀκταμήνων. Περὶ τῶν ὀκταμήνων εἰσί τινες οἵ φασιν οὐθὲν ζῆν· τοῦτο δ' ἐστὶ ψεῦδος· ζῇ γάρ, καὶ τοῦτο μάλιστα μὲν ἐν Αἰγύπτῳ δῆλον διὰ τὸ τρέφειν τε πάντα τὰ γινόμενα τοὺς Αἰγυπτίους. … οὐ μὴν ἀλλὰ καὶ ἐν τῇ Ἑλλάδι τηροῦσιν ἔστιν ἰδεῖν οὕτως ἔχειν, ὥστε τὸ μὲν ἅπαντα τὰ ὀκτάμηνα μὴ ζῆν οὐκ ἀληθές ἐστιν, ὅτι μέντοι ὀλίγα καὶ ἧττον τῶν ἑπταμήνων τε καὶ τῶν ἐκ τοῦ πλείονος ἀριθμοῦ γενομένων ἀληθές. … πονοῦσι δ' αἱ γυναῖκες μάλιστα τὸν μῆνα τὸν δ καὶ τὸν η, καὶ ἐὰν διαφθείρωσι η ἢ δ μηνί, διαφθείρονται καὶ αὐταὶ ὡς ἐπὶ τὸ πολύ, ὥστε οὐ μόνον τὰ ὀκτάμηνα οὐ ζῆν, ἀλλὰ καὶ διαφθειρομένων αἱ τίκτουσαι κινδυνεύουσιν. (Orib. *Med. Coll. Inc.* 12.1–7.1 (CMG 6.2.2, 94.14–95.9))

ἐπισυνέργειν, κινήσεις δὲ παραλαμβάνειν μόνας τὰς διὰ φορείου ἢ μακρὰς καθέδρας, πλὴν εἰ μὴ μέχρι διεκλύσεως ὀρεχθείη τις τοῦ περιπατῆσαι. Πλείονος δὲ οὔσης τῆς δυσφορίας καὶ ἀνατείνειν ἁρμόσει πρὸς μίαν ἡμέραν, ὥστε διὰ τῆς ἡρεμίας ἐκλυθῆναι τὸ δυσαρέστημα," Sor. *Gyn.* 1.56.1–2.1 (CMG 4, 40.8–14); trans. Temkin 1956, 56).

87 Solevåg 2013, 207.

88 Cobb 2022.

89 For Hippocrates' influence on other medical authors, see e.g. Bouras-Vallianatos and Xenophontos 2018; Marganne 2015; Constantelos 1999; Temkin 1962. Concerning his influence on non-medical authors, see e.g. Preat 2021; Plati 2020. For Aristotle's influence, see e.g. Constantinou 2022; Becchi 2013; Oehler 1964.

The fragment starts with a criticism against those, namely Hippocrates and his followers, who argue that eighth-month infants are not viable. The examples of Egyptian, but also some Greek, eighth-month children who survive proves the Hippocratic doctrine wrong. However, Aristotle and through him Oribasios do not completely reject the doctrine. Despite their scepticism, Aristotle and Oribasios confirm the established idea that giving birth in the eighth month, as in the fourth month, is extremely painful, causing not only the foetus' death but also that of the mother.

Even if ancient and early Byzantine audiences of the *PPF* might not have treated the survival of Felicity and her baby as miraculous, but as one of those few cases that according to (medical) authorities proved the possibility of a successful eighth-month delivery, the creation of a striking association between the mother's and the martyr's pain ensured the strong Christological, and at the same time poetic, dimension of the episode featuring Felicity's delivery. During her eighth-month delivery, Felicity undergoes such great suffering that it provokes the reaction of a prison officer, who asks her how she will treat the pain caused by the wild animals' attacks in the arena if she is so overcome by the pains of childbirth.

Felicity's reply, however, is unexpected – and one could say unrealistic – considering her grave position. Experiencing pains that medical authorities repeatedly described as some of the harshest ones, Felicity speaks not just confidently, clearly, and calmly, but also poetically: "Now I myself endure what I endure, but in that place is another who endures <within me> on my behalf [he will be in me so that he might endure], since I endure on his behalf" ("Νῦν ἐγὼ πάσχω ὃ πάσχω· ἐκεῖ δὲ ἄλλος ἐστὶν ὁ <ἐν ἐμοὶ> πάσχων ὑπὲρ ἐμοῦ [ἔσται ἐν ἐμοὶ ἵνα πάθῃ], διότι ἐγὼ πάσχω ὑπὲρ αὐτοῦ," *PPF* 15.6; trans. Cobb 2021, 59). In prison, Felicity suffers as a mother, whereas in the arena she will suffer as a martyr of Christ. Both sufferings are equally unbearable, but the first is purely physical, whereas the second acquires a metaphysical dimension. As such, the first is the prerequisite of the second. In Cobb's words, "indeed, it was precisely her labour pains that strengthened Felicitas' faith" in Christ and made her believe that He would suffer for her during her tortures.[90]

Just as the delivery scene points towards death in the arena, the description of Felicitas in the arena refers back to her delivery:

And similarly, Felicitas was rejoicing in the safety of her childbirth so that she could fight the beasts – from blood to blood, from midwife to single combat – being about to bathe after childbirth in a second baptism, that is to say, with her own blood.

Ὁμοίως καὶ ἡ Φηλικιτάτη χαίρουσα ἐπὶ τῇ τοῦ τοκετοῦ ὑγείᾳ ἵνα θηριομαχήσῃ, ἀπὸ αἵματος εἰς αἷμα, ἀπὸ μαίας πρὸς μονομαχίαν, μέλλουσα λούσασθαι μετὰ τὸν τοκετὸν βαπτισμῷ δευτέρῳ, τουτέστιν τῷ ἰδίῳ αἵματι. (*PPF* 18.3; trans. Cobb 2021, 61)

90 Cobb 2022, 17.

In contrast to the other martyrs' bodies, that of Felicity bleeds more and suffers longer. Her bleeding and pain start from the moment of delivery, and two days later, when she is taken to the arena, she still bleeds. During Felicity's tortures, the blood of martyrdom is added to her postpartum bleeding. The narrator, however, refers only to the blood of Felicity's childbirth, which, as he points out, is substituted by the blood of martyrdom, just as the midwife is replaced by the torturer. Yet there is no midwife helping at the delivery – Felicity gives birth alone, attended by a prison officer. The narrator's rhetoric aims at suppressing Felicity's lochia, which is repressed also through the emphasis on her leaking breasts, as will be further discussed in the following section.

The New Mother's First Milk

While Felicity was walking naked in the arena to be killed by "a most savage heifer" ("ἀγριωτάτην δάμαλιν," *PPF* 20.1; trans. Cobb 2021, 61), her nipples were leaking. In the narrator's words, "milk was dripping from her breasts, as she had recently given birth" ("μασθοῖς στάζουσαν γάλα, ὡς προσφάτως κυήσασαν," *PPF* 10.2; trans. with some modifications Cobb 2021, 63). According to Laurence Totelin, whose analysis is based on the Latin version of the text, which presents Felicity's bodily situation in a similar manner,[91] at this very point the new mother's "milk comes in …; it starts to flow abundantly."[92] As Totelin goes on to remark, "her breasts are not 'still leaking'; they leak out for the first time. … Felicity has passed the stage in which her body produces only the thick, cheesy milk that is unfit for consumption."[93]

Despite its attractiveness, this interpretation does not seem to be supported by the text. If Felicity was experiencing an overflow of milk, then a different verbal form would have been used – at least in the Greek text. In place of the participle "στάζουσαν" ("shedding [milk] drop by drop"), the Greek translator would have employed one of the following participles: "(ἐκ)βλύζουσα" ("gushing out [milk]"), "βρύουσα" ("overflowing"), or "ῥέουσα" ("flowing [with milk]"), which are the terms used by our authors to talk about overflowing breasts.[94]

---

91 *partu recentem stillantibus mammis* ("fresh from childbirth, with breasts dripping," *PPF* 20.2, ed. Van Beek 1936; trans. Cobb 2021, 37).

92 Totelin 2021, 249.

93 Totelin 2021, 249. See, however, Chapter 5, where Totelin appears to have a different opinion: Felicity's "milk was flowing on the arena, perhaps for the first time."

94 The verbs "βλύω" ("gush out") and "βρύω" ("overflow") are, for instance, employed in the aforementioned episode from the *Life of Patriarch Eutychios* in which an anonymous woman's breasts start overflowing with milk through Saint Eutychios' miraculous intervention: "my breasts gushed out on the spot and they overflowed for many days continuously" ("παραχρῆμα ἐξέβλυσαν οἱ μαστοί μου καὶ ἐπὶ πολλὰς ἡμέρας ἀδιαλείπτως ἔβρυον," *LE* 1686–1688). As for the word "ῥέοντες" ("flowing"), in a spurious homily of John Chrysostom, for example, it is used to refer to the breasts of the lactating mothers whose infants were killed by King Herod ("when the milk that was flowing from the breasts whitened the earth;" "ὅτε καὶ μαζοὶ ῥέοντες γάλα τὴν γῆν ἐλαύκαινον," *Hom. on Salome's Dancing and the Decapitation of John the Forerunner*, PG 59, 525).

That the liquid leaking from Felicity's nipples is what we today call "colostrum" (foremilk), and not mature milk, is also suggested by the time which elapses between the holy woman's parturition and martyrdom, in association with her premature labour, which could cause the delayed coming in of her milk. In the *PPF*, it is explicitly stated that Felicity gives birth three days before the Christians' execution in the arena (*PPF* 15.4). According to Soranos' *Gynaecology*, which Totelin, too, uses for her argument, it is from the fourth day onwards that a new mother's milk becomes suitable for consumption, suggesting that mature milk comes in at least three days after parturition. Soranos writes:

> If, however, a woman well able to provide milk is not at hand, during the first three days one must use honey alone or mix goat's milk with it. Then one must supply the mother's milk, the first portion having been sucked out beforehand by some stripling (for it is heavy), or squeezed out gently with the hands, since the thick part is hard to suck out and is also apt to clog up in newborn children on account of the softness of their gums.
>
> εἰ δὲ μὴ παρείη τις εὐπόρως τὸ γάλα παρέχειν δυναμένη, ταῖς πρώταις τρισὶν ἡμέραις μόνῳ τῷ μέλιτι χρηστέον ἢ καὶ τὸ αἴγειον αὐτῷ γάλα συμπλεκτέον, εἶτα τὸ μητρῷον ἐπιχορηγητέον τοῦ πρώτου προεκμυζηθέντος διὰ μειρακίου τινός (βαρὺ γάρ ἐστιν) ἢ πράως διὰ χειρῶν ἀποθλιβέντος ἐπεὶ καὶ δυσεκμύζητόν ἐστιν τὸ παχυμερὲς καὶ δυνάμενον ἐπὶ τῶν ἀρτιγενῶν διὰ τὴν τρυφερίαν τῶν οὔλων ἐπινασθῆναι. (Sor. *Gyn.* 2.18.3 (CMG 4, 65.7–13); trans. with minor modifications Temkin 1956, 89)

In Soranos' logic, the liquid dropping from Felicity's nipples on the day of her martyrdom is not mature milk but a first milk (colostrum), and as such it should be avoided. It is, therefore, to her benefit that Felicity's newborn daughter receives the mature milk of a surrogate mother, despite her blood mother's death. Since Felicity's baby is breastfed with mature human milk, ensuring its survival – "a woman well able to provide milk is at hand" – the blood mother's absence is not seen as a problem for medical authors, such as Soranos, Galen, and their early Byzantine followers (Oribasios and Paul of Aegina), who treat the wet nurse's milk as the most suitable nourishment for the newborn.[95]

Similarly, Perpetua's death does not harm her son's upbringing, which is undertaken by her family. In any case, as discussed in the previous part ("Society and Ideology"), it was a common practice in antiquity and Byzantium to entrust children's rearing to surrogate mothers, who often took the foster children into their own homes. In these cases, blood mothers were completely absent from their children's early lives, a fact that does not appear to have been seen as problematic in the examined societies. What is suggested once again is that if we take into

---

95 See Gal. *Hygiene* (*San. Tu.*) 1.9.7–9 (CMG 5.4.2, 22.21–29), ed. Koch 1923; Orib. *Med. Coll. Inc.* 30 (CMG 6.2.2, 121.9–24); Paul Aegin. *Epitome of Medicine* 1.2–3 (CMG 9.1, 9.10–10.4), ed. Heiberg 1921.

consideration these realities, neither Felicity nor Perpetua sacrificed her child, as some modern scholars have pointed out.[96] Both women secured their babies' survival by entrusting them to surrogate mothers. In so doing, they followed a common social practice.

Turning back to Soranos, he strongly condemns the mother's first milk, which today is considered extremely important for the newborn's protection against "allergic and chronic diseases, in addition to long-term metabolic benefits."[97] Soranos advises against the consumption of the first milk because its "heaviness" and "thickness" endanger the newborn's life. In a previous passage, Soranos expresses more eloquently his biases against the first milk:

> [T]he maternal milk is in most cases **bad**, being **thick**, very **cheesy**, and therefore **hard to digest**, **raw**, and **not mature**. Furthermore, it is produced by **bodies** which are in a **bad state**, **agitated** and **changed** to the extent that we see the body altered after delivery when, from having suffered a great discharge of blood, it is **dried up**, **toneless**, **discoloured**, and in the majority of cases it is **feverish** as well. For all these reasons, it is **absurd to prescribe the maternal milk** until the body enjoys stable health.
>
> τὸ γὰρ μητρῷον … εἰκότως ἐπὶ τὸ πλεῖστον **φαῦλόν** ἐστιν ὡς **παχὺ** καὶ **τυρῶδες** ἄγαν καὶ διὰ τοῦτο **δύσπεπτον** καὶ **ἀργὸν** καὶ **ἀκατέργαστον** καὶ ἀπὸ **σωμάτων κεκακοπαθηκότων** καὶ **ἐκτεταραγμένων** φερομένων καὶ τοσαύτην **μετακόσμησιν** εἰληφότων, ὅσην ὁρῶμεν συμβαίνουσαν μετὰ τὴν ἀποκύησιν, **ἰσχνουμένου** καὶ **ἀτονοῦντος** καὶ **ἀχροοῦντος** τοῦ σώματος ὡς πολλὴν αἵματος ἀπόκρισιν ὑπομένοντος, τὰ πολλὰ δὲ καὶ **πυρέττοντος**· ὧν χάριν πάντων **τὸ μητρῷον γάλα**, μέχρις ἂν εὐσταθήσῃ τὸ σῶμα, **συντάσσειν ἄτοπόν ἐστιν.** (Sor. *Gyn.* 2.18.1.2–2.1 (CMG 4, 64.22–65.1); trans. with some modifications Temkin 1956, 89; emphasis added)

According to Soranos, the worst thing that can happen to the newborn is to consume the blood mother's first milk, whose evilness is determined by two factors: its texture and its producer.[98] Being highly concentrated like cheese, the first milk is considered difficult to suck and to digest. Due to its thickness, it might also cause the baby to choke or damage its gums. As for the milk producer, the mother, her bad bodily state after parturition is seen to be reflected in the quality of her first milk. Like her unstable, dried up, exhausted body, tainted with blood, her first milk is changeable, raw, immature, and discoloured. As Soranos explains later in his section "On testing the milk," milk which is suitable for consumption has an unchangeable white colour, a pleasant smell, smoothness, homogeneity, and moderate density (Sor. *Gyn.* 2.22 (CMG 4, 69.19–70.25)). Being yellowish and thick,

---

96 See e.g. Parkhouse 2017, 584; Nelson 2016, 13; Moss 2010, 196; Burnett 2009, 87; Caseau 2009, 142; see also above, n. 63.
97 Bardanzellu et al. 2017, 843.
98 For a discussion of bad and damaging milk, see Constantinou and Skouroumouni-Stavrinou 2022.

the first milk, by contrast, is the exact opposite of the good, mature milk that is aestheticized through Soranos' detailed description.

Behind Soranos' graphic juxtaposition of colostrum and mature milk and his rejection of the first lies an anxiety which was "a widespread cultural phenomenon."[99] The thick liquid, which came from the new mother's breasts while her vagina was bleeding, was considered by Soranos, his contemporaries, and his followers to be a milk tainted with blood. The first milk was "a dangerous aberration"[100]; it was as polluting as the menstrual blood and the lochial bleeding.[101] By emphatically stating that the people in the arena could see the milk which was dripping from Felicity's breasts and by avoiding any mention of her lochia, as stated above, the narrator aims at averting his audiences' gaze from the new mother's "dreadful" and "polluting" lochia.

Breast Inflammation

Being a nursing mother, Perpetua is quite anxious about the reaction of both her baby and her body as soon as her father, wishing to punish her for choosing Christianity instead of the Roman religion, deprives her of the nursling. Her concerns are revealed through the following words, which she enters in her diary after realizing that through divine intervention her fears will never come true: "Just as God ordained, however, thereafter neither did the infant desire the **breasts**, nor did I experience any **inflammation** – probably in order that I would not **be troubled** by both the child's care and the **pain of the breasts**" ("Πλήν, ὡς ὁ θεὸς ᾠκονόμησεν, οὔτε ὁ παῖς **μασθοὺς** ἐπεθύμησεν ἔκτοτε, οὔτε ἐμοί τις προσγέγονεν **φλεγμονή**· ἴσως ἵνα <μὴ> καὶ τῇ τοῦ παιδίου φροντίδι καὶ τῇ τῶν **μασθῶν ἀλγηδόνι καταπονηθῶ**," *PPF* 6.7–8; trans. with modifications Cobb 2021, 53; emphasis added).

As for the effects of the father's act on Perpetua's milky breasts, which concern us here – the nursling's reaction to this forced weaning will be discussed in the next section – our heroine, like the Greek translator when he reports on Felicity's parturition, examined above, employs medical language to present these effects. The words "breasts" ("μασθοί" or "μαστοί"), "inflammation" ("φλεγμονή"), "pain" ("ἀλγηδών"), "hurt" ("ἀλγέω"), and "be troubled" ("καταπονέομαι") are used by our medical authors to talk about the diseases of (lactating) breasts and their symptoms.[102] Soranos, for example, describes as follows a situation similar with that of Perpetua, whose breasts were full but, due to her baby's absence, could not be emptied:

On the intumescence of the breasts. ... For with the influx of the milk, the **breasts** swell greatly and at first become heavy; this is called *chondrōsis* (lumpiness); later on they also **hurt** and become tense and inflamed, and such a state is called *spargēsis* (intumescence). Consequently, one

---

99 Totelin 2017, 7.
100 Totelin 2021, 230.
101 See e.g. Lawrence 2021; Salvo 2021; Pedrucci 2013c.
102 For breast diseases in ancient and early Byzantine medical works, see Tuten 2014.

must carry out treatment as against **inflammation**, and in the beginning one must use mildly contracting things (such as a soft sea sponge moistened in diluted vinegar, with a close-fitting bandage, or tender dates triturated with bread and diluted vinegar). … If, however, the breasts cannot stand the weight one should first apply fomentations and press them down while soaking them with sweet warm olive oil. … <But> if suppuration has set in one must empty the fluid. … And when the inflammation is past its height, one must apply wax salve only.

Περὶ σπαργήσεως μαστῶν. … κατὰ γὰρ τὴν ἐπιφορὰν τοῦ γάλακτος διογκούμενοι συντόνως οἱ **μαστοὶ** βαροῦνται τὸ πρῶτον, ὅπερ λέγεται χόνδρωσις· εἶτα καὶ **ἀλγοῦσιν** καὶ διατεινόμενοι πυροῦνται, καὶ τὸ τοιοῦτον καλεῖται σπάργησις. δεῖ τοίνυν ὡς πρὸς **φλεγμονὴν** ποιήσασθαι τὴν ἐπίστασιν, καὶ κατ᾽ ἀρχὰς μὲν χρῆσθαι τοῖς ἠρέμα στέλλουσιν (ἐξ ὧν σπόγγος ἐστὶν τρυφερὸς ὀξυκράτῳ νενοτισμένος μετὰ προστυποῦς ἐπιδέσεως ἢ φοίνικες λεῖοι μετὰ ἄρτου καὶ ὀξυκράτου λειοτριβηθέντες)·… εἰ δὲ μὴ φέροιεν τὸ βάρος οἱ μαστοί, καταβροχῇ διὰ γλυκέος ἐλαίου. … διαπυήσεως <δὲ> γενομένης ἐκλαμβάνειν τὸ ὑγρόν. … παρακμαζούσης δὲ τῆς **φλεγμονῆς** κηρωτὴν ἐπιβάλλειν καθ᾽ ἑαυτήν. (Sor. *Gyn.* 2.7.2–4 (GMG 4, 55.13–56.14); trans. Temkin 1956, 77; emphasis added)

Soranos terms Perpetua's symptomatology *chondrōsis* (lumpiness) and *spargēsis* (intumescence). The second problem is the result of the first trouble: after swelling and becoming heavy through the accumulation of milk, the breasts start hurting; in a second phase, fever and inflammation are produced, causing further bodily discomfort. Soranos provides different remedies for healing breast engorgement – application of homemade potions and fomentations to the breasts – depending on the seriousness of the disease and the nursing woman's bodily burdens. He also advises avoiding extracting milk from the affected nipples, since the production of more milk might worsen the lactating woman's situation ("one should not … allow the breasts to be sucked. … [M]ore milk streams into the parts in proportion to the sensation of being sucked, and the nipples are irritated in proportion to their being bruised"; "παραιτεῖσθαι … τὴν … τῶν μαστῶν ἐκμύζησιν … πρὸς τὴν τῆς ἐκμυζήσεως συναίσθησιν πλεῖον ἐπὶ τοὺς τόπους συντρέχει, πρὸς τὴν περίθλασιν ἀγανακτοῦσιν αἱ θηλαί," Sor. *Gyn.* 2.8.2.1–5 (CMG 4, 56.20–24); trans. Temkin 1956, 78).

As suggested by Perpetua's use of medical vocabulary, she, or the Greek translator of the *PPF*, was possibly aware of contemporary medical discourses concerning the symptomatology and treatment of breast engorgement. This possibility is also strengthened by Perpetua's anxiety: she is concerned because she knows that breast engorgement causes great pain and distress. In contrast to Soranos' patients, Perpetua understands that her situation as a prisoner does not allow her to receive medical treatment which would reduce her discomfort and cure her breast engorgement.

Soranos' remedies for diseases of lactating breasts are substantially enriched by the early Byzantine medical author Aetios. The sixteenth and last book of his

32 *Stavroula Constantinou and Aspasia Skouroumouni-Stavrinou*

Tetrabiblos (*Tetr.*), which has been described as "the epitome of gynaecological knowledge of the Graeco-Roman world,"[103] includes five chapters (*Tetr.* 16.38–42, 51.1–56.28, ed. Zervos 1901) on breast problems faced by lactating women.[104] For each stage of a breast disease, Aetios provides several remedies, which are mostly applications of mixtures taking time to prepare and consisting of ingredients that are not always easily accessible, such as seaweeds and Asian stone (*Tetr.* 16.38, 51.1–52.2, Zervos). Some of these remedies might have been developed by Aetios himself or might have originated from folk traditions.[105] As for the remaining remedies, Aetios collects them from other medical authors, whom he does not always name.[106] In fact, the sources Aetios chooses to mention are the two important gynaecologists Soranos and Philoumenos.[107] He repeats Soranos' instruction to avoid having painful breasts sucked (*Tetr.* 16.38, 51.12–15, Zervos), while he cites the work of Philoumenos in two separate chapters (*Tetr.* 16.41–42, 54.15–56.28, Zervos).

For the burning breast inflammation which concerned Perpetua, Aetios cites the following remedies from Philoumenos:

Do this, too, as [it is] most suitable for burning breast inflammations: [take] one libra each of wax, pine tree resin, and oil; three unciae of the leaves of the horned opium plant, softened and mixed with chopped leaves. As they say, the rennet of a rabbit dissolved in water wipes out every breast swelling and discomfort [created] by large milk quantity.

ποιεῖ δὲ καὶ τοῦτο κάλλιστα πρὸς τὰς πυρώδεις φλεγμονὰς τῶν μαστῶν· κηροῦ, κολοφωνίας, ἐλαίου ἀνὰ λίτρ. α΄. μήκωνος, κερατίτιδος φύλλων γογ΄. ἤτοι οὐγ. γ΄. τὰ τηκτὰ τοῖς φύλλοις λειωθεῖσι μίσγε· ποιεῖ δὲ φασί, πιτύα λαγωοῦ ὕδατι λειωθεῖσα καὶ καταχριομένη πρὸς πᾶσαν διόγκωσιν καὶ διάθεσιν μαστῶν μάλιστα ὑπὸ πλήθους γάλακτος. (*Tetr.* 16.41, 55.27–56.3; trans. based on Ricci 1950, 46)

103 Ricci 1990, 49.
104 These chapters have the following titles: Chapter 38: "To prevent the curdling of milk in the breasts" ("Πρὸς τὸ μὴ θρομβοῦσθαι τὸ γάλα ἐν μαστοῖς"); Chapter 39: "Concerning *chondriasis* (lumpiness) and *spargēsis* (intumescence) of the breasts" ("Περὶ χονδριάσεως μαστῶν καὶ σπαργανώσεως"); Chapter 40: "Concerning spoiled milk harming the breasts" ("Περὶ κακώσεως γάλακτος βλάπτοντος τοὺς μαστοὺς"); Chapter 41: "Concerning breast inflammations, according to Philoumenos" ("Πρὸς τὰς τῶν μαστῶν φλεγμονὰς Φιλουμένου"); and Chapter 42: "Concerning sclerotic breast inflammations according to Philoumenos" ("Πρὸς τὰς σκληρυνόμενας φλεγμονὰς μαστῶν Φιλουμένου").
105 As long as no trustworthy edition of *Tetr.* is available, it is difficult, if not impossible, to draw secure conclusions about the origins of Aetios' remedies.
106 For the sources of the sixteenth book of Aetios' *Tetr.*, see Ricci 1950, 5–6.
107 Even though Philoumenos' work is now lost – it has partly survived in the work of Aetios – it seems to have been influenced by that of Soranos (see Temkin 1956, xliii, xliv). According to Sir Clifford Allbutt, Aetios' access to Soranos' work was through Philoumenos (Clifford Allbutt 1913, 428); see also Green 1985, 79. For Soranos and Philoumenos, see also Hummel 1999, 15–17 and 43.

Philoumenos via Aetios gives two recipes for the treatment of breast inflammation. The first recipe provides instructions for the creation of a kind of wax cream composed of plants and plant products that is to be applied to the afflicted breasts. The second recipe, which has an oral source ("they say") and probably originated from folk medicine,[108] is a potion based on animal substances. Both recipes are presented as equally effective. Obviously, the choice of one recipe over the other was determined by the availability of the ingredients. For an imprisoned mother, such as Perpetua, however, neither of the two recipes could be easily executed. Miraculous cure thus becomes the only possible solution for both Perpetua's breast engorgement and lactation cessation.

Lactation Cessation and Weaning

As mentioned in the previous part ("Breast Inflammation"), Perpetua is very anxious also about her nursling's reaction to its sudden removal from the maternal breast. In fact, the Greek term used for weaning, *apogalaktismos* ("ἀπογαλακτισμός"), as Totelin reminds us, means literally the "act of taking away (*apo*) the breastmilk (*gala*)."[109] The inherent negative meaning of the term *apo-galaktismos* reflects the infant's disapproval of loosing the mother's breast, a reality authors contemporary to Perpetua – but also later moralists – did not fail to point out.

For instance, Origen (ca. AD 185–254) wrote that "the infant which is weaned bewails. It does not get away from the mother, suffering for being deprived of her milk" ("ἀπογαλακτισθέντα … παιδία, τὴν θλῖψιν δηλῶν· οὐ γὰρ ἀφίσταται τῆς μητρός, ὀδυνώμενος ἐπὶ τῷ στερηθῆναι τοῦ γάλακτος," Orig. *Psalm* 130.2.5–8, ed. Pitra 1883). One or two centuries later, John Chrysostom remarked in one of his homilies that even if the infant that has been weaned has all kinds of gifts, it does not cease to "seek after the nipple" ("τὸ παιδίον τὴν θηλὴν ἐπιζητεῖ," John Chrys. *Hom. in Colossians*, PG 62, 4.4, 330). Under these circumstances, abrupt weaning, as Perpetua also fears, can provoke a stronger reaction and suffering on the nursling's part.

The negative effects of sudden weaning on nurslings were also acknowledged by medical authorities. Soranos, for example, who devotes a whole section of his *Gynaecology* to weaning ("When and how to wean the infant"; "Πότε καὶ πῶς ἀπογαλακτιστέον τὸ βρέφος," Sor. *Gyn.* 2.46–48 (CMG 4, 85.27–87.29); trans. Temkin 1956, 117–119), advises a well-designed weaning involving a slow transition from breastmilk to other types of food.

[O]ne must stealthily and gradually take it [infant] off the breast and wean it by adding constantly to the amount of other food but diminishing the quantity of milk. For thus the infant will be weaned without harm, getting away little by little from the first habit. At the same time the milk of the child's

---

108   For the adaptation of folk medicine in classical medicine, see Scarborough 2013.
109   See Chapter 5.

nurse will simply dry up because of the gradual elimination of sucking. For it is harmful to anoint the nipple with some bitter and ill-smelling things and thus wean the infant suddenly, because the sudden change has an injurious effect and because sometimes the infant becomes ill when the stomach is damaged by the drugs.

λεληθότως καὶ κατ' ὀλίγον ἀποσυνεθίζειν αὐτὸ τοῦ μαστοῦ καὶ ἀπογαλακτίζειν τῷ προστιθέναι μὲν ἀεὶ τῷ πλήθει τῆς ἄλλης τροφῆς, ὑποσπᾶν δὲ τῆς ποσότητος τοῦ γάλακτος. οὕτω γὰρ ἂν μᾶλλον τὸ βρέφος ἀποσυνεθισθήσεται ἀλύπως κατὰ βραχὺ τῆς πρώτης ἀποχωροῦν συνηθείας, ἅμα δὲ ἀπεριέργως σβεσθήσεται τὸ γάλα τῆς τιτθευούσης τὸ νήπιον τῇ κατὰ μικρὸν ὑφαιρέσει τῆς ἐκμυζήσεως. τὸ γὰρ πικροῖς τισι καὶ δυσώδεσι περιχρίειν τὰς θηλὰς καὶ ἀθρόως ἀπογαλακτίζειν αὐτὸ βλαβερὸν διὰ τὸ τὸν ἐν τῇ ἀθρόᾳ μεταβολῇ ξενισμὸν ἐμποιεῖν καὶ διὰ τὸ κακούμενον ὑπὸ τῶν φαρμάκων τὸν στόμαχόν ποτε πάσχειν. (Sor. *Gyn.* 2.47.1.4–2 (CMG 4, 86.27–87.4); trans. Temkin 1956, 118)

Soranos presents breastfeeding as the infant's first and most central habit, serving both nutritional and emotional needs. As such, breastfeeding cannot be easily and quickly replaced by eating habits belonging to a subsequent state of human development. Exclusive breastfeeding cannot be interrupted before the age of six months, when the infant's body is ready to tolerate other types of food. Soranos lists the types of food that can be gradually introduced in the nursling's diet and until its teeth grow, explaining how they can be prepared and combined.[110] While adding more and more types of food to the infant's diet, the mother or wet nurse is asked to reduce the provision of breastmilk. As the infant becomes acquainted with new nutritional habits, the milk quantity produced by the lactating woman diminishes gradually without causing any breastfeeding complications.

According to Soranos, an infant's weaning could begin around 18–24 months, but again this should not be accomplished suddenly by smearing the nipple with some unpleasant and foul-smelling stuff. Byzantine sources attest to the continuation of this practice beyond antiquity.[111] In the systematic collection of the *Apophthegmata Patrum* (*Apoph. Pat. Syst. Coll.*; 4th/5th c. AD), for instance, we read the following: "when a mother wants to wean her child, she applies squill on her breast, and when the child comes to nurse according to habit it is driven away by

---

110 Like Soranos, the other medical authors under discussion propose at least the first six months as a period of exclusive breastfeeding and two or three years of a combination of breastmilk with solid food. See e.g. Gal. *San. Tu.* 1.10.1 (CMG 5.2.2, 23.4–9). These time frames for exclusive breastfeeding and weaning are confirmed also by hagiographical sources and stable carbon and nitrogen isotope ratio analysis. See Bourbou et al. 2013; Bourbou and Garvie-Lok 2009; Dupras and Tocheri 2007; Dupras et al. 2001; see also Chapter 5 in this volume.

111 In some places, this practice did survive until the twentieth century. For example, women in rural Cyprus of the last century used to apply to their breasts a cream-like potion consisting of hot pepper. Antonia Tsolaki, the mother of Stavroula Constantinou, informed us that she used this method when she wanted to wean the latter.

the bitterness" ("Ὅταν θέλῃ ἡ μήτηρ ἀπογαλακτίσαι τὸ παιδίον αὐτῆς, σκίλλαν βάλλει εἰς τὸν μασθὸν αὐτῆς καὶ ἔρχεται τὸ παιδίον κατὰ τὸ ἔθος θηλάσαι καὶ ἀπὸ τῆς πικρίας φεύγει," *Apoph. Pat. Syst. Coll.* 5.35.3–5, ed. Guy 1993).[112]

Abrupt and early weaning in premodern times was dangerous, because it could cause the baby's death.[113] Perpetua, however, does not appear to worry about the child's life, a fact suggesting that the boy was old enough to be weaned. For Thomas Heffernan, Perpetua's infant must have been 18 months old when it was deprived of the maternal breast.[114] As Totelin rightly points out in Chapter 5 ("Weaning and Lactation Cessation in Late Antiquity and the Early Byzantine Period: Medical Advice in Context"), "there is very little to substantiate this claim in Perpetua's narrative. All we can tell is that the child was not a very small infant when his mother was arrested."[115] Starting from Perpetua's lactation cessation, Totelin's chapter focusses on infant weaning and lactation cessation in early Byzantine medical works. The chapter stresses that whereas, as already remarked, our medical authors explained when to initiate weaning, they did not precisely prescribe when to stop it. Altogether, the chapter examines the cultural expectations that are involved in physicians' recipes concerning the termination of milk production. In contrast to the *PPF*, medical treatises, as Totelin notes, never discuss the bodily and psychological effects of weaning on lactating women.

As for the other two chapters of the volume's second part (Chapter 4: "Breastmilk as a Therapeutic Agent in Ancient and Early Byzantine Medical Literature" and Chapter 6: "'Galaktology' and Genre: Simple Literary Forms on Milk and Breastfeeding in Ancient and Early Byzantine Medical Treatises"), they deal with milk itself, the lactating woman's precious product. Chapter 4 provides a critical investigation of the therapeutic uses of milk in medical and magico-medical works from the fifth century BC to the seventh century AD, both in Greek and Latin. The chapter indicates that the medical uses of human milk were originally related to the treatment of gynaecological issues. By the early centuries AD, however, human milk was employed for different diseases, including eye and ear infections and *phthisis*. Finally, Chapter 6 explores the literary articulation of ancient and early Byzantine milk debates. It shows how the same *galaktology* themes take on various shapes and meanings in different medical authors. It also brings to the fore the ways in which these authors employ short literary forms, and for what purposes. As it argues, the elucidation of medical (re)writing in terms of literary transformations proves essential for a better understanding of both premodern *galaktology* and the composition of scientific works, such as medical treatises.

As the above discussion on medicine and practice has revealed, there was a fertile interchange of medical, philosophical, theological, and hagiographical

---

112   For more examples, see Chapter 5 in this volume.
113   For infants' mortality in connection with weaning times, see e.g. Bourbou et al. 2013, 3911; Parkin 2013; Sallares 1991, 231.
114   Heffernan 2012, 151.
115   Chapter 5, p. 131.

discourses concerning maternal health that was considered essential for the infant's survival and well-being.[116] Hagiography, and in this case the *PPF*, incorporates prevalent social ideologies and practices with a medical background, which it both serves and subverts. At the same time, medical doctrines were used by hagiographers to support their texts' religious meanings. Through the comparative reading attempted here, ancient and Byzantine ideologies on childbirth and lactation have been illuminated, while the *PPF*'s rhetoric and theological arguments have been elucidated and better understood.

Art and Literature

The *PPF*'s various voices and perspectives (the redactor's, Perpetua's, and Saturos'), as Marco Formisano rightly remarks, "create a tension between the autobiographical and biographical narratives."[117] Even though the text's hybrid and polyphonic status renders its generic classification difficult, we would describe it as an hagio/auto/biography. The suggested label constitutes a combination of two generic terms also characterized by hybridity: "hagio-autobiography" and "auto/biography," which were coined to describe texts from different literatures. The first term was introduced to Byzantine studies by Alexander Kažhdan to refer to hagiographical works whose authors added autobiographical information to their accounts of saints' lives.[118] Of course, the *PPF* represents a different form of hagio-autobiography. Instead of providing elements of his own autobiography, the anonymous redactor creates a text that is to a large extent based on the autobiographical accounts of two martyrs (Perpetua and Saturos). Texts such as the *PPF*, which have escaped Kažhdan's notice, are much less common in the Byzantine hagiographical tradition.[119]

As for auto/biography, it was coined by Liz Stanley to talk about all forms of contemporary women's life writing: autobiography, biography, diary, and letter.[120] Stanley's auto/biography and general approach follows feminist criticism which challenges traditional generic distinctions that are mainly created by male theorists and are based on men's literary works.[121] Hagio/auto/biography, therefore, is a useful category for our purposes, as it reflects the life genres forming the *PPF* (hagiography, diary, visionary account, and biography), while at the same time it challenges the widely used categories of *Passio* and hagiography that erase the

---

116   See e.g. Rawson 1991, 15; Rousselle 1988, 47; Moffatt 1986.
117   Formisano 2019, 218.
118   Kažhdan 1983, 546.
119   Another example similar to and possibly a bit later than the *PPF* is the *Passion of Pionios* (last decades of the 3rd c. AD), which incorporates Pionios' arrest and prison speeches (see Castelli 2004, 92–102). An example of an early Byzantine hagiographical text including the protagonist's autobiographical account is the *Life of Mary of Egypt* (7th c. AD). Mary, who is probably not a historical personality, relates her former lives as a prostitute and penitent to the monk Zosimas, who discovers her in the desert (see Constantinou 2005, 59–85).
120   Stanley 1992.
121   Kažhdan's hagio-autobiography, too, refers to male-authored texts with male protagonists.

text's uniqueness and strong female perspective. But let us return to the two hagio/auto/biographical narratives that concern us here: Perpetua's diary and Felicity's biographical account.

The two narratives in question, which establish the maternal self and subjectivity through the acts of breastfeeding, mothering, and childbirth, constitute some of the oldest specimens of maternal literature. According to Elizabeth Podnieks and Andrea O'Reilly, who coined the term "maternal literature," it involves "mother subjects and mother writers, women who produce auto/biography, fiction, and poetry about mothering, motherhood, and being mothered, who thus engage in the process or act of textual mothering."[122] Perpetua's diary and Felicity's biography are also matrifocal narratives – another term introduced by O'Reilly to describe specifically narrative maternal literature. In matrifocal narratives, the mother and her mothering are "thematically elaborated and valued, and [are] structurally central to the plot."[123] Matrifocal narratives, as Podnieks elaborates,

> are written and narrated by mothers in the first-person or limited third-person voice, rendering maternal identity and experience from subjective perspectives. Further, they (re)value the significance and meaning of maternal figures in cultural, social, and national arenas and often contest or negotiate traditional ideologies of the "good" mother as self-sacrificing, nurturing … with her antithesis, the "bad" mother.[124]

Perpetua's diary is written in the first person and "with her own hand" ("αὐτῆς … τῇ χειρὶ συγγράψασα," *PPF* 2.3), as the redactor remarks. Even though it is written in the third person, Felicity's short biographical account focusses – uncommonly for martyrdom accounts – on the maternal experiences of premature childbirth and first lactation. Furthermore, Felicity's poetic voice, which is heard after the prison official's challenge concerning the pains of parturition in relation to her battle with the beasts, discussed above ("Medicine and Practice"), is so strong, decisive, and authoritative that it renders her guard speechless.

Through their willingness to die for their religion, Perpetua and Felicity challenge the maternal ideals of their society, as shown in section "Society and Ideology." In short, the two women's accounts break taboos about maternal corporeality by explicitly and graphically discussing breast engorgement, parturition, blood, and leaking breasts, which are aestheticized and thus become essential literary elements. The diary and the biographical account are thus exemplary matrifocal narratives. In what follows, the matrifocal character of the diary, which is the longest, will be explored in terms of genre and narrative. Like the previous two sections, this final section will close with a short presentation of the chapters included in this volume's last part.

122 Podnieks and O'Reilly 2010, 1.
123 O'Reilly 2020, 54.
124 Podnieks 2020, 176.

Genre

Taking into consideration other martyrs' Greek autobiographical writings that have come down to us, either as self-standing texts or as parts of other longer works,[125] two essential things come to the fore: first, with the single exception of Perpetua's diary, these autobiographical writings are male-authored; and second, they take various forms, such as letters,[126] speeches, testaments, and visionary texts, but they are never written in a diary form. We would, therefore, argue that there is an interrelationship between gender and genre in Christian martyrs' autobiographical writings which is also manifested in the *PPF*, where the female-authored autobiographical text is a diary, while its male counterpart is a visionary text.

We can thus conclude that the autobiography of martyrdom, like all hagiographical genres, is a male-dominated genre.[127] Perpetua's text is the exception that confirms this rule. Furthermore, the facts that no male martyr writings took the form of a diary and that the only autobiographical writing produced by a woman martyr was a diary suggest that the diary is a female rather than a male genre.[128] Finally, Perpetua's text belongs to the subgenre of the mothering diary,[129] since, as will be further discussed below, her maternal behaviour and experience shape its form and structure.

The diary has been defined as the genre of the domestic and everyday detail, as well as the genre of privacy, intimacy, and inner life that imprints the thoughts, feelings, and experiences of its author.[130] As such, the diary is closer to women's lives, which have been traditionally associated with domesticity, the private realm, and emotionality.[131] The diary has also been described as an informal, repetitive, fragmentary, and open-ended genre with a loose and episodic structure.[132] It is possibly due to these inherent qualities of the diary that male martyrs chose other autobiographical genres for their writings, which were produced as public documents promoting their authors' theology and martyrdom theory.

Addressing his letter to the Christians of his diocese, Phileas, for example, focussed on the martyrs' steadfastness and heroism before horrendous tortures, with the intention of encouraging his audiences to "hold firmly to their faith in Christ,

---

125   To the first category belong, for instance, the seven letters which Ignatios the Bishop of Antioch wrote as a captive on his way to Rome, where he was martyred at some point between AD 108 and 140 (for Ignatios' letters, see e.g. Castelli 2004, 78–85; Perkins 1995, 189–192). An example of the second category is the letter which Phileas the Bishop of Thmuis (Thebaid) composed, while he was imprisoned in Alexandria (probably in AD 303/304) awaiting martyrdom (for Phileas, see Bremmer 2021; Musurillo 1972, xlvi). This letter is quoted in the fourth-century *Ecclesiastical History* of Eusebios (Eus. *EH* 8.10.2–10; ed. Schwartz 1908).

126   The letter is the most common genre of martyrdom autobiography; see McLarty 2013.

127   Constantinou 2004.

128   The contemporary diary is also treated as a female genre; see e.g. Hogan 1991; Huff 1989.

129   For the genre of the mothering diary or memoir, see e.g. Hewett 2020; Podnieks and O'Reilly 2010, 4, 7.

130   See e.g. Lejeune (1999) 2009; Bunkers and Huff 1996.

131   See e.g. Constantinou and Meyer 2019.

132   See e.g. Popkin and Rak 2009; Hogan 1991, 95–100.

even after his own death" ("τὸ ἀπρὶξ ἔχεσθε καὶ μετ᾽ αὐτὸν ... τελειωθησόμενον τῆς ἐν Χριστῷ θεοσεβείας," Eus. *EH* 8.10.11; trans. Musurillo 1972, 325). Similarly, Ignatios' letters recorded "the historical experience of martyrdom and the emergent Christian theology of suffering and persecution."[133] Advocating a public selfhood with apostolic dimensions through their theological and highly rhetorical letters, these bishops worked towards the spread of Christianity and sought to guide and support contemporary Christian communities – including their own flocks – that were threatened by persecution.

Perpetua, by contrast, being an imprisoned nursing mother having also to endure the ordeals of both her father and torturers, finds herself in a completely different situation: our heroine does not and cannot share the heroism and majesty of either Phileas or Ignatios. In Perpetua's case, the diary is the most suitable form of expression, allowing her to confide her bodily and emotional condition, along with her personal experiences with the divine. According to the important diary (and autobiography) theorist Philippe Lejeune, "people keep a diary in times of crisis, during a phase of life."[134] Indeed, Perpetua undergoes a personal crisis, having to oppose her father, who loves her more than her brothers and who also suffers because of her decision to follow an illegal religion that leads to the family's defamation. Yet her greatest personal crisis is the result of her vacillation between Roman ideals about good and bad motherhood in association with the dilemma her father puts her into, that is, to choose between her baby boy and her faith.[135] For Perpetua, diary writing becomes a meaningful and supportive activity in her attempt to come to terms with her multiple crises. Diary writing allows Perpetua "to release, to unload the weight of [her] emotions and thoughts," thus "purifying and cleansing" herself before her premature and violent death.[136]

In terms of language, style, form, and structure, Perpetua's diary has all the generic characteristics that have been identified by diary theorists. Her language and style are simple and paratactic in both the Latin and the Greek versions of the *PPF*. Based on the Latin version, scholars have commented on Perpetua's language and style in relation to her education and the characteristics of earlier and contemporary Latin literature. For Erich Auerbach,

> there is no rhetorical art in Perpetua's narrative. The careful education she had received is hardly reflected in her style. Her vocabulary is limited; her sentence structure is clumsy, the connectives are not always clear. A specialist cannot help noting the many vulgarisms and typically Christian locutions. The language in general is brittle, quite unliterary, naïve, almost childlike.[137]

---

133 Castelli 2004, 78.
134 Lejeune and Bogaert 2020, 25; see also Lejeune 2009, 193 and (1999) 2009, 34.
135 See also above.
136 Lejeune 2009, 194.
137 Auerbach (1958) 1965, 63.

Nevertheless, individuals undergoing Perpetua's many anxieties, which are the primary reasons and motivations for, as well as the material of, her diary would be
interested in expressing and coming to terms with those very anxieties rather than
displaying their education and writing skills. As Auerbach himself emphatically
remarks, despite her "almost childlike" language, Perpetua "is expressive." "She
speaks of ... the first hours in prison, in the stifling darkness, among the soldiers,
with her famished child; the happiness she comes to experience in prison."[138]

Much more recently, Walter Ameling, on the other hand, has argued that Perpetua's style reveals that her "education did not extend to literary composition, and
[that] active literary composition was alien to her education."[139] As Ameling further
elaborates, "Perpetua's faults in composition, the predominance of colloquialisms,
the departure from syntax and grammar – all of this would have been completely
unacceptable to the public of an educated ... author (and to the author himself,
too)."[140] Indeed, the above-mentioned martyr bishops, who produced public rhetorical texts, would never author such "faulty" compositions. For Perpetua, by contrast,
who wrote a text with different aspirations, faultless composition was not important.

In other words, Perpetua's language and style are not necessarily indicative of
her education or writing abilities but reflect those of diary writing. This view could
be further supported through a twentieth-century example, that of Virginia Woolf,
who was both an accomplished literary author and a diarist. When she rereads her
own diary, Woolf is bothered by her style, while she recognizes that a diary has a
loose form, including "everything that comes into ... mind." In diary writing, she
continues, "the main requirement ... is not to play the part of censor, but to write as
the mood comes or of anything whatever. ... I went for things put in haphazard."[141]
What is suggested here is that Perpetua's language and style are better understood
and evaluated in the light of the diary's generic conventions rather than in the
framework of ancient education and in relation to ancient canonical genres.

Concerning form and structure, Perpetua's diary, too, is characterized by frag-
mentariness and has an episodic structure. The diary's first entry is introduced
abruptly, depicting a scene that enacts Perpetua's intense confrontation with her
father, which takes place some days before the martyrs' imprisonment and while
they are kept under surveillance. This scene is followed by a number of relatively
short episodes running through the passing days. Each episode is introduced with
a time conjunction or with a reference to time or to the elapsing of time (mostly
the passing of days). Such time markers are the following: "while" ("ἔτι," *PPF*
1.1; trans. Cobb 2021, 49), "then" ("τότε," *PPF* 4.1),[142] "and immediately, on the
evening in which" ("καὶ εὐθὺς ἐν τῇ ἑσπέρᾳ ἐν ᾗ," *PPF* 8.1; trans. Cobb 2021, 53),
"o terrible day" ("ὦ δεινὴν ἡμέραν," *PPF* 3.6; trans. Cobb 2021, 49), "and on

138 Auerbach (1958) 1965, 64.
139 Ameling 2012, 92.
140 Ameling 2012, 93.
141 Woolf 1953, 13; see also Hogan 1991, 102–104; Huff 1989, 7–9.
142 Cobb erroneously translates "τότε" with "and" (trans. Cobb 2021, 49).

the day in which" ("καὶ τῇ ἡμέρᾳ ἐν ᾗ," *PPF* 6.1; trans. Cobb 2021, 51 with a modification), "a day before" ("πρὸ μιᾶς," *PPF* 10.1; trans. Cobb 2021, 55), "to-morrow" ("αὔριον," *PPF* 4.2; trans. Cobb 2021, 49), and "after a few days" ("μετὰ δὲ ἡμέρας ὀλίγας," *PPF* 5.1; trans. Cobb 2021, 51).

The heroine stops her writing activity a day before her death and after adding her longest diary entry, which includes her last prison dream and her understanding of it. In this dream, Perpetua sees herself overcoming her temptations, which take the form of an enormous Egyptian man whom she conquers in a single battle. Even though Perpetua still has some time until her execution to add more entries to her diary, at this point she decides to put an end to her writing activity. Having gained full control of her passions and having solved all her personal and maternal crises, she no longer needs to keep the diary. If, according to Lejeune, people "keep a jour-nal for … one reason,"[143] Perpetua no longer has a reason to write, as she knows that she has already won all her contests.

The open-endedness and incompleteness of Perpetua's diary are defied by her invitation to "whoever wishes [to] write down what will happen in the amphi-theater" ("Τὰ ἐν τῷ ἀμφιθεάτρῳ γενησόμενα ὁ θέλων συγγραψάτω," *PPF* 10.15; trans. Cobb 2021, 55). Thus, Perpetua's final moments and the way of her dying are recorded by someone else, our redactor. The redactor, however, takes more ini-tiative. He brings to a conclusion not only Perpetua's diary and life story but also the autobiographical account and life of Saturos, as well as the lives of the other Christians who were martyred with them.

Narrative

Perpetua's diary is a matrifocal narrative not just because its author, protagonist, and narrator is a mother character who confesses her maternal experiences in the first person, thus giving a unique voice to the complexities of mothering while challenging ancient social ideologies about motherhood. As will be further shown, the diary is a matrifocal narrative also because maternity and mothering, both bod-ily and spiritual, literal and metaphorical, human and divine, provide it with mean-ing, structure, (emotional) power, and the expressivity detected by Auerbach.

In most of the diary's episodes, the action is fuelled by maternal agony, crisis, and care (*PPF* 3, 6, 7, 8). In one episode in which the action is prompted by a dif-ferent dynamic – a fellow prisoner prompting Perpetua to ask for a prophetic dream that would reveal her future – maternal status and affection play a central role (*PPF* 4). Finally, in two of the three episodes in which the plot develops around Perpetua's conflict with her father (*PPF* 3, 5, 9), the maternal role influences the two characters' behaviour and emotional reactions. It is only in the last episode, the diary's aforementioned final entry, that – for the reasons discussed in the previous part ("Genre") – maternity or any maternal issues are totally absent. In sum, mater-nity and the maternal perspective pervade Perpetua's narrative.

---

143 Lejeune 2009, 193.

Our diarist appears to experience her first maternal anxiety as soon as she is sent to a depressing prison – it is uncommonly dark, excessively hot, and overpopulated; its many guards suppress the prisoners – that is totally unsuitable for the practice of breastfeeding, but also for a baby. Perpetua's concerns for the nursling are communicated to two free Christians, the deacons Tertios and Pomponios, who are immediately spurred to action. Seeking ways to improve the imprisonment's conditions, the two heroes contribute to the development of the episode's plot, which is initiated by an imprisoned nursing mother's sad feelings, needs, and desires.

After the deacons bribe the prison officials, Perpetua and the other Christian prisoners are taken to a more habitable space where the heroine can receive and nurse her hungry infant. Perpetua's mother and brother take the fed baby back to the paternal house once they receive her instructions on how to take good care of the boy. Yet, the episode's maternal plot reaches a climax when Perpetua's great sadness returns due to the nursling's absence. The heroine's separation anxiety drives her once again to take initiative. This time she asks to be allowed to have the nursling in prison with her. The episode's plot reaches its closure when Perpetua's anguish is transformed into a great happiness as she can uninterruptedly breast-feed her baby, who in the meantime has fully recovered from hunger. Perpetua's exhilaration is reflected in the words with which she closes her entry: "the prison became for me a palace" ("ἡ φυλακὴ ἐμοὶ γέγονεν πραιτώριον," *PPF* 3.9; trans. Cobb 2021, 49).

In the following episode, which is introduced with the time marker "then" ("τότε," *PPF* 4.1), and thus appears to take place on the same day on which Perpetua's infant fully recovers, causing her emotional transformation, we hear the words of a fellow prisoner, who describes the heroine as someone who "already has a very privileged position" ("ἤδη ἐν μεγάλῳ ἀξιώματι ὑπάρχεις," *PPF* 4.1).[144] As a privileged individual, Perpetua could, according to the anonymous fellow prisoner, ask for a divine dream. The heroine responds by simply saying: "I will report to you tomorrow" ("αὔριόν σοι ἀπαγγελῶ," *PPF* 4.2; trans. Cobb 2021, 49), yet she confides to her diary the following: "and I … knew that I conversed with God – from whom I possessed such great benefits" ("Κἀγὼ … ᾔδειν με ὁμιλοῦσαν θεῷ, οὗ γε δὴ τοσαύτας εὐεργεσίας εἶχον," *PPF* 4.2; trans. Cobb 2021, 49).

Several important questions arise here which seem to be related to Perpetua's experience as a breastfeeding mother: for what reason does the anonymous Christian prisoner consider Perpetua's position as "very privileged"? How does she know that she can converse with the divine? Why is she closer to God than her fellow prisoners? Could her assumed ability to communicate with the divine be the result of her experiences as a nurturing mother suffering for her faith, including the transformation of her prison into a palace? The last question might be answered in the affirmative if one takes into consideration the fact that the reference to Perpetua's special privilege surfaces immediately after the episode which centres around the

---

144 Once again Cobb's translation is not followed – she translates the phrase as "already you have great honor" (Cobb 2021, 49).

heroine's maternal feelings, which are transformed from anxiety into exhilaration. Moreover, the divine dream sent to Perpetua on the same night further reinforces the argument that the heroine's supernatural experience is strongly associated with her breastfeeding and mothering self.

Perpetua's first dream, which includes a scene of parental nurturing and affection that is enacted after a scene of violence, can be read as an allegory of the daily life of an imprisoned nursing mother awaiting punishment. In her dream, Perpetua sees herself arriving in a huge garden as soon as she overcomes temptation in the form of a huge dragon and a long series of deathly obstacles through her sacrifice. In the middle of the garden, there is an enormous divine figure that is embodied by an elderly shepherd who, surrounded by innumerable martyrs dressed in white, is milking the sheep. Once the shepherd notices Perpetua's presence, he addresses her as a parent: "welcome, child" ("Καλῶς ἐλήλυθας, τέκνον," *PPF*, 4.9; trans. with a modification Cobb 2021, 51). He then summons the heroine, to give her some of the sustenance he is milking. When she puts the sacred food in her mouth, Perpetua becomes a member of the garden's uniform population, who glorify this sacred union. When Perpetua wakes up from the dream, the taste of something sweet is still in her mouth, testifying to the reality of her sacred communion.

By feeding Perpetua with a milk product, the dream's divine figure imitates her role as a nursing mother. The paradisiacal milk He distributes to the individuals entering the garden establishes a bond between Himself and the consumers, as well as among the consumers themselves, just as breastfeeding creates a bond between the mother and her nursing infant(s) and between the nurslings themselves, as is also attested by Basil's testimony, discussed above ("Society and Ideology"). God's motherly behaviour divinizes the suffering maternity of Perpetua, who through the dream communicates with God and identifies with Him. This is a privilege possessed only by the nursing mother about to die as a martyr.

In the next episode, Perpetua's maternal joy is interrupted by her father, who, after returning from his trip, visits her in prison imploring her in tears to give up her Christianity. The heroine's feelings for her father in this scene recall her negative emotional situation when she was separated from her nursling. She writes in her diary: "And I myself felt pain on account of my father's disposition" ("Ἐγὼ δὲ περὶ τῆς διαθέσεως τοῦ πατρὸς ἤλγουν," *PPF* 5.6; trans. Cobb 2021, 51). Yet Perpetua finds the courage to console her father. Their roles as daughter and father are at this point overturned. The father behaves like a child that cries because his desires are not satisfied. Perpetua, on the other hand, undertakes the role of the child's mother who explains why his wishes cannot be fulfilled. She tells him: "Whatever the Lord wills shall happen. ... For we know that we will be not in our power but in that of God" ("γενήσεται ... <ὃ> ἐὰν θέλῃ ὁ κύριος· γνῶθι γὰρ ὅτι οὐκ ἐν τῇ ἡμετέρᾳ ἐξουσίᾳ, ἀλλ' ἐν τῇ τοῦ θεοῦ ἐσόμεθα," *PPF* 5.6; trans. Cobb 2021, 51).

Since Perpetua insists on her religion, she is sentenced with the other Christians to be thrown to the beasts, a decision that fills all the prisoners with joy. Perpetua's delight, however, does not last: her father refuses to give her the baby back despite her pleas that it needs her breastmilk and affection. The baby's abrupt weaning and the milky breasts' discomfort, which have been discussed above ("Medicine and

Practice"), fill Perpetua once again with desperate anxiety which due to divine intervention turns soon into respite. Even though she is no longer allowed to mother her infant, she does not give up her maternal role. Having fulfilled the bodily requirements of the nursing mother, Perpetua is now ready to perform the spiritual and symbolic tasks of maternity.

In the diary's next entry, Perpetua reports that a few days later while she was praying, she suddenly said the name Dinokrates, which belonged to her seven-year-old brother that had died years earlier. The memory of Dinokrates, who died from facial gangrene, a terribly painful and disfiguring disease, causes Perpetua a pain that equals the suffering she experiences every time her baby is taken away from her. As she writes in her diary, "I felt pain coming to a recollection of his death" ("ἤλγησα … εἰς μνήμην ἐλθοῦσα τῆς αὐτοῦ τελευτῆς," *PPF* 7.1; trans. Cobb 2021, 53). Realizing that Dinokrates was carried away from his mother before receiving the holy baptism, Perpetua decides that he needs her intercession to achieve salvation. She immediately begins to pray. As an answer to her continuous and fervent prayers, she receives another divine dream, which reveals her brother's otherworldly suffering, thus confirming her fears for the boy.

In the dream, as in reality, Perpetua is kept away from the object of her motherly affection. As is the case with her infant boy, Perpetua cannot approach Dinokrates. She watches her brother from a distance while he comes from a dark place populated with burnt and thirsty people – a place resembling the heroine's first prison. Just as the first prison was unfit for Perpetua's baby, so this place is unhealthy for her brother. Wearing dirty clothing, Dinokrates is pale and still has the grotesque facial wound with which he died. Even though a pool full of water stands in front of the boy, who suffers from great thirst, his low height prevents him from reaching the water he desperately needs. Witnessing her brother's torture and being unable to assist him, Perpetua suffers: "and I felt pain" ("Ἐγὼ δὲ ἤλγουν," *PPF* 7.1; trans. Cobb 2021, 53).

Like her own infant, Dinokrates needs to be fed in order to be saved. Perpetua knows that even though she can no longer offer physical nurturing to her own baby, she has the power to help Dinokrates to obtain spiritual nurturance. As an answer to her new and intensifying prayers that last for days and nights, she receives a follow-up dream. On the day when she receives this dream, however, Perpetua experiences a double discomfort. Next to her agony about her brother, she is stressed by the chains that are added to her body. The dream, by contrast, is redemptive. Dinokrates appears redeemed: his facial wound is healed and restored, he is clean and no longer thirsty, and he is playing happily in a beautiful and refreshing place. Dinokrates' transformation constitutes a further indication of the sacred status of Perpetua's maternity, which is both material and spiritual, distressing and uplifting.

The next and penultimate entry in Perpetua's diary concerns an episode taking place some days after the heroine's second dream with Dinokrates and shortly before the day of public honours, a time when she feels encouraged and supported. Her positive feelings are once again overturned when her father comes to see her for a last time. At this final meeting, the father undertakes the mother's role and Perpetua becomes his child again. Treating his daughter as already dead, the father performs his mourning, which Perpetua describes thus: "he began to pluck out his own beard and to cast it on the ground, and, lying face down, to revile himself, speaking against his age and saying such words as to be able to shake all creation" ("ἤρξατο τὸν πώγωνα τὸν ἴδιον ἐκτίλλειν ῥίπτειν τε ἐπὶ γῆς, καὶ πρηνὴς κατακείμενος κακολογεῖν, τὰ ἑαυτοῦ ἔτη κατηγορῶν καὶ λέγων τοιαῦτα ῥήματα ὡς πᾶσαν δύνασθαι τὴν κτίσιν σαλεῦσαι," *PPF* 9.2; Cobb 2021, 55).

This motherly mourning, which replicates mothers' lamentations in ancient literature and particularly in tragedy, where they are presented tearing their hair and clothes and giving themselves up to heartbreaking lamentations for their dead sons,[145] proves overwhelming for Perpetua, who deals differently with her own losses. Unlike her pagan father, she turns to God and to her diary to heal her wounds. The father's "maternal" pathos makes the heroine speechless, but also very sad: she is unable to offer her previous consolation. The entry ends with a short reference to Perpetua's own mourning for her old father.

As the preceding discussion of Perpetua's diary has revealed, maternity, spirituality, and creativity coexist and are mutually generative in this matrifocal narrative. The mother's role and the experiences associated with it provide our diarist with power, faith, inspiration, motivation, and literary vision. Diary writing, in turn, relieves Perpetua's maternal anxieties and crises while at the same it allows her to share her divine experiences. At Perpetua's hands, maternity is transformed from a silent and submissive role into an expressive, authoritative, generative, and spiritual selfhood. As a mother/author, Perpetua does not just challenge patriarchal ideologies and establish herself as creative and powerful but also sanctifies maternity and the lactating body.

So far, we have been investigating literary representations of breastfeeding and mothering. What about their visual counterparts? As noted in this chapter's introductory section, there is no visual parallel of Perpetua and Felicity's lactation and maternity. In fact, according to the conclusions of Chapter 7 ("Images of Breastfeeding in Early Byzantine Art: Form – Context – Function"), human breastfeeding and mothering were rarely represented in early Byzantine art. They were, nevertheless, introduced into different media and settings: funerary, secular, and religious. Furthermore, rather than being treated as a simple genre scene, breastfeeding served symbolic or allegorical functions, whether to identify a woman as a mother in funerary portraiture, to promote dynastic claims on imperial coinage, or to articulate ideas about fertility, nurture, vulnerability, dependency, and protection.

Chapter 8 ("Empowering Breasts: Women, Widows, and Prophetesses-with-Child at Dura-Europos"), on the other hand, focusses on prophetesses-with-child. These figures exhibit their maternal status through their naked breasts and babies, affirming their ability to discern meaning in life, resist hardship, and enact salvific processes. Jochebed, Miriam, the daughter of Pharaoh, and the widow of Sarepta as represented in the paintings at the Dura synagogue are analysed as cases in

---

145 See Loraux 1998.

point. The paintings are interpreted according to midrash, applying the version of the story of Moses' rescue from Ezekiel the Tragedian, and linking images with performances by actresses. Further, these women's independence is considered in comparison to real-life Durene women. The chapter also puts forward the hypothesis that seat inscriptions in the "salles à gradins" of temples dedicated to goddesses were connected to childbirth.

Visual representations of breastfeeding are also discussed in Chapter 9 ("Roman Charity: Nonnos of Panopolis, Support for Parents, and Questions of Gender"), though here the focus is on literary depictions of the legendary story of the daughter who breastfeeds her imprisoned father who is starving to death. This chapter examines this theme, which has often been called "Roman charity" because of its classical origins, before turning to what is one of its most intriguing aspects: the father's replacement by the mother in some versions of the tale. The chapter considers the evidence for this gender shift, its significance, and the possible reasons underlying it.

Finally, Chapter 10 ("Children in Distress: Agonizing Mothers as Intercessors in Early Byzantine Miracle Collections") constitutes a first attempt to approach the interaction of children and mothers in early Byzantine healing miracles. Taking its cue from the different treatment observed in structure and plot when the patient is a child, the chapter focusses on three important parameters: the ritualistic miracle structure, the role of the mother as an intercessor between the child and the saint(s), and the body of the child as a locus of cure. The study of these parameters shows that miracles involving children constitute a special category in which mothers and children form narrative pairs and that this pairing was consciously acknowledged and narratively exploited by Byzantine hagiographers.

In this volume, as its contents reveal, the lactating woman and the work of mothering are approached through the study of a great variety of sources, mainly works of Greek-speaking cultures, penned and visual, anonymous and eponymous, which were mostly produced between the first and the seventh century AD.[146] The textual works include biblical texts, apocrypha, magical papyri, legal documents, medical treatises, philosophical works, homiletics, hagiography, epic poetry, and paradoxography. As for the visual works under discussion, they comprise frescoes, mosaics, icons, tapestries, tombstones, medallions, and figurines. Beyond doubt, the wide generic, chronological, and geographical span of the studied material imposes its own limitations. The diverse forms of evidence, however interactive and interdependent, belong to different genres, each governed by its own rhetorical, generic, or artistic conventions, at different stages of its development.

---

146 Some of this volume's chapters (2, 4, and 6) also discuss earlier texts, to bring to the fore continuities and discontinuities from antiquity to early Byzantium in the treatment of wet nurses (Chapter 2) and in medical approaches to milk (Chapters 4 and 6). Chapter 3, on the other hand, uses later visual evidence from the ninth to fourteenth centuries, as there are no earlier images depicting mothers' punishment for not breastfeeding their infants.

Equally diverse also are regional customs and their different enactments over a long period of time amounting to seven centuries. What is more, produced mainly, if not exclusively, by upper-class, urban males, the written material is unavoidably doubly biased. In terms of gender, the lactating woman's own voice is very rarely articulated. In terms of class, the large populations of lower-class citizens and slaves are hardly visible. Evidently, these sources tell us much more about the anxieties, preoccupations, and ideologies of the societies that produced them and much less about actual contemporary mothering. Still, exploring the cross-fertilization of those concerns and ideologies from one context to another, and from one period to the next in an investigation roughly encompassing the first seven centuries of our common era, provides an essential comparative understanding of principles and cultural products that have not been considered together before.

Concerning the chronology of most examined sources, the first century of our common era has been taken as our starting point because the large majority of the ancient works thematizing breastfeeding with the greatest impact on Byzantine authors, as the volume's ten chapters also manifest, were produced from the first century onwards. The seventh century AD, on the other hand, provides a good end point, as it is situated before the rise of the Arab and Islamic civilization, which gave a new impetus to ancient and Byzantine science and philosophy through which the lactating woman could be approached. Of course, the volume does – and could – not offer an exhaustive analysis of the examined period's lactating woman and her work of mothering, yet we believe that it will lead to more investigations enhancing our understanding of mothering practices, both in the period under discussion and in later times.

References

Texts: Editions and Translations

Argyriou, A. ed. 1996. *Μακάριου τοῦ Μακρῆ συγγράμματα*. Βυζαντινά Κείμενα και Μελέται 25. Thessaloniki: Centre for Byzantine Research.

Baggarly, J.D., and C.A. Kühn. eds. 2007. *Anastasius of Sinai Hexaemeron*. Orientalia Christiana Analecta 278. Rome: Pontifico Istituto Orientale.

Beckby, H. ed. 1965–1968. *Anthologia Graeca*. 4 vols. 2nd ed. Munich: Heimeran.

Beek, C.I.M. van. 1936. *Passio sanctarum Perpetuae et Felicitatis: Textum graecum et latinum ad fidem codicum Mss. 1.* Nijmegen: Deeker and Van de Vegt S.A.

Berger, A. ed. 2002. "Die alten Viten des Heiligen Mamas von Kaisareia mit einer Edition der Vita *BHG* 1019," *Analecta Bollandiana* 120: 280–308.

Chiesa, P. ed. 1990. *Le versioni latine della Passio Sanctae Febroniae: Storia, metodo, modelli di due traduzioni agiographiche altomedievali*. Spoleto: Centro Italiano di Studi sull'Alto Medioevo, 368–395.

Cobb, S.L. ed. and trans. 2021. *The Passion of Perpetua and Felicitas in Late Antiquity*. Oakland: University of California Press, 43–65.

Courtonne, Y. ed. and trans. 1957. *Saint Basile, Lettres*. Vol. 1. Paris: Belles Lettres.

Dagron, G. ed. 1978. *Vie et miracles de Sainte Thècle*. Brussels: Société des Bollandistes.

De Lacy, P.H., and B. Einarson. trans. 1959. *Plutarch Moralia*. Vol. 3. Cambridge, MA and London: Harvard University Press.

Deferrari, R.J. trans. 1926. *St. Basil: The Letters*. Vol. 1. Cambridge, MA and London: Harvard University Press.

Delehaye, H. ed. (1902) 1984. "Synaxarium ecclesiae Constantinopolitanae" ("e codice Sirmondiano nunc Beroninensi"). *Acta Sanctorum* 62: 437–496.

Dieten, J. van. ed. 1972. *Nicetae Choniatae orationes et epistulae*. Berlin: De Gruyter.

Duffy, J.M. ed. 1992. *Michaelis Pselli philosophica minora*. Leipzig: Teubner.

Farquharson, A.S.L. ed. (1944) 1968. *The Meditations of the Emperor Marcus Aurelius*. Vol. 1. Reprint, Oxford: Clarendon Press.

Festugière, A.J., and L. Rydén. eds. 1974. *Léontios de Néapolis, Vie de Syméon le Fou et Vie de Jean de Chypre*. Paris: Paul Geuthner, 55–104.

Gaisford, T. ed. 1823. *Poetae minores Graeci [Scholia ad Hesiodum]*. Vol. 2. Leipzig: Kühn, 448–459.

Gill, C. trans. 2013. *Marcus Aurelius: Meditations, Books 1–6*. Oxford: Oxford University Press.

Guy, J.-C. ed. and trans. 1993. *Les Apophtegmes des Pères, collection systématique*. Vol. 1. Sources Chrétiennes 387. Paris: Editions du Cerf.

Halkin, F. ed. 1973. *Légendes grecques de martyres romaines*. Subsidia Hagiographica 55. Brussels: Société des Bollandistes, 185–204.

———. 1987–1989. "Eloge de Saint Cyr et de sa mère Julitte (*BHG* 318)," Ἐπετηρὶς Ἑταιρείας Βυζαντινῶν Σπουδῶν 47: 34–41.

Hansen, D.U. ed. 1998. *Das attizistische Lexikon des Moeris*. Berlin and New York: De Gruyter.

Harl, M., H.-I. Marrou, C. Matray, and C. Mondésert. eds. 1960. *Clément d'Alexandrie: Le pédagogue*. Vol. 1. Sources Chrétiennes 70. Paris: Editions du Cerf.

Harris, J.R., and S.K. Gifford. eds. 1890. *The Acts of the Martyrdom of Perpetua and Felicitas: The Original Greek Text Now First Edited from a Ms. in the Library of the Convent of the Holy Sepulchre at Jerusalem*. London: C.J. Clay and Sons, Cambridge University Press Warehouse.

Heiberg, J.L. ed. 1921. *Paulus Aegineta, Libri I–IV*. Leipzig and Berlin: Teubner.

Heylbut, H. 1887. "Ptolemaeus Περὶ διαφορᾶς λέξεων," *Hermes* 22: 388–410.

Holstenius, L. [corr. by H. de Valois]. ed. 1664. *Passio SS. Perpetuae et Felicitatis*. Paris: Carolus Savreux.

Ilberg, J. ed. 1927. *Sorani Gynaeciorium libri IV, De signis fracturarum, De fasciis, Vita Hippocratis secundum Soranum edidit J. Ilberg*. Leipzig and Berlin: Teubner.

Koch, K., G. Helmreich, C. Kalbfleisch, and O. Hartlich. eds. 1923. *Galeni De sanitate tuenda libri IV, edidit K. Koch. De alimentorum facultatibus libri III, edidit G. Helmreich. De bonis malisque sucis liber, edidit idem. De victu attenuante liber, edidit C. Kalbfleisch. De ptisama liber, edidit O. Hartlich*. Leipzig and Berlin: Teubner.

Kühn, C. G. ed. 1822. *Claudii Galeni Opera omnia*. Vol. 4. Leipzig: Knobloch.

Laga, C. ed. 1992. *Eustratii presbyteri vita Eutychii patriarchae Constantinopolitani*. Turnhout: Brepols.

Latte, K. ed. 1953–1966. *Hesychii Alexandrini lexicon*. Vols 1–2. Copenhagen: Munksgaard.

Lutz, C.E. ed. 1947. *Musonius Rufus "The Roman Socrates."* New Haven: Yale University Press.

Maraval, P. ed. 1971. *Grégoire de Nysse, Vie de Sainte Macrine: Introduction, texte critique, traduction, notes et index*. Sources Chrétiennes 178. Paris: Editions du Cerf.

Marshall, P.K. ed. 1969. *Aulus Gellius, Noctes Atticae*. Vol. 2. Oxford: Clarendon Press.

May, M.T. trans. 1968. *Galen on the Usefulness of the Parts of the Body/Peri chreias morion/De usu partium*. Ithaca, NY: Cornell University Press.

Migne, J.-P. ed. 1857–1866. *Patrologiae cursus completus. Series Graeca (MPG)*. Paris: Migne.

Musurillo, H. ed. and trans. 1972. *Acts of the Christian Martyrs*. Vol. 2. Oxford: Clarendon Press.

Papadopoulos-Kerameus, A. ed. 1909. "*Miracles of Artemios (BHG* 173–173c)," in *Varia graeca sacra*. St Petersburg: Kirschbaum, 1–75.

Pitra, J.B. ed. 1883. *Analecta sacra spicilegio Solesmensi parata*. Vol. 3. Paris: Tusculum.

Potter, P. ed. and trans. 2010. *Hippocrates, Coan Prenotions, Anatomical and Minor Clinical Writings*. Vol. 9. Cambridge, MA and London: Harvard University Press.

Rackham, H. trans. 1938. *Pliny. Natural History*, vol. 1: *Books 1–2*. Cambridge, MA and London: Harvard University Press.

Raeder, J. ed. 1933. *Oribasii Collectionum medicarum reliquiae, libri XLIX–L, libri incerti, eclogue medicamentorum, edidit J. Raeder*. Leipzig and Berlin: Teubner.

Ricci, J.V. trans. 1950. *Aetios of Amida: The Gynaecology and Obstetrics of the VIth Century, A.D.* Philadelphia and Toronto: The Blakiston Company.

Sandbach, F.H. ed. 1972. *Menandri reliquiae selectae*. Oxford: Clarendon Press, 231–265.

Schmidt, M. 1861–1862. *Hesychii Alexandrini Lexicon*. 4 vols. Halle: Jenae, Sumptibus Hermanni Dufftii (Libraria Maukiana).

Schwartz, E. ed. 1908. *Eusebius, Kirchengeschichte. Kleine Ausgabe*. Leipzig: J.C. Hinrichs'sche Buchhandlung.

Sieveking, W. ed. (1929) 1972. *Plutarchi Moralia*. Vol. 3. Reprint, Leipzig: Teubner.

Sigalas, A. ed. 1925. "Ἀνωνύμου Βίος καὶ ἀνατροφὴ τοῦ ἁγίου Θεοδώρου τοῦ Τήρωνος," Ἐπετηρὶς Ἑταιρείας Βυζαντινῶν Σπουδῶν 2: 220–226.

Sturz, F.W. ed. 1820. *Orionis Thebani Etymologicon*. Leipzig: Weigel.

Temkin. O. trans. 1956. *Soranus' Gynecology*. Baltimore: Johns Hopkins University Press.

Theodoridis, C. ed. 1976. *Die Fragmente des Grammatikers Philoxenos*. Berlin: De Gruyter.

Tsames, D.G. ed. 1980. Ἰωσὴφ Καλόθετου συγράμματα. Θεσσαλονικεῖς Βυζαντινοί Συγγραφεῖς 1. Thessaloniki: Centre for Byzantine Research.

Ven, P. van den. ed. 1962. *La vie ancienne de S. Syméon Stylite le Jeune (521–592)*, vol. 1: *Introduction et texte grec*. Subsidia Hagiographica 48. Brussels: Société des Bollandistes.

Zervos, A. ed. 1901. *Gynaekologie des Aëtios*. Leipzig: Fock.

Secondary Works

Abou Aly, A. 1996. "The Wet Nurse: A Study in Ancient Medicine and Greek Papyri," *Vesalius* 2 (2): 86–97.

Aboul, A. A. 1998. "Testing Women's Milk," *Sciences exactes et sciences appliquées à Alexandrie* 16: 207–215.

Ameling, W. 2012. "*Femina liberaliter instituta* – Some Thoughts on a Martyr's Liberal Education," in Bremmer and Formisano 2012a, 78–102.

Anagnostakis, I., and A. Pellettieri. eds. 2016. *Latte e latticini: Aspetti della produzione e del consumo nelle società mediterranee dell'Antichità e del Medioevo*. Lagonegro: Grafica Zaccara.

Ariantzi, D. 2012. *Kindheit in Byzanz: Emotionale, geistige und materielle Entwicklung im familiären Umfeld vom 6. bis zum 11. Jahrhundert*. Berlin: De Gruyter.

Atkinson, C. 1991. *The Oldest Vocation: Christian Motherhood in the Middle Ages*. Ithaca, NY and London: Cornell University Press.

Auerbach, E. (1958) 1965. *Literary Language and Its Public in Late Latin Antiquity and in the Middle Ages*, trans. R. Manheim. New York: Bollingen Foundation.

Augoustakis, A. 2010. *Motherhood and the Other: Fashioning Female Power in the Flavian Epic.* Oxford: Oxford University Press.

Bacalexi, D. 2005. "Female Responsibilities: Midwives, Nannies and Mothers in Some Physicians of Antiquity and the Renaissance," *Gesnerus* 62: 5–32.

Bal, M. (1991) 2012. "Perpetual Contest," in Bremmer and Formisano 2012a, 139–149.

Bardanzellu, F., V. Fanos, and A. Reali. 2017. "'Omics' in Human Colostrum and Mature Milk: Looking to Old Data with New Eyes," *Nutrients* 9: 843.

Beaucamp, J. 1982. "L'allaitement: Mère ou nourrice?," *Jahrbuch der Österreichischen Byzantinistik* 32: 549–558.

Bécares Rodríguez, L. 2019. "Alimentación infantil al margen de la lactancia materna: El hallazgo de biberones en el mundo clásico," in Reboreda Morillo 2019a, 113–130.

Becchi, M. 2013. "Plutarch, Aristotle, and the Peripatetics," in M. Beck (ed.) *A Companion to Plutarch.* Malden, MA and Oxford: Wiley Blackwell, 73–87.

Bennett, D. 2000. "Medical Practice and Manuscripts in Byzantium," *Society for the Social History of Medicine* 13: 279–291.

Beth Rose, M. 2017. *Plotting Motherhood in Medieval, Early Modern, and Modern Literature.* London: Palgrave Macmillan.

Bleek, M. 2017. *Motherhood and Meaning in Medieval Sculpture: Representations from France, c. 1100–1500.* Woodbridge: Boydell Press.

Bolman, E.S. 2004. "The Coptic Galaktotrophousa Revisited," in M. Immerzeel, and J. van de Vliet (eds) *Coptic Studies on the Threshold of a New Millennium: Proceedings of the Seventh International Conference of Coptic Studies.* Louvain: Peeters, 1173–1184.

———. 2015. "The Enigmatic Coptic Galaktotrophousa and the Cult of the Virgin Mary in Egypt," in M. Vassilaki (ed.) *Images of the Mother of God: Perceptions of the Theotokos in Byzantium.* Aldershot: Ashgate, 13–22.

Bonfante, L. 1997. "Nursing Mothers in Classical Art," in Koloski-Ostrow and Lyons 1997, 173–196.

Boswell, J. 1988. *The Kindness of Strangers: The Abandonment of Children in Western Europe from Late Antiquity to the Renaissance.* New York: Pantheon Books.

Bouras-Vallianatos, P., and S. Xenophontos. eds. 2018. *Greek Medical Literature and Its Readers: From Hippocrates to Islam and Byzantium.* London and New York: Routledge.

Bourbou, C. 2016. "Breasts and Bottles: The Contribution of Bioarchaeology to the Study of Infant Feeding Practices in Byzantine Greece (6th–15th c. AD)," in Anagnostakis and Pellettieri 2016, 93–102.

———. 2017. "Être un enfant à Aventicum," *Aventicum-Nouvelles de l'Association Pro Aventico* 32: 10–12.

Bourbou, C., and V. Dasen. 2018. "Enfance en peril: Les maladies infantiles à l'époque romaine," *Archéologia* 564: 58–65.

Bourbou, C., and S.J. Garvie-Lok. 2009. "Breastfeeding and Weaning Patterns in Byzantine Times: Evidence from Human Remains and Written Sources," in Papaconstantinou and Talbot 2009, 65–83.

Bourbou, C., B.T. Fuller, S.J. Garvie-Lok, and M.P. Richards. 2013. "Nursing Mothers and Feeding Bottles: Reconstructing Breastfeeding and Weaning Patterns in Greek Byzantine Populations (6th–15th Centuries AD) Using Carbon and Nitrogen Stable Isotope Ratios," *Journal of Archaeological Science* 40: 3903–3913.

Bradley, K.R. 1978. "The Age at Time of Sale of Female Slaves," *Arethusa* 11: 243–251.

———. 1980. "Sexual Regulations in Wet-Nursing Contracts from Roman Egypt," *Klio* 62 (2): 321–325.

———. 1986. "Wet-Nursing at Rome: A Study in Social Relations," in B. Rawson (ed.) *The Family in Ancient Rome: New Perspectives*. London: Croom Helm, 201–229.

———. 1987. *Slaves and Masters in the Roman Empire: A Study in Social Control*. New York and Oxford: Oxford University Press.

———. 1991. "The Social Role of the Nurse in the Roman World," in K.R. Bradley (ed.) *Discovering the Roman Family: Studies in Roman Social History*. New York: Oxford University Press, 13–36.

———. 1994a. *Slavery and Society in Rome*. Cambridge: Cambridge University Press.

———. 1994b. "The Nurse and the Child at Rome: Duty, Affect and Socialisation," *Thamyris* 1: 137–156.

———. 2003. "Sacrificing the Family: Christian Martyrs and Their Kin," *Ancient Narrative* 3: 150–181.

Bremmer, J.N. 2000. "The Passion of Perpetua and the Development of Early Christian Afterlife," *Nederlands Theologisch Tijdschrift* 54: 97–111.

———. 2002. "Perpetua and Her Diary: Authenticity, Family, and Visions," in W. Ameling (ed.) *Märtyrer und Märtyrerakten*. Stuttgart: Steiner, 97–111.

———. 2003. "The Vision of Saturus in the *Passio Perpetuae*," in F. García Martínez, and G.P. Luttikhuizen (eds) *Jerusalem, Alexandria, Rome: Studies in Ancient Cultural Interaction in Honour of A. Hillhorst*. Leiden: Brill, 55–73.

———. 2004. "The Motivation of Martyrs: Perpetua and the Palestinians," in B. Luchesi, and K. von Stuckrad (eds) *Religion im kulturellen Diskurs*. Berlin and New York: De Gruyter, 535–554.

———. 2021. "Roman Judge vs. Christian Bishop: The Trial of Phileas during the Great Persecution," in H.O. Maier, and K. Waldner (eds) *Desiring Martyrs: Locating Martyrs in Space and Time*. Berlin and Boston: De Gruyter, 81–118.

Bremmer, J.N., and M. Formisano. eds. 2012a. *Perpetua's Passions: Multidisciplinary Approaches to the Passio Perpetuae et Felicitatis*. Oxford: Oxford University Press.

———. 2012b. "Perpetua's Passions: A Brief Introduction," in Bremmer and Formisano 2012a, 1–13.

Bretin-Chabrol, M. 2015. "Du lait de la nourrice aux *alimenta* du père nourricier: Des liens fragiles dans la Rome Imperiale," *Cahiers du Genre* 58: 21–39.

Bunkers, S.L., and C.A. Huff. 1996. *Inscribing the Daily: Critical Essays on Women's Diaries*. Amherst: University of Massachusetts Press.

Burnett, C.M.C. 2009. "Mother-Child Bonding in the Greek and Latin Fathers of the Church," in C.B. Horn, and R.R. Phenix (eds) *Children in Late Ancient Christianity*. Tübingen: Mohr Siebeck, 75–101.

Burrus, V. 2008. "Torture and Travail: Producing the Christian Martyr," in A.-J. Levine (ed.) *A Feminist Companion to Patristic Literature*. New York: T&T Clark, 56–71.

Butler, R.D. 2006. *The New Prophecy and "New Visions": Evidence of Montanism in the Passion of Perpetua and Felicitas*. Washington, DC: Catholic University of America.

Cairns, D.M. Hinterberger, A. Pizzonne, and M. Zaccarini. eds. 2022. *Emotions through Time: From Antiquity to Byzantium*. Emotions in Antiquity 1. Tübingen: Mohr Siebeck

Cardoso, K.S. 2015. "Reverberações culturais e criação de identidade no cristianismo primitivo: Análise retórica e iconográfica de *Passio Perpetua*," *Revista Oracula* 11 (16): 15–28.

Caseau, C.B. 2009. "Childhood in Byzantine Saints' Lives," in Papaconstantinou and Talbot 2009, 127–166.

Castelli, E.A. 2004. *Martyrdom and Memory: Early Christian Culture Making*. New York: Columbia University Press.

Centlivres Challet, C.-E. 2016. "Tires-lait ou biberons romains? Fonctions, fonctionalités et affectivité," *L'Antiquité Classique* 85: 157–180.

———. 2017. "Feeding the Roman Nursling: Maternal Milk, Its Substitutes, and Their Limitations," *Latomus* 17: 895–909.

Chirban, J. ed. 1991. *Health and Faith: Medical, Psychological, and Religious Dimensions*. Lanham: University Press of America.

———. ed. 2010. *Holistic Healing in Byzantium*. Brookline: Holy Cross Orthodox Press.

Clifford Allbutt, T. 1913. "Byzantine Medicine: The Finlayson Memorial Lecture," *Glasgow Medical Journal* 80 (5): 321–439.

Cobb, S.L. 2019. "Suicide by Gladiator? The *Acts of Perpetua and Felicitas* in Its North African Context," *Church History* 88 (3): 597–628.

———. ed. and trans. 2021. *The Passion of Perpetua and Felicitas in Late Antiquity*. Oakland: University of California Press.

———. 2022. "The Other Woman: Felicitas in Late Antiquity," *Journal of Late Antiquity* 15 (1): 1–27.

Coccagna, H.A. 2014. "Manipulating *mastoi*: The Female Breast in the Sympotic Setting," in A. Avramidou, and A.D. Demetriou (eds) *Approaching the Ancient Artifact: Representation, Narrative, and Function*. Berlin: De Gruyter, 399–412.

Cohen, B. 1997. "Divesting the Female Breast of Clothes in Classical Sculpture," in Koloski-Ostrow and Lyons 1997, 66–92.

Congourdeau, M.-H. 2009. "Les variations du désir d'enfant à Byzance," in Papaconstantinou and Talbot 2009, 35–63.

Constantelos, D.J. 1999. "Medicine and Social Welfare in the Byzantine Empire," *Medicina nei Secoli* 11 (2): 337–355.

Constantinou, S. 2004. "Subgenre and Gender in Saints' Lives," in P. Odorico, and P.A. Agapitos (eds) *Les vies des saints à Byzance: Genre littéraire ou biographie historique?* Dossiers Byzantins 4. Paris: Centre d'études byzantines, néo-helléniques et sud-est européennes, École des hautes études en sciences sociales, 411–423.

———. 2005. *Female Corporeal Performances: Reading the Body in Byzantine Passions and Lives of Holy Women*. Studia Byzantina Upsaliensia 9. Uppsala: Acta Universitatis Upsaliensis.

———. 2015. "The Saints' Two Bodies: Sensibility under (Self-)Torture in Byzantine Hagiography," *Classica et Mediaevalia* 66: 285–320.

———. 2022. "Angry Warriors in the Byzantine *War of Troy*," in Cairns, Hinterberger, Pizzone, and Zaccarini 2022, 339–358.

———. 2023a. "Monastic 'Gynealogy': The Maternal-Feminine Structure of Byzantine Women's Asceticism," in A. Purpura, and T. Arentzen (eds) *Orthodoxy, Women, and Gender*. Eugene, OR: Wipf & Stock, in press.

———. 2023b. "The Martyr's Body: Sanctification through Blood, Milk, and Water," in P. Sarris (ed.) *Blood in Byzantium*. London and New York: Routledge, in press.

———. 2023c. "Mothers' Time: The Temporality of Motherhood in the *Life of Martha* and the *Life of Symeon Stylite the Younger*," in M. Dell'Isola (ed.) *Female Authority and Holiness in Early Christianity and Byzantium*. Berlin and Boston: De Gruyter, in press.

Constantinou, S., and M. Meyer (eds) 2019. *Emotions and Gender in Byzantine Culture*. London: Palgrave Macmillan.

Constantinou, S., and A. Skouroumouni-Stavrinou. 2022. "Premodern *Galaktology:* Reading Milk in Ancient and Early Byzantine Medical Treatises," *Journal of Late Antique, Islamic and Byzantine Studies* 1 (1–2): 1–40.

———. 2024. "The Other Mother: Ancient and Early Byzantine Approaches to Wet Nursing and Mothering," *Journal of Hellenic Studies*, in press.

Cooper, K. 2007. *The Fall of the Roman Household*. Cambridge: Cambridge University Press.

———. 2011. "A Father, a Daughter and a Procurator: Authority and Resistance in the Prison Memoir of Perpetua of Carthage," *Gender and History* 23: 685–702.

Corbier, M. 2001. "Child Exposure and Abandonment," in S. Dixon (ed.) *Childhood, Class and Kin in the Roman World*. London and New York: Routledge, 52–73.

Corrington, G.P. 1989. "The Milk of Salvation: Redemption by the Mother in Late Antiquity and Early Christianity," *Harvard Theological Review* 82: 393–420.

Cotter-Lynch, M. 2016. *Saint Perpetua across the Middle Ages: Mother, Gladiator, Saint*. New York: Palgrave Macmillan.

Dasen, V. 2010. "Des nourrices Grecques à Rome?," *Paedagogica Historica* 46: 699–713.

———. 2012a. "Bibliographie sélective, I: La nourrice et le lait: Antiquité–Moyen Age,'" in V. Dasen and M.-C. Gérard-Zai (eds) *Art de manger, art de vivre: Nourriture et société de l'Antiquité à nos jours*. Gollion: Infolio, 314–324.

———. 2012b. "Construire sa parenté par la nourriture à Rome," in V. Dasen, and M.-C. Gérard-Zai (eds) *Art de manger, art de vivre: Nourriture et société de l'Antiquité à nos jours*. Gollion: Infolio, 40–59.

De Beauvoir, S. 1949. *Le deuxième sexe*. 2 vols. Paris: Gallimard.

De Forest, M.M. 1993. "Clytemnestra's Breast and the Evil Eye," in D. Raymond Deklavon (ed.) *Woman's Power, Man's Game: Essays on Classical Antiquity in Honor of Joy K. King*. Wauconda, IL: Bolchazy-Carducci, 129–148.

Demand, N. 1994. *Birth, Death, and Motherhood in Classical Greece*. Baltimore: Johns Hopkins University Press.

Dixon, S. 1988. *The Roman Mother*. Norman: University of Oklahoma Press.

Dockray-Miller, M. 2000. *Motherhood and Mothering in Anglo-Saxon England*. New York: St Martin's Press.

Dova, S. 2017. "Lactation Cessation and the Realities of Martyrdom in 'The Passion of Saint Perpetua,'" *Illinois Classical Studies* 42: 245–265.

Dunn, S. 2010. "The Female Martyr and the Politics of Death: An Examination of the Martyr Discourses of Vibia Perpetua and Wafa Idris," *Journal of the American Academy of Religion* 78 (1): 202–225.

Dupras, T.L., H.P. Schwarcz, and S.I. Fairgrieve. 2001. "Infant Feeding and Weaning Practices in Roman Egypt," *American Journal of Physical Anthropology* 115: 204–212.

Dupras, T.L., and M.W. Tocheri. 2007. "Reconstructing Infant Weaning Histories at Roman Period Kellis, Egypt Using Stable Isotope Analysis of Dentition," *American Journal of Physical Anthropology* 134: 63–74.

D-Vasilescu, E.E. 2018. *Heavenly Sustenance in Patristic Texts and Byzantine Iconography: Nourished by the Word*. London: Palgrave.

Engelbrecht, E. 1999. "God's Milk: An Orthodox Confession of the Eucharist," *Journal of Early Christian Studies* 7 (4): 509–526.

Evans Grubbs, J. 2009a. "Church, State, and Children: Christian and Imperial Attitudes Toward Infant Exposure in Late Antiquity," in A. Cain, and N. Lenski (eds) *The Power of Religion in Late Antiquity*. Burlington, VT: Ashgate, 119–131.

———. 2009b. "Marriage and Family Relationships in the Late Roman West," in P. Rousseau (ed.) *A Companion to Late Antiquity*. Malden, MA and Oxford: 201–219.

———. 2010. "Hidden in Plain Sight: *Expositi* in the Community," in V. Dasen, and T. Späth (eds) *Children, Memory, and Family Identity in Roman Culture*. Oxford: Oxford University Press, 293–310.

———. 2011. "The Dynamics of Infant Abandonment: Motives, Attitudes and (Un)intended Consequences," in K. Mustakallio, and C. Laes (eds) *The Dark Side of Childhood in Late Antiquity and the Middle Ages*. Oxford: Oxbow Books, 21–36.

———. 2013a. "Infant Exposure and Infanticide," in J. Evans Grubbs, and T. Parkin (eds) *Childhood and Education in the Classical World*. Oxford and New York: Oxford University Press, 83–107.

———. 2013b. "Between Slavery and Freedom: Disputes over Status and the Codex Justinianus," *Roman Legal Tradition* 9: 31–93.

Evans Grubbs, J., and T. Parkin. eds. 2013. *The Oxford Handbook of Childhood and Education in the Classical World*. Oxford: Oxford University Press

Farina, W. 2009. *Perpetua of Carthage: Portrait of a Third Century Martyr*. Jefferson, NC: MacFarland.

Fildes, V. A. 1986. *Breasts, Bottles, and Babies: A History of Infant Feeding*. Edinburgh: Edinburgh University Press.

———. 1988. *Wet Nursing: A History from Antiquity to the Present*. Oxford: Basil Blackwell.

Formisano, M. 2012. "Perpetua's Prisons: Notes on the Margins of Literature," in Bremmer and Formisano 2012a, 329–347.

———. 2019. "Perpetua's Alibi: Image Control, Visions and Death in the *Passio Perpetuae et Felicitatis*," in G. Blamberger, and D. Boschung (eds) *Competing Perspectives: Figures of Image Control*. Leiden and New York: Brill, 215–233.

French, V. 1986 "Midwives and Maternity in the Greco-Roman World," *Helios* 13 (2): 69–84.

Galinsky, K. 1996. *Augustan Culture: An Interpretive Introduction*. Princeton, NJ: Princeton University Press.

Gardner, J.F. 1998. *Family and Familia in Roman Law and Life*. Oxford: Oxford University Press.

Gerber, D. 1978. "The Female Breast in Greek Erotic Literature," *Arethusa* 11: 203–212.

Giladi, A. 1999. *Infants, Parents and Wet Nurses: Medieval Islamic Views on Breastfeeding and Their Social Implications*. Leiden: Brill.

Gkegkes I., D. Darla, M. Vassiliki, and C. Iavvazo. 2007. "Breastfeeding in Byzantine Icon Art," *Archives of Gynecology and Obstetrics* 286: 71–73.

Glancy, J.A. 2006². *Slavery in Early Christianity*. Minneapolis: Fortress Press.

Gold, B.K. 2018. *Perpetua: Athlete of God*. New York: Oxford University Press.

Goldhill, S. 2012. "Forms of Attention: Time and Narrative in Ecphrasis," *Cambridge Classical Journal* 58: 88–104.

Gonzalez, E. 2014. *The Fate of the Dead in Early Third Century North African Christianity: The Passion of Perpetua and Felicitas and Tertullian*. Tübingen: Mohr Siebeck.

Gourevitch, D. 1990. "Les tire-lait antiques et l'utilisation médicale du lait humain," *Histoire des sciences médicales* 24: 93–98.

———. 1992. "Femme nourrisant son enfant au biberon," *Antike Kunst* 35: 78–81.

Green, M.H. 1985. *The Transmission of Ancient Theories of Female Physiology and Disease through the Early Middle Ages*. Princeton: Princeton University Press.

Guazzelli, G.A. 2009. "Gli 'Acta brevia sanctarum Perpetuae et Felicitatis': Una proposta di rilettura," *Cristianesimo nella storia* 30: 1–38.

Günther, R. 1987. *Frauenarbeit – Frauenbindung: Untersuchungen zu unfreien und freige-lassenen Frauen in den stadtrömischen Inschriften*. Munich: W. Fink.

Habermehl, P. 2004. *Perpetua und der Ägypter oder Bilder des Bösen im frühen afrikanis-chen Christentum: Ein Versuch zur Passio Sanctarum Perpetuae et Felicitatis*. Berlin and New York: De Gruyter.

Hadjinicolaou-Marava, A. 1950. *Recherches sur la vie des esclaves dans le monde byzantin*. Athens: French Institute of Athens.

Hadot, P. 1998. *The Inner Citadel: The Meditations of Marcus Aurelius*. Translated by M. Chase. Cambridge, MA and London: Harvard University Press.

Hanson, A.E. 1987. "The Eight Months' Child and the Etiquette of Birth: *Obsit omen!*," *Bulletin of the History of Medicine* 61: 589–602.

———. 2003. "'Your Mother Nursed You with Bile': Anger in Babies and Small Children," *Yale Classical Studies* 32: 185–207.

Harman, K.V. 2013. "Motherhood and Life Writing," in M. Jolly (ed.) *Encyclopedia of Life Writing: Autobiographical and Biographical Forms*. London and New York: Routledge, 617–618.

Harper, K. 2011. *Slavery in the Late Roman World, AD 275–425*. Cambridge: Cambridge University Press.

Hatlie, P. 2009. "Images of Motherhood and Self in Byzantine Literature," *Dumbarton Oaks Papers* 63: 41–57.

Heffernan, T.J. 1988. *Sacred Biography: Saints and Their Biographers in the Middle Ages*. New York and Oxford: Oxford University Press.

———. 2012. *The Passion of Perpetua and Felicity*. New York: Oxford University Press.

Henten, J.W. van. 2012. "Maternity and Sainthood in the Medieval Perpetua Legend," in Bremmer and Formisano 2012a, 118–133.

Hermann, J. 1959. "Die Ammenverträge in den graeko-aegyptischen Papyri," *Zeitschrift der Savigny-Stiftung für Rechtsgeschichte (Romanistische Abteilung)* 76: 490–499.

Hernández Lobato, J. 2005. "*Repraesentatio rerum*: Hacia un análisis narratológico de la *Passio Perpetuae*," *Voces* 16: 75–95.

Hewett, H. 2020. "Mothering Memoirs," in O'Brien Hallstein, O'Reilly, and Vandenbeld Giles 2020, 191–201.

Hill, G., G. Johnston, S. Campbell, and J. Birdsell. 1987. "The Medical and Demographic Importance of Wet-Nursing," *Canadian Bulletin of Medical History* 3: 183–193.

Hogan, R. 1991. "Engendered Autobiographies: The Diary as a Feminine Form," *Prose Studies* 14: 95–107.

Holman, S.R. 1997. "Molded as Wax: Formation and Feeding of the Ancient Newborn," *Helios* 24: 77–95.

Huff, C. 1989. "'That Profoundly Female, and Feminist Genre': The Diary as Feminist Practice," *Women's Studies Quarterly* 17 (3/4): 6–14.

Hummel, C. 1999. *Das Kind und seine Krankheiten in der griechischen Medizin: Von Aretaios bis Johannes Aktuarios (1. bis 14. Jahrhundert)*. Frankfurt am Main: Peter Lang.

Hunink, V. 2012. "'With the Taste of Something Sweet Still in My Mouth': Perpetua's Visions," in B. Koet (ed.) *Dreams as Divine Communication in Christianity: From Hermas to Aquinas*. Leuven: Peeters, 77–91.

Jensen, A. 2002. *Gottes selbstbewußte Töchter: Frauenemazipation im frühen Christentum?* Freiburg: Herder.

Joly, R. 1976. "La structure du *Foetus de huit mois*," *L'Antiquité Classique* 45: 173–180.

Joshel, S.R. 1986. "Nurturing the Master's Child: Slavery and the Roman Child-Nurse," *Signs* 12: 3–32.

Joshel, S.R., and S. Murnaghan (eds) 1998. *Women and Slaves in Greco-Roman Culture: Differential Equations*. London and New York: Routledge.
Karydas, H.P. 1998. *Eurykleia and Her Successors. Female Figures of Authority in Greek Poetics*. Lanham, MD: Rowman & Littlefield.
Kažhdan, A. 1983. "Hagiographical Notes: Two Versions of the *Vita Athanasii*," *Byzantion* 53 (2): 538–558.
Keith, A. 2011. "Slavery and the Roman Family," in K. Bradley, and P. Cartledge (eds) *The Cambridge World History of Slavery*, vol. 1: *The Ancient Mediterranean World*. Cambridge: Cambridge University Press, 337–361.
Kitzler, P. 2015. *From Passio Perpetuae to Acta Perpetuae: Recontextualizing a Martyr Story in the Literature of the Early Church*. Berlin and Boston: De Gruyter.
Klein, E. 2020. "Perpetua, Cheese, and Martyrdom as Public Liturgy in the *Passion of Perpetua and Felicity*," *Journal of Early Christian Studies* 28 (2): 175–202.
Kokoszko, M., K. Jagusiak, Z. Rzeźnicka, and J. Dybałac. 2018. "Pedanius Dioscorides' Remarks on Milk Properties, Quality and Processing Technology," *Journal of Archaeological Science Reports* 19: 982–986.
Köpstein, H. 1966. *Zur Sklaverei im ausgehenden Byzanz*. Berlin: Akademie-Verlag.
Koloski-Ostrow, A.O., and C.L. Lyons. eds. 1997. *Naked Truths: Women, Sexuality, and Gender in Classical Art and Archaeology*. London: Routledge.
———. 1976. "Zur Novelle des Alexios Komnenos zum Sklavenstatus (1095)," in *Actes du XVe Congrès international d'études byzantines*. Vol. 4. Bibliothēkē tēs en Athēnais Archaiologikēs Hetaireias 92. Athens: Association Internationale des Etudes Byzantines, 160–172.
———. 1993. "Sklaven in der 'Peira,'" in L. Burgmann (ed.) *Fontes minores* 9. Vorschungen zur byzantinischen Rechtsgeschichte 19. Frankfurt: Löwenklau-Gesellschaft, 1–33.
Kraemer, R.S. 2008 "When Is a Text About a Woman?: The Cases of Aseneth and Perpetua," in A.-J. Levine, and M. Mayo Robbins (eds) *A Feminist Companion to Patristic Literature*. New York: T&T Clark, 156–172.
Kraemer, R.S., and S.L. Lander. 2000. "Perpetua and Felicitas," in P.F. Esler (ed.) *The Early Christian World*. Vol. 2. London: Routledge, 1048–1068.
Langener, L. 1996. *Isis lactans–Maria lactans: Untersuchungen zur koptischen Ikonographie*. Altenberge: Oros Verlag.
Laskaris, J. 2008. "Nursing Mothers in Greek and Roman Medicine," *American Journal of Archaeology* 112: 459–464.
LaValle, D. 2015. "Divine Breastfeeding: Milk, Blood, and 'Pneuma' in Clement of Alexandria's *Paedagogus*," *Journal of Late Antiquity* 8 (2): 322–336.
Lawrence, T. 2021. "Breastmilk, Breastfeeding, and the Female Body in Early Imperial Rome," in M. Bradley, V. Leonard, and L. Totelin (eds) *Bodily Fluids in Antiquity*. London: Routledge, 224–239.
Lefkowitz, M.R. 1976. "The Motivations for Perpetua's Martyrdom," *Journal of the American Academy of Religion* 44 (3): 417–421.
Lejeune, P. (1997) 2009. "The Diary on Trial," in Popkin and Rak 2009, 147–167.
———. (1999) 2009. "The Practice of the Private Journal: Chronicle of an Investigation (1986)–(1998)," in Popkin and Rak 2009, 29–50.
———. 2009. "How Do Diaries End?," in Popkin and Rak 2009, 187–200.
Lejeune, P., and C. Bogaert 2020. "The Practice of Writing a Diary," trans. D. Meijers-Troller, in B. Ben-Amos, and D. Ben-Amos (eds) *The Diary: The Epic of Everyday Life*. Bloomington: Indiana University Press, 25–38.
Leyser, C., and L. Smith. eds. 2011. *Motherhood, Religion, and Society in Medieval Europe, 400–1400*. London: Routledge.

Liveley, G. 2012. "*Mater Amoris*: Mothers and Lovers in Augustan Rome," in Petersen and Salzman-Mitchell 2012, 185–204.

Lloyd, G. 1979. *Magic, Reason and Experience: Studies in the Origin and Development of Greek Science*. Cambridge: Cambridge University Press.

———. 1983. *Science, Folklore and Ideology*. Cambridge: Cambridge University Press.

———. 2003. *In the Grip of Disease: Studies in the Greek Imagination*. Oxford: Oxford University Press.

Long, A.A. 2012. "The Self in the *Meditations*," in M. van Ackeren (ed.) *A Companion to Marcus Aurelius*. Malden, MA and Oxford: Blackwell, 465–480.

Loraux, N. 1998. *Mothers in Mourning*. Translated by C. Pache. Ithaca, NY and London: Cornell University Press.

Lössl, J. 2000. "Augustine in Byzantium," *Journal of Ecclesiastical History* 51 (2): 267–295.

Maher, V. ed. 1992. *Anthropology of Breast-Feeding: Natural Law or Social Construct*. London: Routledge.

Marganne, M.-H. 2015. "Hippocrate dans un monde de chrétiens: La réception des traités hippocratiques dans la *chôra* égyptienne à la période byzantine (284–641)," in J. Jouanna, and M. Zink (eds) *Hippocrate et les hippocratismes: Médecine, religion, société. Actes du XIVᵉ Colloque international Hippocratique*. Paris and Leuven: Peeters, 284–641.

Marshall, C.W. 2017. "Breastfeeding in Greek Literature and Thought," *Illinois Classical Studies* 42 (1): 185–201.

Matthews Grieco, S.F. 1991. "Breastfeeding, Wet Nursing and Infant Mortality in Europe (1400–1800)," in S.F. Matthews Grieco, and C.A. Corsini (eds) *Historical Perspectives on Breastfeeding*. Florence: Unicef, 15–62.

McLarty, J. 2013. "The Function of the Letter Form in Christian Martyrdom Accounts: 'I Would Like My Community, My Church, My Family, to Remember,'" in O. Hodkinson, P. Rosenmeyer, and E. Bracke (eds) *Epistolary Narratives in Ancient Greek Literature. Mnemosyne* Supplement 359. Leiden and Boston: Brill, 371–385.

Meyer, M. 2009. *An Obscure Portrait: Imagining Women's Reality in Byzantine Art*. London: Pindar.

———. 2012. "Divine Nourishment: On Breasts and Bottles in the Miniatures of Iakobos Kokkinobaphos," *Δελτίον Χριστιανικῆς Ἀρχαιολογικῆς Ἑταιρείας* 33: 265–276.

Miller, T. 1997. *The Birth of the Hospital in the Byzantine Empire*. Baltimore, MD: Johns Hopkins University Press.

———. 2003. *The Orphans of Byzantium: Child Welfare in the Christian Empire*. Washington, DC: Catholic University of America Press.

Milnor, K. 2008. *Gender, Domesticity, and the Age of Augustus: Inventing Private Life*. Oxford: Oxford University Press.

Moffatt, A. 1986. "The Byzantine Child," *Social Research* 53 (4): 705–723.

Moss, C.R. 2010. "Blood Ties: Martyrdom, Motherhood, and Family in the *Passion of Perpetua and Felicitas*," in S.P. Ahearne-Kroll, P.A. Holloway, and J.A. Kelhoffer (eds) *Women and Gender in Ancient Religions: Interdisciplinary Approaches*. Tübingen: Mohr Siebeck, 189–208.

Muehlberger, E. 2022. "Perpetual Adjustment: The *Passion of Perpetua and Felicity* and the Entailments of Authenticity," *Journal of Early Christian Studies* 30 (3): 313–342.

Mulder, T. 2017. "Adult Breastfeeding in Ancient Rome," *Illinois Classical Studies* 42 (1): 227–243.

Mulder-Bakker, A. ed. 1995. *Sanctity and Motherhood: Essays on Holy Mothers in the Middle Ages*. New York: Routledge.

Myers, A.D. 2017. *Blessed among Women?: Mothers and Motherhood in the New Testa-ment*. Oxford: Oxford University Press.

Nelson, B. 2016. "A Mother's Martyrdom: Elite Christian Motherhood and the Martyrdom of Domnina," *Journal of Feminist Studies in Religion* 32 (2): 11–26.

Newbold, R. 2000. "Breasts and Milk in Nonnus' *Dionysiaca*," *Classical World* 94: 11–23.

Nutton V. 1992. "Healers in the Medical Market Place: Towards a Social History of Graeco-Roman Medicine," in A. Wear (ed.) *Medicine in Society: Historical Essays*. Cambridge: Cambridge University Press, 15–58.

———. 2013². *Ancient Medicine*. London and New York: Routledge.

O'Brien Hallstein, L., A. O'Reilly, and M. Vandenbeld Giles. eds. 2020. *The Routledge Companion to Motherhood*. London and New York: Routledge

O'Neill, K. 1998. "Aeschylus, Homer, and the Serpent at the Breast," *Phoenix* 52 (3–4): 216–229.

O'Reilly, A. 2020. "Matricentric Feminism: A Feminism for Mothers," in O'Brien Hallstein, O'Reilly, and Vandenbeld Giles 2020, 51–60.

Oberhelman, S. ed. 2013. *Dreams, Healing, and Medicine in Greece: From Antiquity to the Present*. Farnham: Ashgate.

Oehler, K. 1964. "Aristotle in Byzantium," *Greek, Roman, and Byzantine Studies* 5: 133–146.

Ortner, S., and H. Whitehead. 1981. "Accounting for Sexual Meaning," in S. Ortner, and H. Whitehead (eds) *Sexual Meanings: The Cultural Construction of Gender and Sexuality*. Cambridge: Cambridge University Press, 1–27.

Osiek, C. 2002. "Perpetua's Husband," *Journal of Early Christian Studies* 10: 287–290.

Palmer, G. 2009³. *The Politics of Breastfeeding: When Breasts Are Bad for Business*. London: Pinter & Martin.

Papaconstantinou, A., and A.-M. Talbot. eds. 2009. *Becoming Byzantine: Children and Childhood in Byzantium*. Washington, DC: Dumbarton Oaks Research Library and Collection.

Parca, M. 2013. "Children in Ptolemaic Egypt: What the Papyri Say," in Evans Grubbs and Parkin 2013, 465–483.

———. 2017. "The Wet Nurses of Ptolemaic and Roman Egypt," *Illinois Classical Studies* 42 (1): 203–226.

Parkhouse, S. 2017. "The Fetishization of Female 'Exempla': Mary, Thecla, Perpetua and Felicitas," *New Testament Studies* 63 (4): 567–587.

Parkin, T. 1992. *Demography and the Roman Society*. Baltimore and London: Johns Hopkins University Press.

———. 2013. "The Demography of Infancy and Early Childhood in the Ancient World," in Evans Grubbs and Parkin 2013, 40–61.

Parsons, C., and B. Wheeler. eds. 1996. *Medieval Mothering*. New York: Routledge.

Patlagean, E. 1977. *Pauvreté économique et pauvreté sociale à Byzance, 4ᵉ–7ᵉ siècles*. Paris and The Hague: Mouton.

———. 1981. "Ancienne hagiographie byzantine et histoire sociale," in E. Patlagean (ed.) *Structure sociale, famille, chrétienté à Byzance, IVᵉ–XIᵉ siècle*. London: Variorum Reprints. Vol. 5, 106–126.

———. 1987. "Byzantium in the Tenth and Eleventh Centuries," in P. Veyne (ed.) *A History of Private Life: From Pagan Rome to Byzantium*, vol 1: *From Pagan Rome to Byzantium*. Translated by A. Goldhammer. Cambridge, MA and London: Belknap Press, 551–641.

Pedrucci, 2013a. *L'allattamento nella Grecia di epoca arcaica e classica*. Rome: Scienze e Lettere.

———. 2013b. *L'isola delle madri: Una rilettura della documentazione archeologica di donne con bambini in Sicilia*. Rome: Scienze e Lettere.

———. 2013c. "Sangue menstruale e latte materno: Riflessioni e nuove proposte intorno all'allattamento nella Grecia antica," *Gesnerus* 70 (2): 260–291.

———. 2016. "Breastfeeding Animals and Other Wild 'Nurses' in Greek and Roman Mythology," *Gerión* 34: 307–323.

———. 2017. "Motherhood, Breastfeeding and Adoption: The Case of Hera Suckling Herakles," in P. Johnston, A. Mastrocinque, and L. Takács (eds) *Hera and Juno: The Functions of the Goddesses in Prehistoric and Historic Greece and Rome, Symposium Classicum Peregrinum, June 16–19, 2015, Budapest (Hungary)*. Acta Ant Hung 57: 325–326.

———. 2018. *Maternità e allattamenti nel mondo greco e romano: Un percorso fra scienza delle religioni e studi sulla maternità*. Rome: Scienze e Lettere.

———. 2019a. "Allaitements 'transgressifs' dans l'Antiquité gréco-romaine," in Reboreda Morillo 2019a, 131–146.

———. 2019b. "Allattamento e co-allattamento nel mondo greco e romano," in C. Lambrugo (ed.) *Una favola breve: Archeologia e antropologia per la storia dell'infanzia*. Florence: All'insegna del Giglio, 21–27.

———. ed. 2019c. *Maternità e monoteismi/Motherhood(s) and Monotheisms*. Rome: Quasar.

———. ed. 2019d. *Breastfeeding(s) and Religions: Normative Prescriptions and Individual Appropriation of Them. A Cross-cultural and Interdisciplinary Perspective from Antiquity to the Present. Proceedings of the International Workshop Held at the Max-Weber-Kolleg (University of Erfurt), July 11–12, 2018*. Rome: Scienze e Lettere.

———. 2020a. "La nutrice come figura vicaria e 'di attaccamento' all'interno della famiglia greca e romana," in *Proceedings of the IV Seminario Internacional del Grupo Deméter. Familias, edades y género: Perspectivas histórico-jurídicas. Oviedo, 9–10 de noviembre de 2017*. Oviedo: Silex.

———. 2020b. "Mothers for Sale: The Case of the Wet Nurse in the Ancient Greek and Roman World: An Overview," *Arenal* 27 (1): 127–140.

———. 2020c. "On the Use of Human Milk and Menstrual Blood between Medicine and Magic in the Greek and Roman Worlds," in E. Sanzo, A. Mastrocinque, and M. Scapini (eds) *Ancient Magic: Then and Now*. Nordhausen: Verlag T. Bautz, 287–302.

Penna, D. 2022. "The Role of Slaves in the Byzantine Economy, 10th–11th Centuries: Legal Aspects," in F. Rosu (ed.) *Slavery in the Black Sea Region, c. 900–1900: Forms of Unfreedom at the Intersection between Christianity and Islam*. Studies in Global Slavery 11. Leiden and Boston: Brill, 63–89.

Penniman, J.D. 2015. "Fed to Perfection: Mother's Milk, Roman Family Values, and the Transformation of the Soul in Gregory of Nyssa," *Church History* 84 (3): 495–530.

———. 2017. *Raised on Christian Milk: Food and the Formation of the Soul in Early Christianity*. New Haven, CT: Yale University Press.

Perkins, J. 1995. *The Suffering Self: Pain and Narrative Representation in the Early Christian Era*. London and New York: Routledge.

———. 2007. "The Rhetoric of the Maternal Body in the *Passio of Perpetua*," in T. Penner, and C. Vadner Stichele (eds) *Mapping Gender in Ancient Religious Discourses*. Biblical Interpretation Series 84. Leiden and Boston: Brill, 312–333.

Perry, M.J. 2014. *Gender, Manumission, and the Roman Freedwoman*. Cambridge: Cambridge University Press.

Petersen, L.H., and P. Salzman-Mitchell. eds. 2012. *Mothering and Motherhood in Ancient Greece and Rome*. Austin: University of Texas Press.

Pfister, E.J. 1964. "A Biographical Note: The Brothers and Sisters of St. Gregory of Nyssa," *Vigiliae Christianae* 18 (2): 108–113.

Pillet, A. 1885. *Histoire de Sainte Perpétue et de ses compagnons*. Lille: Librairie de J. Lefort.

Pitarakis, B. 2009. "The Material Culture of Childhood in Byzantium," in Papaconstantinou and Talbot 2009, 167–251.

Plati, E. 2020. "Medical Allusions and Intertext of *Physis* in Plutarch's *Comp. Cim. et Luc.* 2.7," in T.S. Schmidt, M. Vamvouri, and R. Hirsch-Luipold (eds) *The Dynamics of Intertextuality in Plutarch*. Brill's Plutarch Studies 5. Leiden and Boston: Brill, 376–387.

Podnieks, E. 2020. "Matrifocal Voices in Literature," in O'Brien Hallstein, O'Reilly, and Vandenbeld Giles 2020, 176–190.

———. 2022. *Maternal Modernism: Narrating New Mothers*. Cham: Palgrave Macmillan.

Podnieks, E., and A. O'Reilly. 2010. "Maternal Literatures in Text and Tradition: Daughter-centric, Matrilineal, and Matrifocal Perspectives," in E. Podnieks, and A. O'Reilly (eds) *Textual Mothers/Maternal Texts: Motherhood in Contemporary Women's Literatures*. Waterloo, ON: Wilfrid Laurier University Press, 1–27.

Poirier, M. 1970. "Note sur le *Passio Sanctarum Perpetuae et Felicitatis*: Felicitas était-elle vraiment l'esclave de Perpetua?," *Studia Patristica* 10: 306–309.

Popkin, J.D., and J. Rak. eds. 2009. *Philippe Lejeune, On Diary*. Translated by K. Durnin. Honolulu: University of Hawaii Press.

Preat, R. 2021. "From the Womb to the Page: Gynaecology and History in John of Lydia," *Ágora: Estudos Clássicos em Debate* 23 (1): 91–115.

Prinzig, G. 2010. "On Slaves and Slavery," in P. Stevenson (ed.) *The Byzantine World*. London: Routledge, 92–102.

———. 2014. "Hausbedienstete oder -sklaven in Byzanz zwischen tödlicher Repression und grösßter Hochschätzung: Ein Streiflicht anhand von vier konkreten Fällen," in S. Hanß and J. Schiel (eds) *Mediterranean Slavery Revisited (500–1800)/Neue Perspektiven auf mediterrane Sklaverei (500–1800)*. Zurich: Chronos Verlag, 187–199.

Räuchle, V. 2022. "The Terrible Power of Giving Birth: Images of Motherhood from Antiquity to Byzantium," in Cairns, Hinterberger, Pizzonne, and Zaccarini 2022, 407–432.

Rawson, B. 1991. "Adult–Child Relationships in Roman Society," in B. Rawson (ed.) *Marriage, Divorce and Children in Ancient Rome*. Oxford: Oxford University Press, 7–30.

Ray, A.-L. 2004. "Autour des nourrissons byzantins et de leur regime," in V. Dasen (ed.) *Naissance et petite enfance dans l'Antiquité*. Fribourg and Göttingen: Vandenhoeck & Ruprecht, 363–375.

Rea, J.A. 2016. "Transforming Civic Space into Sacred Space in the 'Passio' of Perpetua and Felicitas," *Classical Outlook* 91 (2): 46–50.

Reboreda Morillo, S. ed. 2019a. *Lactación, corpo e sexualidades: Olladas históricas. International Workshop*, 29–30 October 2015, Ourense (Spain). Dialogues d'histoire ancienne Supplement 19. Besançon: Presses Universitaires de Franche-Comté.

———. ed. 2019b. *Visiones sobre la lactancia en la Antigüedad: Permanencias, cambios y rupturas. Dialogues d'histoire ancienne*. Besançon: Presses Universitaires de Franche-Comté.

Reiss, R.E., and A.D. Ash 1988. "The Eighth-Month Fetus: Classical Sources for a Modern Superstition," *Obstetrics and Gynecology* 71 (2): 270–287.

Ricci, J.V. 1990. *The Development of Gynaecological Surgery and Instruments*. San Francisco: Norman Publishing.

Rich, A. 1995. *Of Woman Born: Motherhood as Experience and Institution*. New York: Norton.

Rio, A. 2017. *Slavery after Rome, 500–1100*. Oxford: Oxford University Press.

Rodger, A. 2007. "A Very Good Reason for Buying a Slave Woman?," *Law Quarterly Review* 123: 446–454.

Ronsse, E. 2006. "Rhetoric of Martyrs: Listening to Saints Perpetua and Felicitas," *Journal of Early Christian Studies* 14 (3): 283–327.

Rotman, Y. 2000. "Formes de la non-liberté dans la campagne byzantine," *Mélanges de l'Ecole française de Rome: Moyen Age* 112 (2): 499–510.

———. 2004. *Les esclaves et l'esclavage: De la Méditerranée antique à la Méditerranée médiévale, VIe–XIe siècles*. Paris: Belles Lettres.

Rousselle, A. 1988. *Porneia: On Desire and the Body in Antiquity*. Translated by F. Pheasant. Eugene, OR: Wipf & Stock.

Rühfel, H. 1988. "Ammen und Kinderfrauen im klassischen Athen," *Antike Welt* 19 (4): 43–57.

Rzeźnicka, Z., and M. Kokoszko. 2020. *Milk and Dairy Products in the Medicine and Culinary Art of Antiquity and Early Byzantium (1st–7th Centuries AD)*. Łódź and Kraków: Łódź University Press and Jagiellonian University Press.

Sallares, R. 1991. *The Ecology of the Ancient Greek World*. Ithaca, NY: Cornell University Press.

Saller, R. 1994. *Patriarchy, Property, and Death in the Roman Family*. Cambridge: Cambridge University Press.

Salvo, I. 2021. "Uterine Bleeding, Knowledge, and Emotion in Ancient Greek Medical and Magical Representations," in M. Bradley, V. Leonard, and L. Totelin (eds) *Bodily Fluids in Antiquity*. London: Routledge, 57–74.

Salzman-Mitchell, P. 2012. "Tenderness or Taboo: Images of Breast-Feeding Mothers in Greek and Latin Literature," in Petersen and Salzman-Mitchell 2012, 141–164.

Scarborough, J. 2013. "Adaptation of Folk Medicines in the Formal 'Materia Medica' of Classical Antiquity," *Pharmacy in History* 55 (2/3): 55–63.

Schechner, R. 2002. *Performance Studies: An Introduction*. London: Routledge.

Scheffler, J. ed. 2002². *Wall Tappings: An International Anthology of Women's Prison Writings 200 to the Present*. New York: Feminist Press at the City University of New York.

Scheidel, W. 1997. "Quantifying the Sources of Slaves in the Early Roman Empire," *Journal of Roman Studies* 87: 156–169.

Schöllgen, G. 1985. *Ecclesia sordida? Zur Frage der sozialen Schichtung frühchristlicher Gemeinden am Beispiel Karthagos zur Zeit Tertullians*. Jahrbuch für Antike und Christentum Ergänzungband 12. Munster: Aschendorff.

Schulze, H. 1998. *Ammen und Paedagogen: Sklavinnen und Sklaven als Erzieher in der antiken Kunst und Gesellschaft*. Mainz am Rhein: Philipp von Zabern.

Severy, B. 2003. *Augustus and the Family at the Birth of the Roman Empire*. London and New York: Routledge.

Shanzer, D. 2009. "Literature, History, Periodization, and the Pleasures of the Latin Literary History of Late Antiquity," *History Compass* 7 (3): 917–954.

Shaw, B.D. 2020. "Doing It in Greek: Translating Perpetua," *Studies in Late Antiquity* 4 (3): 309–345.

Sigismund-Nielsen, H. 2012. "Vibia Perpetua – An Indecent Woman," in Bremmer and Formisano 2012a, 103–117.

Skinner, P. 1997. "'The Light of my Eyes': Medieval Motherhood in the Mediterranean," *Women's History Review* 6 (3): 391–410.

Solevåg, A.R. 2013. *Birthing Salvation: Gender and Class in Early Christian Childbearing Discourse*. Leiden and Boston: Brill.

Sparreboom, A. 2014. "Wet-Nursing in the Roman Empire," in M. Carroll, and E.-J. Graham (eds) *Infant Health and Death in Roman Italy and Beyond. Journal of Roman Archaeology* Supplement 96. Portsmouth, RI: Journal of Roman Archaeology, 145–158.

Sperling, J. 2013. ed. *Medieval and Renaissance Lactations: Images, Rhetorics, Practices*. Aldershot: Routledge.

Spieser, C. 2012. "Les nourrices égyptiennes," in V. Dasen, and M.-C. Gérard-Zai (eds) *Art de manger, art de vivre: Nourriture et société de l'Antiquité à nos jours*. Gollion: Infolio, 19–39.

Stafford, E.J. 2005. "Viewing and Obscuring the Female Breast: Glimpses of the Ancient Bra," in L. Cleland, M. Harlow, and L. Llewellyn-Jones (eds) *The Clothed Body in the Ancient World*. Oxford: Oxbow Books, 96–111.

Stanley, L. 1992. *The Auto/Biographical I: The Theory and Practice of Feminist Auto/Biography*. Manchester and New York: Manchester University Press.

Syme, R. 1960. *The Roman Revolution*. Oxford University Press.

Talbot, A.-M. 1997. "Women," in G. Cavallo (ed.) *The Byzantines*. Translated by T. Dunlap, T. Lavender Fagan, and C. Lambert. Chicago. London: Thames and Hudson, 117–143.

———. 2017. "Childhood in Middle and Late Byzantium: Ninth to Fifteenth Centuries," in R. Aasgaard and C. Horn (eds) *Childhood in History: Perceptions of Children in the Ancient and Medieval Worlds*. London and New York: Routledge, 240–256.

Tawfik, Z. 1997. "Wet-Nursing Stipulations in Greek Papyri and Arabic Sources," in B. Kramer, L. Wolfgan, H. Maehler, and G. Poethke (eds) *Akten des 21. Internationalen Papyrologen-kongresses, Berlin, 13–19. 8. 1995*. Vol. 2. Stuttgart and Leipzig: Teubner, 939–53.

Temkin, O. 1962. "Byzantine Medicine: Tradition and Empiricism," *Dumbarton Oaks Papers* 16: 95–115.

Töpfer, R. 2020. *Kinderlosigkeit: Ersehnte, verweigerte und bereute Elternschaft im Mittelalter*. Stuttgart: J.B. Metzler.

Totelin, L. 2017. "Milk: The Symbolism and Ambivalence of a Substance," *Viewpoint: The Magazine of the British Society for the History of Science* 112: 6–7.

———. 2021. "Breastmilk in the Cave and on the Arena: Early Christian Stories of Lactation in Context," in M. Bradley, V. Leonard, and L. Totelin (eds) *Bodily Fluids in Antiquity*. London: Routledge, 240–257.

Treggiari, S. 1979. "Questions on Women Domestics in the Roman West," in M. Capozza (ed.) *Schiavitù, manomissione e classi dipendenti nel mondo antico*. Università degli Studi di Padova, Pubblicazioni dell'Instituto di Storia Antica 13. Rome: "L'Erma" di Bretschneider, 185–201.

Trovato, S. 2023. *Julian the Apostate in Byzantine Culture*. Translated by S. Knipe. London and New York: Routledge.

Tuten, B.S. 2014. "Lactation and Breast Diseases in Antiquity: Medical Authorities on Breast Health," *Quaestiones Medii Aevi novae* 19: 159–186.

Velten, H. 2010. *Milk: A Global History*. London: Reaktion Books.

Vierow, H. 1999. "Feminine and Masculine Voices in the Passion of Saints Perpetua and Felicitas," *Latomus* 58: 600–619.

Vikan, G. 1984. "Art, Medicine, and Magic in Early Byzantium," *Dumbarton Oaks Papers* 38: 65–86.

Vuolanto, V. 2013. "Elite Children, Socialization, and Agency in the Late Roman World," in Evans Grubbs and Parkin 2013, 580–599.

Walker, H. ed. 2000. *Milk beyond the Dairy: Proceedings of the Oxford Symposium on Food and Cookery 1999*. Totnes: Prospect Books.

Warner, M. 2012. "Memories of the Martyrs: Reflections from a Catholic Girlhood," in Bremmer and Formisano 2012a, 348–365.

Weitbrecht, J. 2012. "Maternity and Sainthood in the Medieval Perpetua Legend," in Bremmer and Formisano 2012a, 150–166.

Wet, C.L. de. 2015. *Preaching Bondage: John Chrysostom and the Discourse of Slavery in Early Christianity*. Oakland: University of California Press.

Williamson, B. 1998. "The Virgin Lactans as Second Eve: Image of the Salvatrix," *Studies in Iconography* 19: 107–138.

Woodacre, E., and C. Fleiner. eds. 2015. *Royal Mothers and Their Ruling Children: Wielding Political Authority from Antiquity to the Early Modern Era*. New York: Palgrave Macmillan.

———. eds. 2016. *Virtuous or Villainess? The Image of the Royal Mother from the Early Medieval to the Early Modern Era*. New York: Palgrave Macmillan.

Woolf, V. 1953. *A Winter's Diary*, ed. L. Woolf. New York: Harcourt Brace Jovanovich.

Yalom, M. 1997. *A History of the Breast*. New York: Ballantine Books.

Zellmann-Rohrer, M. 2019. "The Woman Who Gave Her Breast for Hire: Notes on a Christian Wall-Painting from Tebtunis," *Journal of Egyptian Archaeology* 105 (2): 297–303.

Part I
Society and Ideology

2 Breast Rules

The Body of the Wet Nurse in Ancient and Early Byzantine Discourses*

*Stavroula Constantinou and
Aspasia Skouroumouni-Stavrinou*

Introduction

In premodern societies, such as antiquity and Byzantium, in which there was no formula milk, wet nursing was the securest and most widespread substitute for the biological mother's breastfeeding.[1] Contemporary medical, philosophical, theological, and other authorities strongly advised ancient and Byzantine families to choose under strict guidelines their newborn's wet nurse, whose work, body, lifestyle, and ethics they were invited to supervise, control, and regulate. In so doing, these authorities gave voice to their societies' anxieties about the wet nurse's work and her impact on the (elite) nursling.

This chapter explores some ancient and early Byzantine discourses on wet nurses, focusing mainly on the representation of these lactating women in texts of the broader Greek medical tradition dating from the second century BC to the seventh century AD. Our discussion covers the examined texts' recommendations on how to choose a suitable wet nurse, and the advice found, mostly in the same texts, about her diet and on how to monitor her way of life and work. Through our analysis, we have a double aim: to trace the early history of sociomedical attitudes towards the wet nurse and her desired profile; and to bring to the fore this lactating woman's ambiguous status: she was treated as both an inferior servant and a female philosopher. In our attempt to achieve these purposes, we also discuss the examined texts' intertextual relationships, showing how they are based upon one another.

For reasons of space, we concentrate only on a particular category of surrogate mother, the hired wet nurse, in our attempt to understand how this form of

* The research for this chapter was co-funded by the European Regional Development Fund and the Republic of Cyprus through the Foundation of Research and Innovation (Project: EXCELLENCE/1216/0020), as well as by the University of Cyprus within the framework of an internal research project. Some of the ideas that inform the article's arguments were developed within the framework of the project "Network for Medieval Arts and Rituals" (NetMAR), which received funding from the European Union's Horizon 2020 research and innovation programme under grant agreement nr 951875. The opinions expressed in this document reflect only the authors' views and, in no way, reflect the European Commission's opinions. The European Commission is not responsible for any use that may be made of the information it contains.

1 For a history of wet nursing, see Fildes 1988. For wet nursing within this volume, see Chapters 3–7.

DOI: 10.4324/9781003265658-3

motherhood was constructed in some of the examined period's dominant discourses. Of course, a parallel treatment of wet nurses offering unpaid services could have offered a much better understanding of the ideologies around ancient and early Byzantine wet nursing. Such an endeavour, however, would have been very difficult if not impossible within the framework of the research undertaken for this chapter. Most of our sources do not make a distinction between mercenary and free wet nursing. In addition, the references to free wet nursing that we could find were extremely few.[2] However, a more systematic investigation of free wet nursing, including also earlier and later periods, could yield more results that would lead to some valid conclusions which could, in turn, allow an even better understanding of the socio-ideological position of both mercenary and biological motherhood.

In the Milk Market: How to Choose the "Right" Wet Nurse

A Neopythagorean philosopher of the second century AD or later,[3] who presents themselves as the daughter of the philosopher Pythagoras (ca. 570–ca. 495 BC), "Myia," writes a Letter addressing a certain Phyllis (*Myia to Phyllis* (*Epist. Phyl.*)), a mother with a newborn baby, advising her to choose a wet nurse with the following characteristics:[4]

> **Choose for yourself a wet nurse** who is most well-disposed and **clean**, and, what is more, modest and **not inclined to sleep** nor indeed **to strong drink**. For this is the kind of woman who might be judged best for raising free children – if, that is, she has **nutritious milk** and is **not an easy conquest for bedding down with a man**. A great help in this is that **for her whole life she is first and primarily directed to their upbringing** by nursing them well. For she will do everything well at the appropriate time. She will offer the breast and

---

2 A case in point is Plutarch's unique account in his biography of Cato the Elder that his wife Licinia breastfed both their own son and their slaves' children: "the mother … often gave suck also to the infants of her slaves, that so they might come to cherish a brotherly affection for her son" ("αὐτὴ γὰρ ἔτρεφεν ἰδίῳ γάλακτι· πολλάκις δὲ καὶ τὰ τῶν δούλων παιδάρια τῷ μαστῷ προσιεμένη, κατεσκεύαζεν εὔνοιαν ἐκ τῆς συντροφίας πρὸς τὸν υἱόν") Plut. *Life of Cato the Elder* 20.5.1–4, ed. Ziegler 1969; trans. Perrin 1914, 361.

3 The Letter's latest editor, Städele (1980, 269), has convincingly shown that, due to its strong affinities with medical discourses of the second century, it cannot have been composed earlier, despite the fact that it appears as the work of Pythagoras' daughter, Myia. However, other scholars date the composition of the Letter earlier. According to Pomeroy (2013, 111), who follows the first editor of the Letter (Thesleff 1965), it was composed in the third or second century BC; see also Thesleff 1961, 115. For the philosophical dimension of this and other similar Letters addressed to women, see Bourland Huizenga 2013, 31–213; Harper 2013.

4 As suggested by Bourland Huizenga (2013, 368), Neopythagorean philosophers of the Hellenistic and later periods who wrote letters and treatises addressed to women assumed the names of famous female Pythagorean philosophers, such as Melissa, Myia, and Theano, with the intention of increasing the authority of their works' contents. Bourland Huizenga believes that these works were most probably composed by men who employed the names of famous paradigmatic women to render their teachings on female virtue more effective.

suckling and nourishment not whenever it crosses her mind, but with some forethought, for that is how she will lead the infant to health. **She will not succumb whenever she herself wishes to sleep**, but whenever the newborn has a desire of rest; for she will offer no little relief to the child. The nurse should **never be inclined to anger** nor talkative *nor indifferent to food consumption* but should be orderly and **sōphrōn;** if it is possible, she should not be a barbarian, but a **Greek.** (Emphasis added)

τίτθαν μὲν **ἐκλέξασθαι** τὰν ἐπιταδειοτάταν καὶ **καθάριον**, ἔτι δὲ αἰδήμονα καὶ μὴ **ὕπνῳ προσοικειουμέναν** μηδὲ μὴν **μέθᾳ.** ἁ τοιάδε γὰρ ἂν κρίνοιτο κρατίστα ποττὸ ἐκτρέφειν ἐλευθέρως παῖδας, ἐάν γε δὴ **γάλα τρόφιμον** ἔχῃ καὶ **μὴ ταῖς πρὸς ἄνδρα κοίταις εὐνίκατος πέλῃ.** μεγάλα γὰρ μερὶς ἐν τῷδε καὶ πρῶτα καὶ προκαταρκτικωτέρρα ἐς **ὅλαν τὰν βιοτὰν πέλει ἐν τᾷ τρεφοίσᾳ** ποττὸ καλῶς τραφῆμεν· ποιήσει γὰρ πάντα καλὰ ἐν τῷ ποτεοικότι καιρῷ. τὸν τιτθόν τε καὶ μαζὸν καὶ τροφὰν δόμεν μὴ καττὸ ἐπενθόν, ἀλλὰ μετά τινος προνοίας· οὕτως γὰρ ἐς ὑγίειαν ἄξει τὸ βρέφος. **μὴ ὅτε αὐτὰ θέλοι καθεῦδεν νικῆται,** ἀλλ᾽ ὁπότε ἂν τὸ νεογνὸν ἀναπαύσιος ἔρον ἔχοι· οὐ μικκὸν γὰρ ἄκος τῷ παιδὶ προσοίσει. ἔστω δὲ **μήτ᾽ ὀργίλα** τιθάνα μήτε πρόγλωσσος *μήτε ἐν ταῖς τῶν σιτίων λήψεσιν ἀδιάφορος,* ἀλλὰ τεταγμένα καὶ **σώφρων,** δυνατῶν δὲ ὄντων μὴ βάρβαρος ἀλλὰ Ἑλληνίς. (*Epist. Phyl.* 162, 164 Städele, ed. Städele 1980; trans. with slight modifications Bourland Huizenga 2013, 62–63; emphasis added)

The pseudonymous author appears to summarize passages from medical works that were circulating in their time in which advice is given concerning the type of the wet nurse that should be chosen for an elite nursling. A case in point is the influential *Gynaecology* (*Gyn.*) of Soranos (1st–early 2nd c. AD), whose chapter on the selection of a wet nurse comprises almost 100 printed lines in Ioannes Ilberg's edition (Sor. *Gyn.* 2.19–20 (CMG 4, 66.5–69.5), ed. Ilberg 1927); in bold below are Soranos' words, phrases, and concepts borrowed by "Myia,"[5] which are also highlighted in bold in the previous extract; in different colours are Soranos' words, phrases, and concepts used by later medical authors who are cited below:[6]

On the selection of a wet nurse. **One should choose a wet nurse** not younger than twenty nor older than forty years, who has already given birth twice or thrice, who is healthy, of good habitus, of large frame, and of a good colour. Her breasts should be of medium size, lax, soft and unwrinkled, the nipples

---

5 According to Bourland Huizenga (2014, 249), "the *Gynecology* is not dependent upon *Myia to Phyllis*, nor vice versa; instead, these credentials are simply part and parcel of the dominant cultural discourse." Since the ideas and vocabulary found in "Myia" are very similar to the ones detected in earlier and contemporary medical, philosophical, and biographical works (see below), we agree with Städele 1980 that the Letter in question is dependent on Soranos and earlier authors whose works were circulating in "Myia's" times.

6 For the impact of Soranos' *Gynaecology* in antiquity, through the Middle Ages, and into the sixteenth century, see Temkin 1956, xxv–xxx, xli, xliv–xlv.

neither big nor too small and neither too compact nor too porous ... **She should be sōphrōn**, sympathetic and **not ill-tempered, a Greek**, and **tidy**. ... <'Healthy': because healthful> and **nourishing <milk>** comes from a healthy body. ... And the wet nurse should be **'sōphrōn' so as to abstain from coitus, drinking**, lewdness, and any other such pleasure and incontinence. ... In regard to drinking, first the wet nurse is harmed in soul as well as in body and for this reason the milk also is spoiled. Secondly, **seized by a sleep from which she is hard to awaken**, she leaves the newborn untended. ... 'Sympathetic' and affectionate, that she may fulfil her duties without hesitation and without murmuring. ... And **not 'ill-tempered'**: since by nature the nursling becomes similar to the nurse and accordingly grows sullen **if the nurse is ill-tempered**, but of mild disposition if she is even-tempered. ... For the same reason the wet nurse should not be superstitious and prone to ecstatic states so that she may not expose the infant to danger when led astray by fallacious reasoning, sometimes even trembling like mad. And the wet nurse should be **tidy-minded** lest the odor of the swaddling clothes cause the child's stomach to become weak and it lie awake on account of itching or suffer some ulceration subsequently. And she should be **a Greek** so that **the infant nursed by her** may become accustomed to the best speech.

Περὶ ἐκλογῆς τιτθῆς. Ἐκλεκτέον δὲ τὴν **τιτθὴν** οὔτε νεωτέραν ἐτῶν εἴκοσιν οὔτε πρεσβυτέραν ἐτῶν τεσσαράκοντα, προκεκυηκυῖαν δὶς ἢ τρίς, ἄνοσον, εὐεκτοῦσαν, εὐμεγέθη τῷ σώματι καὶ εὐχρουστέραν, μαστοὺς ἔχουσαν συμμέτρους, χαύνους, μαλακούς, ἀρρυσώτους, καὶ θηλὰς μήτε μεγάλας μήτε μικροτέρας καὶ μήτε πυκνοτέρας μήτε ἄγαν σηραγγώδεις ..., **σώφρονα,** συμπαθῆ καὶ **ἀόργιστον, Ἑλληνίδα, καθάριον** ... <ἄνοσον δέ, ὅτι ὑγιὲς μὲν **τὸ γάλα**> καὶ **τρόφιμον** ἐξ ὑγιεινοῦ σώματος ... **σώφρονα** δέ, **πρὸς τὸ συνουσίας** ἀπέχεσθαι καὶ **μέθης** καὶ λαγνείας καὶ τῆς ἄλλης ἡδονῆς καὶ ἀκρασίας ... διὰ δὲ τὰς μέθας πρῶτον μὲν ἡ γαλουχοῦσα βλάπτεται καὶ τῇ ψυχῇ καὶ τῷ σώματι, διὰ τοῦτο δὲ καὶ τὸ γάλα διαφθείρει· δεύτερον δὲ **ὕπνῳ δυσδιεγέρτῳ κατεχομένη** καταλείπει τὸ βρέφος ἀνεπιμέλητον ... συμπαθῆ δὲ καὶ **φιλόστοργον**, ἵνα καὶ **τὰ τῆς ὑπηρεσίας ἀόκνως παρέχῃ** καὶ ἀγογγύστως ... **ἀόργιστον** δέ, ὅτι φύσει συνεξομοιοῦται τὰ τρεφόμενα ταῖς τρεφούσαις καὶ διὰ τοῦτο βαρύθυμα μὲν **ἐξ ὀργίλων**, ἐπιεικῆ δὲ ἐκ μετρίων γίνεται· ... διόπερ οὐδὲ δεισιδαίμονα δεῖ καὶ θεοφόρητον εἶναι τὴν γαλοῦχον, ἵνα μὴ παραλογισθεῖσά ποτε καὶ μανιωδῶς σαλευθεῖσα κινδύνῳ τὸ βρέφος περιβάλῃ. **καθάριον** δὲ δεῖ εἶναι τὴν τιτθήν, ἵνα μὴ διὰ τὴν τῶν σπαργάνων ὀσμὴν ὁ στόμαχος ἐκλύηται τῶν νηπίων ἀγρυπνῇ τε διὰ τοὺς ὀδαξησμοὺς ἢ τιν' ὕστερον ἕλκωσιν ὑπομένῃ. Ἑλληνίδα δέ, χάριν τοῦ τῇ καλλίστῃ διαλέκτῳ ἐθισθῆναι **τὸ τρεφόμενον** ὑπ' αὐτῆς. (Sor. *Gyn.* 2.19 (CMG 4, 66.5–68.25); trans. with a modification Temkin 1956, 90–94; emphasis added)

The underlined phrase in the above-quoted passage from the Letter of "Myia," "ποιήσει γὰρ πάντα καλὰ ἐν τῷ ποτεοικότι καιρῷ. τὸν τιτθόν τε καὶ μαζὸν καὶ τροφὰν δόμεν μὴ καττὸ ἐπενθόν, ἀλλὰ μετά τινος προνοίας" ("For she will do everything well at the appropriate time. She will offer the breast and suckling and nourishment not whenever it crosses her mind, but with some forethought, for that is how she will lead the infant to health"), seems to be a two-sentence summary of Soranos' Chapters 38–39 in the second book of his *Gynaegology*, which deal with "How and when to give the newborn the breast" (CMG 4, 81.1–82.29; trans. Temkin 1956, 108).[7] As for the phrase in italics in the same passage, "μήτε ἐν ταῖς τῶν σιτίων λήψεσιν ἀδιάφορος" ("[The nurse] should never be … indifferent to food consumption"), at first glance, it recalls a phrase from the work of Mnesitheos of Kyzikos (ca. 180 BC) in which, as the following discussion will demonstrate, it has a different meaning, determined by the author's medical interest and approach.

Mnesitheos' treatise has come down to us in a fragmentary form and not as an independent work, but as part of a much later text, the *Medical Collections Incerti* (*Med. Coll. Inc.*) of Oribasios (4th c. AD). We read the following in Oribasios:[8]

> From the writings of Mnesitheos of Kyzikos. One should hire as a wet nurse for childrearing a Thracian or Egyptian or any other woman who is similar to the aforesaid ones. Let her be sizable, with strong lungs, corpulent, with good appearance, tolerant to all kinds of food, without suffering from stomach upsets. Let her be free from every suffering … Let her wear **clean** clothes and be clean in the rest of her conduct, without having an ill-smelling skin. Let her have a cheerful thinking, be uncomplicated, **gentle**, simple, and not older than thirty years old, but she could be one or two years younger, having no menses. Let her also be **harsh concerning intercourse with men**.
>
> Ἐκ τῶν Μνησιθέου τοῦ Κυζικηνοῦ. Εἰς παιδοτροφίαν τροφὸν μὲν γένει λαμβάνειν Θρᾷτταν ἢ Αἰγυπτίαν ἢ ἄλλην παραπλησίαν ταῖς εἰρημέναις. ἔστω δ᾽ *εὐμεγέθης*, εὔπλευρος, *εὔσαρκος*, *καλὴ τὴν ὄψιν, εὔκολος πρὸς ἅπαν σιτίον*, μὴ ἐκταρασσομένη τὴν κοιλίαν. ἀπολελύσθω δὲ παντὸς πάθους …, ἔστω δὲ **καθάριος** κατὰ τὴν ἐσθῆτα καὶ τὴν λοιπὴν δίαιταν, κατὰ τὸν αὐτῆς χρῶτα μὴ δυσώδης, τῇ τε διανοίᾳ ἱλαρά, ῥάθυμος, **πραεῖα**, ἁπλῆ, *ἐτῶν οὖσα* μὴ πλέον τριάκοντα, ἐλάττων δ᾽ ἑνὶ ἢ δυσίν, ᾗ τὰ καταμήνια μὴ φαίνηται. ἔστω δ᾽ **αὐστηρὰ πρὸς ἀνδρῶν ὁμιλίαν**. Orib. *Med. Coll. Inc.* 32.1–5 (CMG 6.2.2, 124.28–125.2), ed. Raeder 1933; emphasis added)[9]

The previous chapter in *Medical Collections Incerti* (Chapter 31) has the title "On the selection of a wet nurse" and is of more or less the same length as Soranos' corresponding chapter. Oribasios rewrites the above-quoted passage from Soranos as follows:[10]

---

7 Parts of this section of the *Gynaecology* are examined below ("Breastfeeding under surveillance and control").

8 In bold are words, phrases, and concepts employed first by Soranos and later by "Myia"; in red are the ones used by Soranos and his medical followers.

9 Unless otherwise stated, translations are our own.

10 In bold is what is found in both Soranos and "Myia"; in red and underlined green are the correspondences between Oribasios and Soranos; and in blue and all green, whether underlined or not, are phrases of Oribasios adopted by later medical authors mentioned below.

On the selection of a wet nurse. Most of all, **one should choose a wet nurse** who has no disease, … and who is neither too young nor too old. She should be no younger than twenty-five and no older than thirty-five years old. … [She should be] of large frame and good habitus, broad-chested, having breasts of medium size, unwrinkled; [having] nipples neither big nor small, neither too narrow nor too broad or porous. … The wet nurse should be such: **sōphrōn, sober, clean, not ill-tempered**, in good condition and not suffering from epilepsy … And she should abstain from lewdness, because the milk is greatly spoiled if the breastfeeding woman has sexual intercourse … The wet nurse's hands and shoulders should ache if she is supposed to do good to the child.

Περὶ ἐκλογῆς τιτθῆς. Πρὸ δὲ τούτων πάντων **ἐκλεκτέον τὴν τιτθὴν** μηδὲ ὁτιοῦν νόσημα ἔχουσαν, … καὶ μήτε ἄγαν νεωτέραν μήτε ἄγαν πρεσβυτέραν. ἔστω δ' ἡ μὲν νεωτέρα ἕως ἐτῶν κε, ἡ δὲ πρεσβυτέρα ἐτῶν λε … εὐμεγέθης δὲ τῷ σώματι καὶ εὐεκτοῦσα, εὔστερνος, μασθοὺς ἔχουσα συμμέτρους, ἀρρυσώτους, θηλὰς μήτε μεγάλας μήτε μικρὰς μήτε στενοτέρας μήτε ἄγαν εὐρυτέρας ἢ σηραγγώδεις … πρὸς τούτοις δὲ χρὴ εἶναι τὴν τιτθὴν [οἷον] **σώφρονα, ἀμέθυσον, καθαράν, ἀόργητον,** εὔχυμον καὶ μὴ ἐπίληπτον … ἀπεχέσθω δὲ καὶ λαγνείων· φθορὰ γὰρ μεγίστη τῷ γάλακτι εἰ μίσγοιτο γυνὴ θηλάζουσα … Πονείτω δ' ἡ τιτθὴ ἀπὸ τῶν χειρῶν καὶ τῶν ὤμων, εἰ μέλλει τι τὸ παιδίον ὠφελεῖν. (Orib. Med. Coll. Inc. 31.1–5, 19–20 (CMG 6.2.2, 121.25–122.15, 123.18–21))

The rest of this chapter of Oribasios, however, focuses on the wet nurse's regimen (Orib. *Med. Coll. Inc.* 31.6–19, 25–34 (CMG 6.2.2, 122.16–123.18, 123.33–124.16)) which in the *Gynaecology* is dealt with in a different series of chapters entitled "How to conduct the regimen of the nurse" ("Πῶς διαιτητέον τὴν τροφόν," Sor. *Gyn.* 2.24–26 (CMG 4, 71.5–73.25); trans. Temkin 1956, 98), and which concern the wet nurse's bodily control, which is discussed in more detail below ("Breastfeeding under Surveillance and Control"). A similar treatment of Soranos' material can also be detected in Oribasios' phrase, "Πονείτω δ' ἡ τιτθὴ ἀπὸ τῶν χειρῶν καὶ τῶν ὤμων" ("The wet nurse's hands and shoulders should ache"), which is taken almost verbatim by the Byzantine physician Paul of Aegina (fl. early 7th c. AD; "ἡ τιτθὴ … πονείτω διὰ τῶν χειρῶν καὶ τῶν ὤμων"; see below). In this case, too, Oribasios reworks a part, albeit a small one, of the said section on the wet nurse's regimen. This part reads as follows: "She should also work her body hard at such exercises as are apt to shake all parts, but particularly **those of the hands and shoulders** because this is where feeding mostly takes place" ("δεῖ δὲ καὶ τοῖς γυμνασίοις ἐκείνοις διαπονεῖν τὸν ὄγκον οἷς δύναται μὲν σαλευθῆναι πάντα τὰ μέρη, ἐπὶ πλεῖον δὲ τὰ **περὶ τὰς χεῖρας καὶ τοὺς ὤμους** ἕνεκα τοῦ τὴν τροφὴν ἐκεῖ φέρεσθαι μᾶλλον," Sor. *Gyn.* 2.24.4.1–4 (CMG 4, 71.21–24); trans. with modifications Temkin 1956, 97; emphasis added). Soranos' instruction that the wet nurse should exercise her hands and shoulders, which frequently remain immovable because they are used for holding the nursling during breastfeeding, is transformed in Oribasios, and Paul who follows him, into a criterion for choosing a suitable wet nurse. What makes a good wet nurse, among other things, are her painful hands and shoulders, which prove her regular and sufficient breastfeeding of the nursling. Her body pain is a sign of her hard mothering work.

Both Soranos' and Oribasios' longer chapters on the selection of a wet nurse are rewritten in a summary form by later medical authors, such as Aetios of Amida (fl. ca AD 530–560) and Paul (mentioned above), revealing a diachronic interest in setting physical and characterological criteria for choosing a wet nurse.[11] Aetios' entry in his *Tetrabiblos* (*Tetr.*) is a mixture of Soranos', Galen's,[12] and Oribasios' discourses.[13] Paul of Aegina's entry in his *Epitome of Medicine* (*Epitome*), on the other hand, constitutes a synoptic rewriting of Oribasios' corresponding chapter.[14]

The writings of Mnesitheos, Soranos, "Myia," Oribasios, Aetios of Amida, and Paul of Aegina concerning the choice of a suitable wet nurse may be divided into two categories according to the factors considered by their authors as essential to the wet nurse's successful performance of the work of mothering.[15] In the first category are the Greco-Roman authors Mnesitheos, Soranos, and "Myia," for whom successful mothering is based on four different factors: the wet nurse's physiology, personality, thinking, and culture. The second category includes the approaches of Oribasios, Aetios of Amida, and Paul of Aegina. For the Byzantine authors of the latter category, the choice of a wet nurse should be primarily determined by her physiology, secondarily by her personality, while her thinking and culture are not taken into account. Yet, in these authors' later discussions concerning, for example, children's diet and the treatment of their diseases, the wet nurse's maternal

---

11　For an introduction to the ways in which early Byzantine medical authors, such as Oribasios, Aetios of Amida, and Paul of Aegina, use earlier medical sources (e.g. Soranos and Galen) and each other's work, see Eijk 2015, 195–204 and 2010.

12　The passage from Galen is not quoted here.

13　"On the selection of a wet nurse. Most of all, **one should choose a wet nurse** not younger than twenty nor older than forty years, who has already given birth twice or thrice, who is healthy, of good habitus, of large frame, broad-chested, having breasts of medium size, unwrinkled; [having] nipples neither big nor small, neither too narrow nor much too broad or porous ... The wet nurse should be such: *sōphrōn*, **sober, not ill-tempered, clean**, in good condition and not suffering from epilepsy" ("Περὶ ἐκλογῆς τιτθῆς. Πρὸ δὲ τούτων πάντων **ἐκλεκτέον τὴν τιτθὴν** οὔτε νεωτέραν ἐτῶν κ οὔτε πρεσβυτέραν ἐτῶν μ, προκεκυηκυῖαν δὶς ἢ τρίς, ἄνοσον, εὐεκτοῦσαν, εὐμεγέθη τῷ σώματι, εὔστερνον, μαστοὺς ἔχουσαν συμμέτρους, ἀρυσώτους, θηλὰς μήτε μεγάλας μήτε **μικρὰς** μήτε στενοτέρας μήτ᾽ ἄγαν εὐρυτέρας ἢ σηραγγώδεις ... πρὸς τούτοις δὲ εἶναι χρὴ τὴν τιτθὴν **σώφρονα ἀμέθυσον ἀόργητον, καθάριον** εὔχυμον καὶ μὴ ἐπίληπτον," Aet. *Tetr.* 4.4.1–18 (CMG 8.1, 361.3–10), ed. Olivieri 1935).

14　"On the wet nurse. **One should** thus **choose a wet nurse** who has no disease, and who is neither too old nor too young. She should be neither younger than twenty-five years old, nor older than thirty-five years old. She should have a big chest and big breasts, and her nipples should be neither prominent nor retracted. The rest of her body should be neither very fat nor very thin ... The wet nurse should abstain from lewdness and her hands and shoulders should ache" ("Περὶ τιτθῆς. **Αἱρεῖσθαι** οὖν **χρὴ τιτθὴν** μηδ᾽ ὁτιοῦν νόσημα ἔχουσαν καὶ μήτε ἄγαν πρεσβυτέραν μήτε νεωτέραν, ἔστω δὲ ἡ μὲν νεωτάτη ἐτῶν κε, ἡ δὲ πρεσβυτάτη ἐτῶν λε· καὶ στῆθος μέγα ἐχέτω καὶ τιτθοὺς μεγάλους καὶ θηλὰς μήτε μεμυκυίας μήτε ἀπεστραμμένας, ἔστω δὲ τὸ ἄλλο σῶμα μήτε πῖον ἰσχυρῶς μήτε ὑπέρλεπτον ... ἀπεχέσθω δὲ ἡ τιτθὴ καὶ λαγνείων καὶ πονείτω διὰ τῶν χειρῶν καὶ τὸν ὤμων," Paul Aegin. *Epitome* 1.2.1 (CMG 9.1, 9.10–20), ed. Heiberg 1921).

15　For the wet nurse's mothering, see also Constantinou and Skouroumouni-Stavrinou 2024, in press.

thinking, even though not explicitly mentioned, constitutes a self-evident prerequisite for efficacious mothering. Since Oribasios, Aetios of Amida, and Paul of Aegina were living and working within the Byzantine Greek culture, it does not make any sense for them and their audiences to stipulate Greekness as a criterion for the selection of a wet nurse.

In contrast to Soranos and "Myia," Mnesitheos, as quoted by Oribasios, appears to place a more or less equal importance on the wet nurse's personality, thinking, and culture, whereas he puts somewhat greater emphasis on her physiology. Of course, we cannot know whether this was the choice of Mnesitheos or whether this is just the impression given by Oribasios' summary. Mnesitheos' recited account starts from the wet nurse's ideal origin and culture (Thracian, Egyptian, or of similar origin). It moves to characteristics of her physiology (a healthy, sturdy, and good-looking body, as well as a good stomach). Then, it mentions qualities of her personality (clean, easy-going, not ill-tempered, and chaste) and thinking (cheerful) and adds further physical characteristics (age: between 28 and 30 years old, without menses, mother of more than one child). In Mnesitheos' short-reported account, the good wet nurse's various features are listed without any explanation. There is, for example, no justification for favouring a Thracian or Egyptian wet nurse,[16] nor is there any explanation of what is meant by the phrase "a woman of similar origin"; possibly Mnesitheos' or Oribasios' contemporaries were aware of the implications of these words.

Furthermore, while Mnesitheos' insistence on the wet nurse's health is plausible, for it is held responsible for the quality of her milk, this is not the case for her bodily beauty and "cheerful thinking." Concerning the latter in particular, it is not quite clear what Mnesitheos understands by "διανοία ἱλαρά" – which does not occur in the other corresponding passages examined here – or how this characteristic or the said beauty contributes to the production of nutritious milk, the main concern of all the medical authors examined here. Possibly Mnesitheos' "cheerful thinking" refers to the wet nurse's positive mindset, her practice of focusing on the goodness of her mothering through undertaking all actions ensuring the good health influencing her milk. If this is the case, "cheerful thinking" appears here to be as important as physiology and good health to the production of the right quantity and quality of milk.

In concluding this section of our discussion, we would like to draw attention to the fact that the extremely long tradition of the right selection of a wet nurse, which starts in antiquity and reaches one of its high points through Soranos' influential approach, did not end with Byzantium but continued to the twentieth century, when wet nursing was still an occupation. Modern job announcements that were posted either by prospective employees or by wet nurses are quite revealing of how persistent the ideologies for and prejudices against wet nurses have been over the centuries. In the following two advertisements, we read the same anxieties about the wet nurse's morals, health (bodily and emotional), age,

---

16 Other sources suggest that Egyptian women were believed to be fond of children, while their Thracian counterparts were considered strong and devoted; see Dasen 2010, 707–708; Bäbler 1998.

mothering experiences, and physiology that we have detected in the ancient and Byzantine texts we have been discussing:

> WANTED immediately, a wet NURSE, with a *good breast of milk* … Any such person that can be well recommended for *honesty, health, cleanliness,* and *care.* [Philadelphia, 1767]
> WANTS a Place, as Wet-Nurse, a *cleanly, healthy, cheerful young Woman,* about 23, whose Husband is not-in England; she has a *good Breast of Milk, two fine Children* about ten Weeks old, and can have a good Recommendation. [London, 1776][17]

As attested by these advertisements posted by parents and prospective wet nurses, an eighteenth-century wet nurse, whether in America or Europe, was chosen according to criteria that were set by ancient and Byzantine physicians and philosophers: the cleanliness emphasized by Mnesitheos, Soranos, "Myia," Oribasios, and Aetios; the bodily health pointed out by Oribasios, Aetios, and Paul; Mnesitheos' "cheerful thinking" and his age limit (under 30 years old); the honesty and sexual abstinence promoted by all the authors discussed; the good breasts and the suitable milk quality of Soranos and his medical followers; Soranos' and Aetios' preference for a mother of two children; and finally, the motherly care advanced by Soranos and particularly "Myia."

Good Food Consumption: The Wet Nurse as a Philosopher

In contrast to our medical authors, "Myia" links the wet nurse's diet to an ethics of motherhood. Her interest in the wet nurse's physical qualities is very limited. She only mentions the wet nurse's "nutritious milk," which is seen as the result of motherhood ethics rather than as the product of a healthy body with particular characteristics; that is mostly the medical authors' approach. According to Mnesitheos, therefore, the wet nurse's stomach should be tolerant of all kinds of food ("εὔκολος πρὸς ἄπαν σιτίον") in order to ensure continuous bodily health and good-quality milk. In "Myia," on the other hand, the good wet nurse is intellectually involved in the consumption of food. She carefully chooses her food according to its nutritious elements and quality that guarantee the nursling's survival, health, and growth, which are under her control. In so doing, she exhibits the moral qualities of an orderly and wise individual ("μήτε ἐν ταῖς τῶν σιτίων λήψεσιν ἀδιάφορος, ἀλλὰ τεταγμένα καὶ σώφρων"). In sum, food becomes for "Myia" an important domain through which the wet nurse's goodness, involving her maternal thinking, goodwill, honesty, moderation, decorum, and self-control, are manifested and assessed.

"Myia's" ethical attitude to food and drink ("μηδὲ μὴν μέθᾳ προσοικειουμέναν") could be exemplified also through the work of Musonius,[18] an important prac-

---

17 Rhodes 2015, 49, 52; emphasis added.
18 That there are affinities between Musonius' *Discourses* and the Neopythagorean letters and treatises addressed to women has been already pointed out by Swain 2013, 311–320, 334–340. Here a further common subject of these two types of philosophical writings (diet) is brought to the fore.

tical philosopher of the Roman Imperial period whose teachings have been transmitted through the writings of his students and have in large part survived because of Stobaios' *Anthology*, which also shows a Byzantine interest in the philosopher's work.[19] Two of Musonius' 21 lectures that have come down to us (*Discourses* 18a and 18b (*Disc.*)) are devoted to the subject of food.[20] That food was important in Musonius' system of practical ethics is illustrated by the textual length he devotes to the subject, as well as by his student's comment with which the first *Discourse* on food is introduced. Taken together, *Discourses* 18a and 18b comprise 143 printed lines, which is the most he allocates to any of the subjects of his reported lectures. As for the comment with which *Discourse* 18a opens, it reads:

> On the subject of food he used to speak frequently and very emphatically too, as a question of no small significance, nor leading to unimportant consequences; indeed he believed that the beginning and foundation of temperance lay in self-control in eating and drinking.
>
> Περὶ δὲ τροφῆς εἰώθει μὲν πολλάκις λέγειν καὶ πάνυ ἐντεταμένως ὡς οὐ περὶ μικροῦ πράγματος οὐδ' εἰς μικρὰ διαφέροντος· ᾤετο γὰρ ἀρχὴν καὶ ὑποβολὴν τοῦ σωφρονεῖν εἶναι τὴν ἐν σίτοις καὶ ποτοῖς ἐγκράτειαν. (Muson. *Disc.* 18a.1–7, ed. and trans. Lutz 1947, 113)

As food had not traditionally been a subject of philosophical discourse, Musonius has to repeatedly and forcefully teach his students on the subject in an attempt to prove its philosophical value and to show how its use could contribute to the practice of virtuous life. If pleasure is a hindrance to virtue, then food and drinking should not be used for providing a context for hedonism, but as vehicles for nourishment, strength, and health:

> And again, just as plants and animals receive nourishment that they may survive and not for their pleasure, so in like manner food is to us the medicine of life. Therefore, it is fitting for us to eat in order to live, not in order to have pleasure.
>
> ὥσπερ τε αὖ τούτοις [φυτόν, ζῷον] διαμονῆς ἕνεκα συμβαίνει τρέφεσθαι καὶ οὐχ ἡδονῆς, παραπλησίως καὶ ἡμῖν ζωῆς καὶ φάρμακον ἡ τροφή ἐστι. διὸ καὶ προσήκει ἐσθίειν ἡμῖν ἵνα ζῶμεν, οὐχ ἵνα ἡδώμεθα. (Muson. *Disc.* 18b.13–16; trans. with slight modifications Lutz 1947, 119)

---

19 Musonius Rufus, the so-called Roman Socrates (Lutz 1947), was the teacher of other famous philosophers, such as Dio Chrysostom and Epictetus (AD 55–135). Among others, Musonius influenced Pliny the Younger (AD 61–113) and Clement of Alexandria (ca. AD 150–215). For a comprehensive study on Musonius Rufus, see Dillon 2004. See also Inwood 2017; Bryan 2013, 139–142; Belliotti 2009, 181–184; Goulet-Gazé 2005; Reydams-Schils 2005, 143–175; Nussbaum 2002; Whitmarsh 2001; Valantasis1999; Geytenbeck 1963; Lutz 1947, 1–30.

20 For food in Musonius, see Stephens 2019; Grimm 2006, 362–363.

Food which serves its appropriate function of survival is described by Musonius as that which is proper to human nature ("σύμφυλον ἀνθρώπῳ," Muson. *Disc.* 18a.10). This includes plants of the earth, grains, and food from domesticated animals that can be eaten without being cooked (Muson. *Disc.* 18a.10–20). Those who follow such a diet, remarks Musonius, are strong and do not get tired easily, they are able to work harder, and they do not require so much sleep (Muson. *Disc.* 18b.35–36, 1–5). All other food, according to Musonius, is heavy and an impediment to reasonable thinking (Muson. *Disc.* 18a.20–21), the innate characteristic of human beings. By choosing and consuming the food that belongs to his or her nature, an individual does not just achieve bodily health but also moral health that is exemplified through three essential virtues: *sōphrosynē* (moderation, wisdom), *taxis* (orderliness), and *katharotēs* (cleanliness, purity):

> For the beginning and foundation of temperance lay **in self-control in eating** and drinking. Exercising **moderation** and decorum in eating, demonstrating one's **self-control** there first of all … Since, then, these and even more vices are connected with eating, if a man wishes **to show self-control**, he must **be clean** of all of them and not be guilty of any of them.
>
> γὰρ ἀρχὴν καὶ ὑποβολὴν τοῦ **σωφρονεῖν** τὴν ἐν **σίτοις** καὶ ποτοῖς ἐγκράτειαν. (Muson. *Disc.* 18a.3–4) **τάξει** καὶ κοσμίως ἐσθίειν, καὶ **σωφροσύνην** ἐνταῦθα ἐπιδείκνυσθαι πρῶτον … Τοσούτων δὴ καὶ ἔτι ἄλλων ἁμαρτιῶν οὐσῶν περὶ τροφήν, δεῖ μὲν ἁπασῶν **καθαρεύειν** αὐτῶν καὶ μηδεμιᾷ ἔνοχον εἶναι τὸν μέλλοντα **σωφρονήσειν**. (Muson. *Disc.* 18b.17–18, 35–37; trans. with some modifications Lutz 1947, 113, 117, 119; emphasis added)

As we read in the passage from "Myia's" Letter cited above, where the terms highlighted here are also present in different lexical forms ("τεταγμένα," "σώφρων," "καθάριον"), *sōphrosynē*, orderliness, and cleanliness also characterize "Myia's" wet nurse, whose treatment of food and drink is similar to that of Musonius. Directed by her virtuous reasoning, the wet nurse in "Myia," as has been stated, chooses her food and drink not for her pleasure, but for the requisite health and power which allow her to successfully perform her demanding mothering tasks. *Sōphrosynē*, which is a repeated term in the passage from Musonius cited above, is "the key virtue" involved in the proper use of food.[21] If for Musonius the practice of *sōphrosynē* and *katharotēs* through the right use of food and drinking is the philosopher's work, then "Myia's" wet nurse is no less a philosopher. She clearly has the profile of the woman philosopher for whom Musonius talks in his third discourse, entitled "That women too should study philosophy," in which he describes the woman philosopher thus:

> Above all a woman must be **chaste and self-controlled**; she must, I mean, **be pure in respect of unlawful love, exercise restraint in other pleasures,**

---

21 Dillon 2004, 19.

not be a slave to desire. ... Such are the works **of a virtuous woman**, and
to them I would add yet these: **to control her temper**, not to be overcome by
grief, and to be superior to uncontrolled emotion of every kind. Now these
are the things which the teachings of philosophy transmit ... And likewise
[she should] not shun hardship and never for a moment **seek ease** and indo-
lence. So it is that a woman is likely to be energetic, strong to endure pain ...
I should not expect **the women who study philosophy** to shirk their ap-
pointed tasks ... Above all, we ought to examine the doctrine which we think
women who study philosophy ought to follow; we ought to see if the study
which presents modesty as the greatest good can make them presumptuous,
if the study which is a guide to the greatest self-restraint accustoms them to
live heedlessly, if what sets forth intemperance as the greatest evil does not
teach self-control ... Finally, the teachings of philosophy exhort the woman
to be content with her lot and to work with her own hands.

δεῖ δὴ καὶ **σώφρονα** εἶναι τὴν γυναῖκα· οἵαν **καθαρεύειν** μὲν **ἀφροδισίων**
παρανόμων, **καθαρεύειν** δὲ τῆς περὶ τὰς ἄλλας **ἡδονὰς ἀκρασίας, μὴ**
δουλεύειν ἐπιθυμίαις ... ταῦτα μὲν ἔργα τῆς **σώφρονός** ἐστι· καὶ ἔτι
πρὸς τούτοις ἐκεῖνα· **κρατεῖν μὲν ὀργῆς,** μὴ κρατεῖσθαι δ᾽ ὑπὸ λύπης,
κρείττονα δὲ πάθους παντὸς εἶναι. ταῦτα δ᾽ ὁ φιλόσοφος παρεγγυᾷ λόγος ...
ὡσαύτως δὲ καὶ τὸν μὲν **πόνον μὴ ἐκτρέπεσθαι,** τὴν δὲ **ἀπονίαν μὴ**
διώκειν ἐξ ἅπαντος. ὅθεν εἰκὸς εἶναι τὴν γυναῖκα ταύτην καὶ αὐτουργικὴν
καὶ κακόπαθον ... ἐγὼ δὲ οὐχ ὅπως τὰς **γυναῖκας τὰς φιλοσοφούσας** ...
ἀξιώσαιμ᾽ ἂν ἀφεμένους τῶν προσηκόντων ἔργων ... πρὸ παντὸς δὲ σκοπεῖν
τὸν λόγον χρή, ᾧ ἕπεσθαι τὰς φιλοσοφούσας ἀξιοῦμεν, εἰ δύναται θρασείας
ποιεῖν ὁ τὴν αἰδῶ μέγιστον ἀποφαίνων ἀγαθόν· εἰ ζῆν ἰταμώτερον ἐθίζει
ὁ καταστολὴν πλείστην ὑφηγούμενος· εἰ μὴ διδάσκει σωφρονεῖν ὁ κακὸν
ἀποδεικνὺς ἔσχατον τὴν ἀκολασίαν· ... καὶ στέργειν δὲ καὶ αὐτουργεῖν ὁ
τῶν φιλοσόφων λόγος παρακαλεῖ τὴν γυναῖκα. (Muson. *Disc.* 3.16–24, 4–6,
16–29; trans. with some modifications Lutz 1947, 41, 43; emphasis added)

Musonius' last sentence is telling: "the teachings of philosophy exhort the woman
to be content with her lot and to work with her own hands." In other words, the
portrait of the female philosopher he sketches is that of a woman confined to her
traditional domestic roles who is both a devoted and a happy worker. With the
hard work of her hands, the woman philosopher fulfils tirelessly all the daily tasks
that "nature" has assigned to her. As a wife, she is faithful to her husband, whom
she serves incessantly; as a mother, she looks after her children, whom she loves
more than her own self; as a mistress, she manages the household economy and
supervises the slaves. The woman who successfully performs these roles and their
associated tasks is by definition the epitome of virtue. She is prudent, just, self-
controlled, moderate, and courageous. Just as food functions as a means to examine
one's character, philosophy operates as a vehicle for scrutinizing women's lives.[22]

---

22 Musonius' approach to women is critically discussed in Nussbaum 2002.

The parallels between Musonius' woman philosopher and the good wet nurse as described in the authors examined here are quite obvious, even though the wet nurse's life is at times stricter.[23] For example, the wet nurse is deprived of sexual life altogether. That the wet nurse was actually expected to avoid sexual intercourse is also manifested in papyrus contracts from Hellenistic and Roman Egypt, where it is clearly stated that she shall not "sleep with a man" (*BGU* 4.1107.G; trans. Lefkowitz and Fant 2016, 347).[24] Furthermore, the wet nurse has to be exclusively devoted to someone else's child, while her body and work are supervised by the nursling's parents, as will be further exemplified below. Yet, like the wife, she is additionally charged with household work. She, too, performs her daily tasks with her own hands, and while doing so she is expected to display the same virtues as the woman philosopher (modesty, loyalty, orderliness, and industriousness).

In fact, Musonius' approach to the female philosopher, along with the wording he uses to describe her profile, has not only been adopted by "Myia" but also by Soranos.[25] There is, then, a triangular intertextual exchange between (a) "Myia" and Musonius; (b) "Myia" and Soranos; and (c) Soranos and Musonius. This is first detectable through "Myia's" Letter, a text of practical philosophy like Musonius' *Discourses* that draws on medical work to outline the profile of the desirable wet nurse in an attempt to provide advice for effective mothering. Concerning the intertextual connection between Soranos' *Gynaecology* and Musonius' work, a parallel reading of the third *Discourse* and the chapter on the selection of a wet nurse is quite revealing:

> But above all a woman must be chaste and self-controlled. She must … be pure in respect of unlawful love and exercise restraint in other pleasures … She would control her temper … She would become an untiring defender of … her children … She would love her children more … She would never for a moment seek … indolence … She would do these without hesitation.
>
> δεῖ δὴ καὶ σώφρονα εἶναι τὴν γυναῖκα· οἵαν καθαρεύειν μὲν ἀφροδισίων παρανόμων, καθαρεύειν δὲ τῆς περὶ τὰς ἄλλας ἡδονὰς ἀκρασίας … κρατεῖν μὲν ὀργῆς … τέκνων ἐπιμελὴς κηδεμών … καὶ τέκνα μᾶλλον ἀγαπᾶν … τὴν δὲ ἀπονίαν μὴ διώκειν ἐξ ἅπαντος … ταῦτα ἀόκνως ποιεῖν. (Muson. *Disc.* 3.16–19, 21, 27, 32, 35, 1, 4–5, 8–9; trans. with some modifications Lutz

---

23 The intersection between Greco-Roman philosophy and medicine is an important chapter in the study of both disciplines that has yet to be written. Some first studies include Jouanna 2012, 121–260; Hankinson 2008a, 2008b, and 2008c; Morison 2008; Tieleman 2008 and 2006; Pellegrin 2006; Gill 2003; Frede 1983, 225–298. The present discussion, despite its different objective, brings to the fore some aspects of the intertextual dialogue between philosophical and medical discourses of Greco-Roman antiquity.

24 For wet-nursing contracts, see Parca 2013, 471; Hermann 1959.

25 Soranos' interest in philosophy is attested in his now lost philosophical work *On Soul*. Furthermore, his *Gynaecology* has been "recognized as the most outstanding representative of the Methodist sect" (Temkin 1956, xxv), which is characterized by its philosophical overtones (Frede 1983, 239–240, 258, 261–278). Since Musonius was an influential contemporary of Soranos, it is highly probable that the physician knew the philosopher's work.

1947, 41, 43; different colours are used for certain words and phrases to mark the correspondences between Musonius and Soranos)

One should choose a **wet nurse** … [who is] self-controlled, **sympathetic** and not ill-tempered …, and tidy … [She should be] self-controlled so as to abstain from coitus, drinking, lewdness, and any other pleasure and incontinence … [She should not] leave the newborn untended … [She should be] affectionate, that she may fulfill **her services** without hesitation and **without murmuring**.

ἐκλεκτέον δὲ τὴν **τιτθὴν** … σώφρονα, **συμπαθῆ** καὶ ἀόργιστον … καὶ καθάριον … σώφρονα δέ, πρὸς τὸ συνουσίας ἀπέχεσθαι καὶ μέθης καὶ λαγνείας καὶ τῆς ἄλλης ἡδονῆς καὶ ἀκρασίας … [μὴ] καταλείπει τὸ βρέφος ἀνεπιμέλητον … καὶ φιλόστοργον, ἵνα καὶ τὰ τῆς **ὑπηρεσίας** ἀόκνως παρέχῃ καὶ **ἀγογγύστως**. (Sor. *Gyn.* 2.19.1.1, 1.6, 2.1, 11.1–2, 12.4, 13.1–2 (CMG 4, 66.6–67.11); trans. with a modification Temkin 1956, 90–93; emphasis added)

As attested in the two passages, Soranos appears to adopt what is considered Musonius' presentation of the woman philosopher, which he rewrites in his own linguistic register, while at times he copies Musonius' exact lexical forms (for example, "σώφρονα" and "ἀκρασίας"). Soranos' major changes to what is considered in the Musonian text include the replacement of the word "γυναῖκα" ("woman") with "τιτθήν" ("wet nurse") and the substitution of certain phrases, along with the addition of words and phrases through which the text is adapted to fit the wet nurse's situation as a surrogate mother. Musonius' descriptions of the biological mother as a tireless guardian of her own children ("τέκνων ἐπιμελὴς κηδεμών") and as someone who loves her offspring more than herself ("τέκνα μᾶλλον ἀγαπᾶν"), two "essential pressure[s]" of the institution of motherhood "on women to validate themselves in maternity,"[26] are transformed in the Soranian text into a portrayal of an "affectionate" ("φιλόστοργον") and child-minded wet nurse ("[μὴ] καταλείπει τὸ βρέφος ἀνεπιμέλητον"), who in turn proves herself through her surrogate mothering.

Soranos also adds some features characterizing the good wet nurse: she is sympathetic ("συμπαθῆ") to her nursling and performs the services assigned to her without complaining ("ὑπηρεσίας … ἀγογγύστως"). Furthermore, she is tidy and clean "lest the odor of the swaddling clothes cause the child's stomach to become weak and it lie awake on account of itching or suffer some ulceration subsequently" ("ἵνα μὴ διὰ τὴν τῶν σπαργάνων ὀσμὴν ὁ στόμαχος ἐκλύηται τῶν νηπίων ἀγρυπνῇ τε διὰ τοὺς ὀδαξησμοὺς ἤ τιν' ὕστερον ἕλκωσιν ὑπομένῃ," Sor. *Gyn.* 2.19.15.1–3 (CMG 4, 68.22–24); trans. Temkin 1956, 93–94). Even though at this very point Soranos employs the term *katharios* ("καθάριος") in its literal meaning, at the same time, he links it symbolically to moral rectitude and mental health ("She should be self-controlled, sympathetic and not ill-tempered … and tidy. … Angry women are like maniacs …, sometimes even trembling like mad. And the wet nurse should be tidy-minded"; "σώφρονα, συμπαθῆ καὶ ἀόργιστον … καὶ καθάριον …. μανιώδεις

26 Rich 1995, ix.

εἰσὶν αἱ θυμούμεναι … ποτε καὶ μανιωδῶς σαλευθεῖσα … καθάριον δὲ δεῖ εἶναι τὴν τιτθήν," Sor. *Gyn.* 2.19.1.6, 2.1, 14.3–4, 14.7, 15.1 (CMG 4, 66.11–68.22); trans. Temkin 1956, 91, 93).

The corresponding word in Musonius, *kathareuein* ("καθαρεύειν"), on the other hand, has an exclusively metaphorical meaning, referring to the philosophical wife's refraining from extramarital affairs and her abstinence.[27] Yet, like Soranos – and here we trace another instance of Musonius' impact on our medical author – Musonius associates bodily with mental and ethical purity. In both authors, as well as in "Myia," the terms *katharios* and *sōphrōn* are used interchangeably.[28] The *katharios* and *sōphrōn* wife of Musonius is honest and faithful to her husband, just as the *katharios* and *sōphrōn* wet nurse of Soranos (and also "Myia") refrains from her conjugal life in an attempt to keep both her milk unspoiled and her mothering services uninterrupted.[29] In other words, Soranos' understanding of the wet nurse's *katharotēs* and *sōphrosynē*, adopted also by Oribasios and Aetios of Amida, is a manifestation of her "uninterrupted practice of mothering" in terms of bodily, mental, and ethical purity,[30] just as the *katharotēs* and *sōphrosynē* of Musonius' wife are manifested in her own continuous practices of wifehood and mothering in the regimen of a pure way of living (sexual, mental, and ethical).

Taking into consideration the high social class of the wife in Musonius' *Discourses* and the low social status of the wet nurse, one could argue that it was most probably much easier for the latter than the former to practise philosophy. Accustomed to being served by slaves and to leading a life of luxury, the elite wife would be reluctant to adopt the philosophical life promoted by Musonius. That was most likely the reason why Musonius exhorted his male audiences to permit and even urge their wives and daughters to study philosophy. The wet nurse, on the other hand, was used to hardship and hard work. Unavoidably, her way of life was the very definition of frugality, simplicity, and abstinence. In sum, it seems to have been much simpler in Imperial Rome to find Soranos' wet nurse rather than to come across Musonius' woman philosopher.

27 As seen above, Musonius uses the term *kathareuein* also in his *Discourses* on food, to refer to the practice of consuming food for survival and not for luxury.

28 The terms *sōphrosynē* and *katharotēs* are employed as synonyms by a number of Greco-Roman and Byzantine authors. See e.g. "*sōphrosynē* is to purify (*kathareuein*) the soul from every passion" ("ἡ δὲ σωφροσύνη τὸ καθαρεύειν παντὸς πάθους τὴν ψυχὴν," Pseudo-Galen, *Medical Definitions* 130, 19.383.14–15K, ed. Kühn 1830); "and [let us] keep ourselves within yet freer from pollution and purer and more temperate" ("ἔχωμεν τὰ δ' ἐντὸς ἔτι μᾶλλον ἀμίαντα καὶ καθαρὰ καὶ σώφρονα," Plut. *Consolation to his Wife* 612.B.12–13, ed. Sieveking (1929) 1972; trans. De Lacy and Einarson 1959, 605); "*sōphrōn*: wise, clean (*katharos*), pure" ("σώφρων· φρόνιμος. καθαρός, ἁγνός," Hesychios, *Lexikon (Π–Ω)* 3107, ed. Schmidt 1861–1862).

29 For Soranos, the best midwife is also *sōphrōn* (*Gyn.* 1.4.4.3 (CMG 4, 5.25)). As far as her character is concerned, Soranos' midwife is presented as the wet nurse's double. Like the wet nurse, the midwife should, for example, be sympathetic, disciplined, sober, and not superstitious (*Gyn.* 1.4 (CMG 4, 5.25.23–30)). The characteristics of the Soranian midwife are discussed in Ecca 2017; Laes 2010.

30 Bourland Huizenga 2010, 382. The *sōphrōn* woman in Greco-Roman culture is also discussed in Bourland Huizenga 2013, 201–213, 329–364; North 1977 and 1966.

Breastfeeding under Surveillance and Control:
Monitoring the Wet Nurse

The second part of "Myia's" Letter informs the elite mother about important characteristics of the right surrogate mothering with which she is advised to become familiar in order to be able to monitor the chosen wet nurse's work. In the first segment of the Letter, as is the case with the corresponding parts in the examined medical works, and as the previous discussion has adequately demonstrated, the employer's need to scrutinize and control the wet nurse becomes part of the selection process.

As suggested in "Myia's" Letter, it is only through the wet nurse's regulation that the elite infant's mothering can be successful. In the author's own words with which the Letter closes: "[I] write down these things for you, inasmuch as good expectation comes from nursing that accords with this guideline" ("ὑπογράψαι τοι τὰς ἐλπίδας ἐκ τροφᾶς [ἢ] καττὸ ὑφαγεόμενον γινομένας," *Epist. Phyl.* 164 Städele; trans. Bourland Huizenga 2013, 64). "Myia's" Letter in its entirety, therefore, acquires a monumental character. It functions as an enduring manual of mothering to which the receiver and its future possessors could always return for (forgotten) guidance concerning the selection and performance of a wet nurse. A similar function is also fulfilled by our medical treatises, yet the Letter's shortness makes the practical application of its precepts easier. As for the good mothering of the nursling, it is presented by "Myia" as follows:

> It is best for the newborn to be directed to sleep in this way, even if it is nicely full of milk …, but if there is any other [sustenance], she must give the most simple. But she must completely abstain from **wine** because it is so strong, or just give a scant quantity mixed into the evening milk. Do not make **baths** frequent, for occasional and temperate baths are a better practice. For the same reasons, suitable **air** also ought to have an equal proportion of heat and cold, and for the **house** not to be too drafty nor too stifling. Nor is it suitable for **water** to be either harsh or soft, nor for **the bedding** to be rough, but it ought to wrap closely, accommodating the body.[31]
>
> ἄριστον, ἐὰν καὶ τοῦ γάλακτος χρηστῶς πιμπλάμενον τὸ νεογνὸν οὕτως ἐς ὕπνον τρέπηται … αἱ δὲ χάτέραν, δόμεν χρὴ ἁπλουστάταν. **οἴνῳ** δὲ τὸ παράπαν ἀπέχεσθαι τῷ δύναμιν ἰσχυρὰν ἔχειν, ἢ καττὸ σπάνιον μεταδιδόμεν τᾷ κράσει δείελον γαλακτῶδες. τὰ δὲ **λουτρὰ** μὴ ποιεῖν συνεχῆ. ἁ γὰρ τῶν σπανίων καὶ εὐκράτων χρᾶσις ἀμείνων. κατταυτὰ δὲ καὶ **ἀὴρ** ἐπιτάδειος θάλπους καὶ ῥίγους ἔχων τὰν συμμετρίαν, καὶ **οἴκησις** δὲ μήτε ἄγαν περιπνεομένα μήτε ἄγαν κατάστεγνος. οὐ μὰν ἀλλὰ καὶ **ὕδωρ** μήτε ἀπόσκληρον μήτε εὐπαράγωγον, καὶ **στρωμνὰ** δὲ οὐ τραχεῖα, ἀλλὰ προσπίπτουσα τῷ χρωτὶ εὐαρμόστως. (*Epist. Phyl.* 164 Städele; trans. with a modification Bourland Huizenga 2013, 63–64)

---

31   For Bourland Huizenga (2013, 63–64), the word "ὕδωρ" refers to drinking water. We think, however, that what is meant here is the water used either for bathing or for washing the bedding.

"Myia's" advice, which once again is largely in accordance with Soranos' precepts,[32] focuses on the factors affecting sleep that, along with milk, are essential to the newborn's health and growth. The biological mother should make sure that the wet nurse puts the nursling to bed after it has suckled its evening milk or consumed some other light dinner. She should also see to it that the wet nurse creates the right air and temperature in the room and prepares appropriate bath water and bedding. By ensuring that the wet nurse fulfils these needs, the biological mother secures her baby's peaceful and uninterrupted sleep, which constitutes the strongest evidence of the wet nurse's good mothering, which, in turn, validates the mother's choice, to which the first part of the Letter is devoted.

As implied earlier, medical treatises discuss at length the regime that the wet nurse has to follow – when and what to eat or drink; what to avoid consuming or doing; when and how to get rest; when and how to exercise her body (for example, Sor. *Gyn.* 2.24–27 (CMG 4, 71.5–74.6); Orib. *Med. Coll. Inc.* 31.7–30, 34 (CMG 6.2.2, 122.18–124.15, 124.25–26); Aet. *Tetr.* 4.6 (CMG 8.1, 362.8–363.3)) – thus suggesting that her bodily life should also be under constant regulation with the intention of ensuring her continuous production of good-quality milk in satisfactory quantity, as well as of confirming her unremitting devotion to the nursling.[33] Along with the surveillance and control of the wet nurse's way of life and diet, her milk should also be regularly tested for its colour, smell, composition, density, and taste in order to assure that the baby always receives healthy milk (for example, Sor. *Gyn.* 2.21–23 (CMG 4, 69.6–71.4); Orib. *Books to Eunapios* (*Eun.*) 1.1.7–8.1 (CMG 6.3, 320.19–23, ed. Raeder 1926), *Med. Coll. Inc.* 32 (CMG 6.2.2, 124.27–126.23); Aet. *Tetr.* 4.5 (CMG 8.1, 361.26–362.7)). If milk quantity and quality did not meet medical standards, the employment of another wet nurse was suggested (for example, Sor. *Gyn.* 2.28 (CMG 4, 74.7–75.9); Gal. *Hygiene* (*San. Tu.*) 1.9.7.1–3 (CMG 5.4.2, 22.21–23, ed. Koch 1923); Orib *Med. Coll. Inc.* 33.2–3, 34.3 (CMG 6.2.2, 126.33–127.3, 128.13–16); Aet. *Tetr.* 4.5.7–10, 4.6.10–15 (CMG 8.1, 362.4–7, 362.17–22)). If this was not possible, it was suggested that the wet nurse's body be investigated and put under stricter control. She had to follow a different and perhaps sterner diet, undertake exercises and baths, rub herself and have her body rubbed by others until she could produce what was considered healthy milk (for example, Sor. *Gyn.* 2.28 (CMG 4, 74.7–75.9); Gal. *San. Tu.* 1.9.1 (CMG 5.4.2, 21.34–22.4); Orib. *Eun.* 1.1 (CMG 6.3, 320.1–29), *Med. Coll. Inc.* 32 (CMG 6.2.2, 124.27–126.23); Aet. *Tetr.* 4.6 (CMG 8.1, 362.8–363.31)).

Once again, Soranos distinguishes himself by his insistence on the minutiae of the wet nurse's mothering. He describes in exact detail, for instance, how breast-feeding should be performed ("Πῶς δεῖ ... διδόναι τῷ βρέφει τὸν μαστόν," Sor.

---

32 Cf. e.g. Soranos' advice about the wet nurse's consumption of wine ("How to Conduct the Regimen of the Nurse," *Gyn.* 2.26.5 (CMG 4, 73.13–23)); the newborn's bath ("On the Bath and Massage of the Newborn," *Gyn.* 2.30 (CMG 4, 76.1–12)); room temperature and bedding ("On Laying the Newborn Down," *Gyn.* 2.16.3–4 (CMG 4, 63.16–24)).

33 For medical authorities' attempt to regulate the wet nurse more generally, see Chapters 4–6 in this volume.

Gyn. 2.36 (CMG 4, 79.18–19)) and how to treat the infant after feeding, thus providing the child's parents with a knowledge that would allow them to better regulate the wet nurse's movements and behaviour. The relevant passage from the *Gynaecology* reads thus:

> Always indeed when giving the breast, the wet nurse should sit down. With her bent arms she should press the newborn against her bosom, letting it lie on its side in a slightly raised position, now on its right, now on its left side, and she should put the nipple between its lips. And she should sit with her head bent forward as if nodding … For the same reason moreover the newborn should lie in a slightly raised position; and not continuously on the right side … Now, having inserted the breast as has been said, and before the child draws on the nipple, the wet nurse should gently express the milk to provoke the appetite.
>
> One must also beware of moving the child about immediately after it is satiated with milk … If, however, the newborn cries constantly after nursing, the wet nurse should hold it in her arms, and soothe its wailing by patting, babbling, and making gentle sounds, without, however, in addition frightening or disquieting it by loud noises or other threats. One ought not then to rock the infant immediately after the meal, but either after the meal has been digested or before the meal.
>
> ἀεὶ μέντοι παρέχουσα τὸν μαστὸν καθεζέσθω καὶ προσστερνισαμένη ταῖς ἀγκάλαις τὸ βρέφος ποσῶς ἀνάρροπον ἐπὶ πλευρὸν ἐσχηματισμένον, ποτὲ μὲν δεξιόν, ποτὲ δὲ εὐώνυμον, ἐντιθέτω τοῖς χείλεσιν αὐτοῦ τὴν θηλήν. Καθεζέσθω μὲν οὖν οἷον ἐπινενευκυῖα, … τοῦ αὐτοῦ δὲ χάριν καὶ τὸ βρέφος ποσῶς ἀνάρροπον ἐσχηματίσθω, μὴ διηνεκῶς δὲ ἐπὶ τὸ δεξιὸν πλευρόν … ἐνθεῖσα μέντοι τὸν μαστόν, ὡς εἴρηται, πρὸ τοῦ τὸ νήπιον ἐπισπᾶσθαι τὴν θηλὴν πράως ἐνθλιβέτω τὸ γάλα πρὸς ὑπόμνησιν τῆς ὀρέξεως …
>
> φυλάττεσθαι δὲ καὶ μετὰ τὸ πληρωθῆναι τοῦ γάλακτος εὐθέως αὐτὸ κινεῖν … εἰ δὲ ἐπιμόνως κλάοι τὸ βρέφος ἀπὸ τῆς γαλακτοποσίας, ἐν ταῖς ἀγκάλαις αὐτὸ διακρατείτω ἐρεθισμοῖς τισιν καὶ ψελλίσμασιν καὶ φωναῖς προσηνέσιν παρηγοροῦσα τὸν κλαυθμόν, μήτε δὲ ἐκφοβοῦσα μήτ' ἐπιταράττουσα ψόφοις τισὶν ἢ ἄλλαις ἀπειλαῖς· … οὐκ εὐθέως οὖν μετὰ τὴν τροφὴν αἰωρητέον, ἀλλὰ ἢ μετ<ὰ τὸ> αὐτὴν ἀναδοθῆναι ἢ πρὸ τροφῆς. (Sor. *Gyn.* 2.37.1–3 (CMG 4, 80.4–17); 2.40.1.1–2, 3.1–4, 4.1–2 (CMG 4, 82.29–83.15); trans. Temkin 1956, 109, 113)

As this passage suggests, the surveillance of the wet nurse should take place also at the very moment of breastfeeding and for some time afterwards. The infant's parents or owners were invited to check the wet nurse's positioning and the way in which she held the nursling, along with her attempts to incite its appetite. The scrutiny of the wet nurse's body and behaviour during nursing, as was the case in the selection process, acquired a pornographic dimension, as it reduced her to an object of the gaze of the spectator, who assumed her or his powerful position over this socially inferior woman who was not trusted in her mothering. As Sandra

Joshel has put it, "the nurse's deleterious influence on the child was limited, and even curtailed, by regulating her as a technical object."[34]

The surveillance of the wet nurse could function as a forceful manifestation of the biological parent's control over surrogate mothering, while at the same time it could diminish the bonding between wet nurse and infant. The biological parent's involvement in the intimate scene of breastfeeding could regulate and restrain the wet nurse's mothering, which was both desired and dreaded. The need for the surveillance of the surrogate breastfeeding reveals an anxiety that the elite parents would be excluded from their child's mothering, which was in the hands of a woman from the lower social strata. A similar anxiety is detected also in contemporary and later nursing contracts, which, through their legal force, trapped the wet nurse physically and financially into a tied relationship with the nursling's parents, who imposed upon her a life of continence.[35]

John Chrysostom's exhortations to parents suggest, in addition to monitoring the wet nurse's feeding and bodily care of the nursling, that parents should also scrutinize the preliminary training she offered. In his homilies, for instance, Chrysostom asked parents not to allow nurses to engage in practices of superstition, such as the hanging on the children's hands of amulets and bells against the evil eye ("τὰ περίαπτα καὶ τοὺς κώδωνας τοὺς τῆς χειρὸς ἐξηρτημένους καὶ τὸν κόκκινον στήμονα ... δέον μηδὲν ... τῷ παιδὶ περιτιθέναι," *Homily on 1 Corinthians* 12.13–14, ed. Field 1854–1862). According to Chrysostom, these practices were ridiculous and moved children away from religious practices with which they were supposed to become familiar, such as the use of the protecting cross, the powerful symbol of Christ's sacrifice for humanity's salvation.[36]

In general, the exhortations towards a continuous surveillance of the wet nurse's body and her performance of mothering had a double aim. First, they sought to convince parents to bring the wet nurse under control, reminding her of her subordination and her obligation to follow established instructions on mothering. Second, the achievement of the first aim ensured that the wet nurse would never assume the place of the biological mother. The need for the monitoring of the wet nurse, as promulgated by medical authors, philosophers, and theologians from antiquity to Byzantium, indicated that despite her social inferiority, this woman, who played such an important role in the nursling's life and development, could overturn the elite family's power dynamics. If, according to ancient and Byzantine sources, milk was thought to influence the infant's character, then the socially inferior woman's breast was affecting the elite family's heirs in ways that were beyond the parents' control. The wet nurse could be seen as threatening because she blurred the boundaries between public and private by selling her mothering services in the family

---

34 Joshel 1986, 8.
35 Parca 2017 and 2013, 471–472; Gale 2009, 182–189; Tite 2009, 378–381; Abou Aly 1996; Bradley 1980.
36 For John Chrysostom's criticism of training offered to children by wet nurses, see De Wet 2015, 130–141.

domain and by having such a long-lasting physical, emotional, and educational contact with the elite child.[37] The only way to reduce her power over the nursling was to place her body and paid work under continuous surveillance and control.

Conclusions: To Become a Wet Nurse Is to Become an Inferior (M)other

According to our sources, the wet nurse, who mothers the elite infant, should be *sōphrōn*, so that her charge grows up according to the moral principles of its social class. At the same time, the wet nurse's low standing allows the *matrona* to assert power over her and to strengthen her own position as the infant's mother. Seen as a threat for the elite nursling, the wet nurse has to be placed from the outset under the control of her employers, even before her employment has begun. Soranos' chapter and those of other medical authors on the selection of the wet nurse, as well as "Myia's" Letter, illustrate in the most graphic way how Greco-Roman and early Byzantine elite families could excuse their total indifference to the wet nurse's situation and difficulties in order to satisfy both their children's and their own interests, needs, and aspirations.

To rephrase Simone de Beauvoir's famous and much-quoted dictum, "one is not born, but rather becomes" a nursing woman,[38] a statement that could be employed as a one-sentence summary of the wet nurse's socio-ideological position in Greco-Roman antiquity and early Byzantium as expressed in the examined sources. Our analysis has shown that the wet nurse was an essential category of the ancient and Byzantine institution of motherhood, in the framework of which she was treated as the elite mother's inferior Other and the nursling's most devoted servant. Despite the fact that in the examined period, there were also biological mothers who undertook to breastfeed and raise their own children, the socio-ideological treatment of wet nurses was quite distinctive, thus validating the separate examination of them that has been attempted here.

References

Texts: Editions and Translations

Bourland Huizenga, A. 2013. *Moral Education for Women in the Pastoral and Pythagorean Letters*. Wissenschaftliche Untersuchungen zum Neuen Testament 263. Leiden: Brill.

De Lacy, P.H., and Einarson, B. trans. 1959. *Plutarch Moralia: On Love of Wealth. On Compliancy. On Envy and Hate. On Praising Oneself Inoffensively. On the Delays of the Divine Vengeance. On Fate. On the Sign of Socrates. On Exile. Consolation to His Wife.* Loeb Classical Library 405. Cambridge, MA: Harvard University Press.

Field, F. ed. 1854–1862. *Ioannis Chrysostomi Interpretatio omnium Epistularum Paulinarum.* 7 vols. Oxford: J.H. Parker.

---

37 For the wet nurse's influence on the nursling, as illustrated and anticipated in other philosophical and medical sources, see Constantinou and Skouroumouni-Stavrinou 2024, in press.

38 De Beauvoir 1997, 295.

Heiberg, J.L. ed. 1921. *Paulus Aegineta, Libri I–IV, edidit J.L. Heiberg.* Corpus Medicorum Graecorum 9.1. Leipzig and Berlin: Teubner.

Ilberg, J. ed. 1927. *Sorani Gynaeciorum libri IV, De signis fracturarum, De fasciis, Vita Hippocratis secundum Soranum, edidit J. Ilberg.* Corpus Medicorum Graecorum 4. Leipzig and Berlin: Teubner.

Koch, K., G. Helmreich, C. Kalbfleisch, and O. Hartlich. eds. 1923. *Galeni De sanitate tuenda libri IV, edidit K. Koch. De alimentorum facultatibus libri III, edidit G. Helmreich. De bonis malisque sucis liber, edidit idem. De victu attenuante liber, edidit C. Kalbfleisch. De ptisana liber, edidit O. Hartlich.* Corpus Medicorum Graecorum 5.4.2. Leipzig and Berlin: Teubner.

Kühn, C.G. ed. 1830. *Claudii Galeni opera omnia.* Vol. 19. Leipzig: Knobloch.

Lefkowitz, M.R., and M.B. Fant. trans. 2016. *Women's Life in Greece and Rome: A Source Book in Translation.* 4th ed. London: Bloomsbury.

Lutz, C.E. ed. and trans. 1947. *Musonius Rufus 'The Roman Socrates.'* New Haven, CT: Yale University Press.

Olivieri, A. ed. 1935. *Aetii Amideni Libri medicinales I–IV, edidit A. Olivieri.* Corpus Medicorum Graecorum 8.1. Leipzig and Berlin: Teubner.

Perrin, B. trans. 1914. *Plutarch's Lives: Themistocles and Camillus, Aristides and Cato Major, Cimon and Lucullus.* Loeb Classical Library 47. Cambridge, MA: Harvard University Press.

Raeder, J. ed. 1926. *Oribasii Synopsis ad Eustathium, Libri ad Eunapium, edidit J. Raeder.* Corpus Medicorum Graecorum 6.3. Leipzig and Berlin: Teubner.

———. ed. 1933. *Oribasii Collectionum medicarum reliquiae, libri XLIX–L, libri incerti, eclogae medicamentorum edidit J. Raeder.* Corpus Medicorum Graecorum 6.2.2. Leipzig and Berlin: Teubner.

Schmidt, M. 1861–1862. *Hesychii Alexandrini Lexicon.* 4 vols. Halle: Jenae, Sumptibus Hermanni Dufftii (Libraria Maukiana).

Sieveking, W. ed. (1929) 1972. *Plutarchi Moralia.* Vol. 3. Reprint. Leipzig: Teubner.

Städele, A. ed. 1980. *Die Briefe des Pythagoras und der Pythagoreer.* Meisenheim am Glan: Hain.

Temkin, O. trans. 1956. *Soranus' Gynecology.* Baltimore, MD: Johns Hopkins University Press.

Thesleff, H. ed. 1965. *The Pythagorean Texts of the Hellenistic Period.* Acta Academiae Aboensis, Humaniora 30 (1). Åbo: Åbo Akademi.

Ziegler, K. ed. 1969. *Plutarchi Vitae Parallelae.* Vol. 1. Leipzig: Teubner.

Secondary Works

Abou Aly, A. 1996. "The Wet Nurse: A Study in Ancient Medicine and Greek Papyri," *Vesalius* 2 (2): 86–97.

Bäbler, B. 1998. *Fleißige Thrakerinnen und wehrhafte Skythen: Nichtgriechen im klassischen Athen und ihre archäologische Hinterlassenschaft.* Beitrage zur Altertumskunde 108. Berlin: Walter de Gruyter.

Beauvoir, S. de. 1997. *The Second Sex.* Translated and edited by H.M. Parshley. London: Vintage.

Belliotti, R.A. 2009. *Roman Philosophy and the Good Life.* Lanham, MD: Lexington Books.

Bourland Huizenga, A. 2010. "*Sōphrosynē* for Women in Pythagorean Texts," in S.P. Ahearne-Kroll, P.A. Holloway, and J.A. Kelhoffer (eds) *Women and Gender in Ancient*

Religion. Wissenschaftliche Untersuchungen zum Neuen Testament 263. Tübingen: Mohr Siebeck, 379–400.

———. 2014. "On Choosing a Wet-Nurse: Physical, Cultural and Moral Credentials," in T.R. Blanton, R.M. Calhoun, and C.K. Rothschild (eds) *The History of Religions School Today: Essays on the New Testament and Related Ancient Mediterranean Texts*. Tübingen: Mohr Siebeck, 241–252.

Bradley, K.R. 1980. "Sexual Regulations in Wet-Nursing Contracts from Roman Egypt," *Klio* 62 (2): 321–325.

Bryan, J. 2013. "Neronian Philosophy," in E. Buckley, and M.T. Dinter (eds) *A Companion to the Neronian Age*. Malden, MA: Wiley-Blackwell, 134–150.

Constantinou, S., and A. Skouroumouni-Stavrinou. 2024. "The Other Mother: Ancient and Early Byzantine Approaches to Wet Nursing and Mothering," *Journal of Hellenic Studies* 145, in press.

Dasen, V. 2010. "Des nourrices grecques à Rome?" *Paedagogica historica* 46: 699–713.

Dillon, J.T. 2004. *Musonius Rufus and Education in the Good Life: A Model of Teaching and Living Virtue*. Lanham, MD: University Press of America.

Ecca, G. 2017. "Fixing Ethical Rules for Midwives in the Early Roman Imperial Period: Soranus, *Gynaecia* I 3–4 [Die Festlegung ethischer Regeln für Hebammen in der frühen römischen Kaiserzeit: Soranos, *Gynaecia* I 3–4]," *Sudhoffs Archiv* 101 (2): 125–138.

Eijk, P. van der. 2010. "Principles and Practices of Compilation and Abbreviation in the Medical 'Encyclopaedias' of Late Antiquity," in M. Horster (ed.) *Condensing Text – Condensed Texts*. Stuttgart: Steiner, 519–554.

Eijk, P. van der, M. Geller, L. Lehmhaus, M. Martelli, and C. Salazar. 2015. "Canons, Authorities and Medical Practice in the Greek Medical Encyclopaedias of Late Antiquity and in the Talmut," in G. Uhlmann (ed.) *Episteme in Bewegung: Wissenstransfer von der Alten Welt bis in die Frühe Neuzeit*. Episteme in Bewegung: Beiträge zu einer transdisziplinären Wissensgeschichte, vol. 1. Wiesbaden: Harrassowitz Verlag, 195–221.

Fildes, V. 1988. *Wet Nursing: A History from Antiquity to the Present*. Oxford: Basil Blackwell.

Frede, M. 1983. *Essays in Ancient Philosophy*. Minneapolis: University of Minnesota Press.

Gale, A.Y. 2009. "'Take This Child and Suckle It for Me': Wet Nurses and Resistance in Ancient Israel," *Biblical Theology Bulletin* 39 (4): 180–189.

Geytenbeck, A.C. van. 1963. *Musonius Rufus and Greek Diatribe*. Assen: Van Gorcum.

Gill, M.L. 2003. "Plato's *Phaedrus* and the Method of Hippocrates," *Modern Schoolman* 80: 295–314.

Goulet-Gazé, M.-O. 2005. "Musonius Rufus," in M.-O. Goulet-Gazé (ed.) *Dictionnaire des Philosophes Antiques*. Vol. 4. Paris: Editions du Centre national de la recherche scientifique, 555–572.

Grimm, V.E. 2006. "On Food and the Body," in D.S. Potter (ed.) *A Companion to the Roman Empire*. Malden, MA: Wiley Blackwell, 354–368.

Hankinson, R.J. ed. 2008. *The Cambridge Companion to Galen*. Cambridge: Cambridge University Press.

Hankinson, R.J. 2008a. "The Man and His Work," in Hankinson 2008, 1–33.

———. 2008b. "Epistemology," in Hankinson 2008, 157–183.

———. 2008c. "Philosophy of Nature," in Hankinson 2008, 210–241.

Harper, L.V. 2013. "The Neopythagorean Women as Philosophers," in Pomeroy 2013, 117–138.

Hermann, J. 1959. "Die Ammenverträge in den graeko-aegyptischen Papyri," *Zeitschrift der Savigny-Stiftung für Rechtsgeschichte: Romanistische Abteilung* 76: 490–499.

Inwood, B. 2017. "The Legacy of Musonius Rufus," in T. Engberg-Pedersen (ed.) *From Stoicism to Platonism: The Development of Philosophy, 100 BCE–100 CE*. Cambridge: Cambridge University Press, 254–276.

Joshel, S.R. 1986. "Nurturing the Master's Child: Slavery and the Roman Child-Nurse," *Signs* 12 (1): 3–22.

Jouanna, J. 2012. *Greek Medicine from Hippocrates to Galen: Selected Papers*. Translated by N. Allies. Studies in Ancient Medicine 40. Leiden: Brill.

Laes, C. 2010. "The Educated Midwife in the Roman Empire: An Example of Differential Equations," in M. Horstmanschoff (ed.) *Hippocrates and Medical Education: Selected Papers Presented at the XIIth International Hippocrates Colloquium, Universiteit Leiden, 24–26 August 2005*. Leiden: Brill, 261–286.

Morison, B. 2008. "Logic," in Hankinson 2008, 66–115.

North, H. 1966. *Sōphrosynē: Self-Knowledge and Self-Restraint in Greek Literature*. Cornell Studies in Classical Philology 35. Ithaca, NY: Cornell University Press.

———. 1977. "The Mare, the Vixen, and the Bee: *Sōphrosynē* as the Virtue of Women in Antiquity," *Illinois Classical Studies* 2: 35–48.

Nussbaum, M. 2002. "The Incomplete Feminism of Musonius Rufus, Platonist, Stoic, and Roman," in M.C. Nussbaum, and J. Sihvola (eds) *The Sleep of Reason: Erotic Experience and Sexual Ethics in Ancient Greece and Rome*. Chicago, IL: University of Chicago Press, 283–326.

Parca, M. 2013. "Children in Ptolemaic Egypt: What the Papyri Say," in J. Evans Grubbs and T. Parkin (eds) *The Oxford Handbook of Childhood and Education in the Classical World*. Oxford: Oxford University Press, 465–483.

———. 2017. "The Wet Nurses of Ptolemaic and Roman Egypt," *Illinois Classical Studies* 42 (1): 203–226.

Pellegrin, P. 2006. "Ancient Medicine and Its Contribution to the Philosophical Tradition," in M.L. Gill, and P. Pellegrin (eds) *A Companion to Ancient Philosophy*. Malden, MA: Northwestern University Press, 664–685.

Pomeroy, S. 2013. *Pythagorean Women: Their History and Writings*. Baltimore, MD: Johns Hopkins University Press.

Reydams-Schils, R. 2005. *The Roman Stoics: Self, Responsibility, and Affection*. Chicago, IL: University of Chicago Press, 143–175.

Rhodes, M.C. 2015. "Domestic Vulnerabilities: Reading Families and Bodies into Eighteenth-Century Anglo-Atlantic Wet Nurse Advertisements," *Journal of Family History* 40 (1): 39–63.

Rich, A. 1995. *Of Woman Born: Motherhood as Experience and Institution*. New York: Norton.

Stephens, W.O. 2019. "Stoicism and Food," in P.B. Thompson, and D.M. Kaplan (eds) *Encyclopedia of Food and Agricultural Ethics*. Heidelberg: Springer, 2245–2251.

Swain, S. 2013. *Economy, Family, and Society from Rome to Islam: A Critical Edition, English Translation, and Study of Bryson's Management of the Estate*. Cambridge: Cambridge University Press.

Thesleff, H. 1961. *An Introduction to the Pythagorean Writings of the Hellenistic Period*. Acta Academiae Aboensis, Humaniora 24.3. Åbo: Åbo Akademi.

Tieleman, T. 1996. *Galen and Chrysippus on the Soul: Argument and Refutation in the 'De placitis' Books II–III*. Philosophia Antiqua 68. Leiden: Brill.

———. 2008. "Methodology," in Hankinson 2008, 49–65.

Tite, P.L. 2009. "Nurslings, Milk and Moral Development in the Greco-Roman Context: A Reappraisal of the Paraenetic Utilization of Metaphor in 1 Peter 2.1–3," *Journal for the Study of the New Testament* 31 (4): 371–400.

Valantasis, R. 1999. "Musonius Rufus and Roman Ascetical Theory," *Greek Roman and Byzantine Studies* 40: 207–231.

Wet, C.L. de. 2015. *Preaching Bondage: John Chrysostom and the Discourse of Slavery in Early Christianity*. California: University of California Press.

Whitmarsh, T. 2001. *Greek Literature in the Roman Empire: The Politics of Imitation*. Oxford: Oxford University Press.

3 The Breast as Locus for Punishment

Dionysios Stathakopoulos

Introduction

There is a penal universe that lies outside earthly law systems: it is where sins are punished in the afterlife. Our information on this place derives mainly from two founts: texts that have been placed outside the canon of Scripture – Apocrypha and prophetic visions of the end of times – and images preserved in various media, but above all monumental painting in churches. Both texts and images describe the punishments that await sinners and include a wide range of sins and sinners. In this chapter, I will focus on punishments that are meted out to women and more specifically to female breasts in this universe. My aim is to untangle the complex processes by which the images emerged and to comment on their function.[1]

The research behind this chapter was undertaken as part of an international project on the representation of hell in Venetian Crete.[2] This has two implications: first, images of infernal punishments gave the impetus to examine the traditions from which they sprang. Second, there is an obvious emphasis on Cretan material. Methodologically, this chapter will work backwards: I will start with presenting and discussing a body of visual evidence that is attested from the ninth/tenth century AD onwards (but reaches its peak in the 14th c. AD) and will move backwards to trace the pictorial and textual traditions on which it was based.

The first piece of evidence I will explore comes from the so-called Church of the Serpents (Yılanlı Kilise) in the Ihlara Valley in Cappadocia. As part of a monumental depiction of the Last Judgement, we can discern a female figure whose breasts are bitten by two serpents. The painted inscription accompanying the figure reads: "She who turns herself away from infants," or "She who turns infants away" ("ΟΠΟΥ ΑΠΟΣΤΡΕΦ[ΕΤΑΙ or ΕΙ] ΤΑ ΝΗΠΗΑ").[3] The combination of the image and the text clearly suggests a woman who does not breastfeed. The dating of the image is debated: Catherine Jolivet-Lévy dates it to the mid- to late eleventh

---

1 Imagery of breastfeeding women in religious and other contexts is also examined in Chapters 7–9 in this volume.
2 The results of this project have been published in two volumes: Lymberopoulou 2020a and Lymberopoulou and Duits 2020.
3 Translations, unless otherwise indicated, are mine.

DOI: 10.4324/9781003265658-4

century AD, without excluding the possibility that it could extend to the early twelfth century.[4] Robert Ousterhout places the church in the ninth century AD;[5] similarly, Sophia Kalopissi-Verti dates the paintings to the late ninth and tenth centuries AD, and Rainer Warland and Mati Meyer to around AD 900.[6]

Another early example comes from a now destroyed, probably monastic, church in the Fayum at Tebtunis.[7] The scene, dated to the early eleventh century AD, shows a female figure whose breasts are bitten by serpents, accompanied by an inscription in Coptic: "The woman who has given her breasts for hire" (trans. Zellmann-Rohrer 2019, 298). It is certainly a similar transgression, although the Tebtunis sinner probably depicts a woman who acted as a wet nurse, as the phrase "for hire" suggests.[8] I will get back to this distinction.

Taking the Cappadocian and Egyptian evidence as our guide, we can explore other depictions of the same motif. We find plentiful evidence on Crete in a number of small, rural churches and chapels dating from late thirteenth century AD onwards, as part of programmes illustrating the fate of sinners after death. It will suffice here to point to some of the examples that preserve both the image of the punished woman and the inscription identifying her transgression (supplied in parenthesis, with the text in restored transcription).

(1) Virgin, Apokoronas, Karydi (Karydaki), Vamos, Chania, dated to AD 1270–1290 ("She who turns infants away"; "ἡ ἀποστρέφουσα τὰ νήπια"); (2) Hagios Georgios, Fres, Apokoronas, Chania, dated to the fourteenth century AD ("ἡ ἀποστρέφουσα τὰ νήπια"); (3) Hagia Pelagia, Ano Vianos, Herakleion, dated to AD 1360 ("ἡ ἀποστρέφουσα τὰ νήπια"); (4) Hagios Panteleimonas, Zymvragou, Kissamos, Chania, ca. AD 1360? ("ἡ ἀποστρέφουσα τὰ νήπια"); (5) Kera, Kardiotissa, Pediada, Herakleion, first half of the fourteenth century AD, ("ἡ ἀποστρέφουσα τὰ νήπια"); (6) Hagia Paraskevi, Kitiros, Selino in Chania, dated to AD 1372–1373 ("She who does not breastfeed"; "ἡ μὴ βυζάνουσα"); (7) Soter, Spili, Hagios Basileios, Rethymnon, dated to the late fourteenth century AD ("She who does not breastfeed infants"; "ἡ μὴ θηλάζουσα τὰ νήπια"); (8) Panagia, Hagia Eirini, Selino (Chania), end of the fourteenth century AD ("She who does not breastfeed another's infant"; "ἡ μὴ θηλάζουσα ξένο βρέφος").[9]

Additionally, there is an example from Cyprus from the church of Asinou dated to AD 1332/1333 bearing the inscription "ἡ ἀποστρέφουσα τὰ νήπια" (Figure 3.1).[10]

---

4 Jolivet-Lévy 1991, 136–137.
5 Ousterhout 2017, 213.
6 Warland 2020, 243; Kalopissi-Verti 2012, 132, n. 82, 146; Meyer 2009, 226.
7 Zellmann-Rohrer 2019; Walters 1989, 202 with plates XXVIII 1–2, 207. I am particularly grateful to Betsy Bolman for drawing my attention to this material.
8 The mercenary aspect and its potential implications for the way wet nurses were received is discussed in Chapters 1 and 2 in this volume. See also Constantinou and Skouroumouni-Stavrinou 2024, in press.
9 References to the monuments from Lymberopoulou and Duits 2020 with catalogue number and pages: (1) Nr 19, 505–508; (2) Nr 7, 468–470; (3) Nr 76, 714–719; (4) Nr 47, 601–607; (5) Nr 86, 755–758; (6) Nr 21, 512–516; (7) Nr 71, 691–696; (8) Nr 10, 477–480.
10 Kalopissi-Verti 2012, 145.

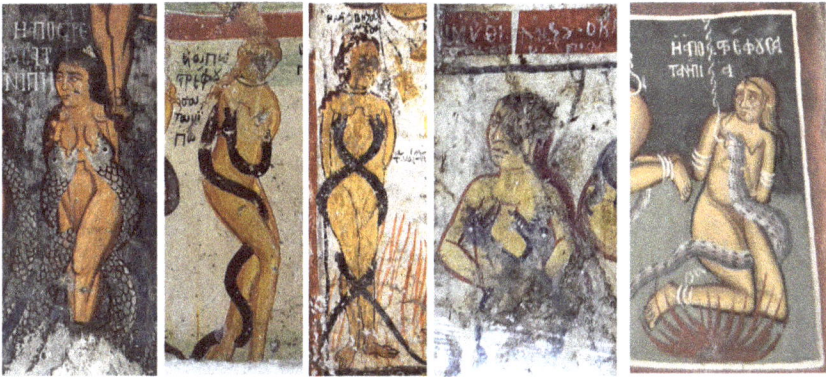

Figure 3.1 A composite image of five scenes depicting female sinners suffering punishment, from left to right: Hagios Georgios, Fres; Hagia Pelagia, Ano Vianos; Hagia Paraskevi, Kitiros; Soter, Spili; Asinou. All photographs by the author.

Even from the selection of examples in Figure 3.1, it is clear that the iconography is largely identical, showing two serpents, each biting one of the woman's breasts (the only difference being that in the Cypriot image there is only one serpent). The inscriptions also bear similar messages about women turning themselves away from infants or, more clearly, not breastfeeding infants, while one case preserves an additional aspect, a woman who refuses to nurse someone else's child.

In a recently published book on *Hell in the Byzantine World*, I undertook a detailed study of the textual sources of these and other similar images of punishments in the afterlife.[11] In many cases, we see punishments meted out by serpents, while the images alongside the accompanying inscriptions suggest that the punishments are applied to the part of the body with which the sin was committed – in our case the breasts that did not nurse infants.[12] This finds a correspondence in the New Testament where Christ provides injunctions on how to treat the parts of the body that sin (Matthew 5:29–30, Mark 9:43–47): "If the hand/foot/eye causes one to sin, then one should cut it off or tear it out instead of risking going into Hell, to the everlasting fire (only in Mark) with one's body whole" ("Καὶ ἐὰν σκανδαλίζῃ σε ἡ χείρ σου, ἀπόκοψον αὐτήν· καλόν ἐστίν σε κυλλὸν εἰσελθεῖν εἰς τὴν ζωὴν ἢ τὰς δύο χεῖρας ἔχοντα ἀπελθεῖν εἰς τὴν γέενναν, εἰς τὸ πῦρ τὸ ἄσβεστον"). This represents the notion of talion (the punishment corresponding to the crime, as suggested by Leviticus 24:19–20: "fracture for fracture, eye for eye, tooth for tooth"; "σύντριμμα ἀντὶ συντρίμματος, ὀφθαλμὸν ἀντὶ ὀφθαλμοῦ, ὀδόντα ἀντὶ ὀδόντος") and more specifically the notion that certain sins are committed by certain body parts.

11 Stathakopoulos 2020. The study explores some of the topics that will be outlined in this chapter in much more depth and detail and should be consulted alongside this text.
12 For the serpent imagery involved in depictions of breastfeeding women, see also Chapter 7 in this volume.

Since Scripture overall is not particularly revealing about the afterlife, the task of providing more ample information on the fate of sinners was taken up in a series of Apocrypha that enumerate and describe (often in gruesome detail) the punishments that await sinners after death. Although it is clear that the two traditions – the earlier textual and the later visual one – are linked, their relationship is not straightforward. It is, therefore, important to look more closely at those texts that record specific punishments inflicted on women's breasts, in order to establish a framework for this investigation.

The earliest text in this respect, and perhaps the oldest of the "tours of Hell" genre, is the Coptic *Apocalypse of Elijah* dated to third-century AD Egypt and most probably based on a lost Greek version.[13] The relevant passage reads as follows: "In that time the [evil] king will command that all nursing women be seized and be brought to him bound to suckle serpents, that their blood be sucked from their breasts to be given as poison for arrows" (at §Dd 35; trans. Frankfurter 1993, 309).[14] A very similar passage is found in a Greek Sibylline oracle now preserved in a sixth-century version but going back to a lost text dated to the fourth century: "And people will seize poisonous asps and suck milk from women with new-born babes and draw blood for the sake of the poison of arrows and the violence of wars" ("καὶ κρατήσουσιν ἀσπίδας καὶ θηλάσουσι τὰς ἐχούσας τὰ βρέφη καὶ αἱμάσσουσι διὰ τὰ φάρμακα τῶν βελῶν καὶ τὰς ἀνάγκας τῶν πολέμων," ed. and trans. Alexander 1967, 28).[15] The connection between the texts is very clear, and it seems safe to assume that this must go back to a common source, perhaps the lost Greek version of the *Apocalypse of Elijah*. I will return to these puzzling passages below. The Greek *Apocalypse of Ezra*, a short text dated roughly between the second and the ninth centuries AD,[16] contains the following description: "And I saw a woman hanging, and four wild beasts sucking upon her breasts. And the angels said to me: She begrudged giving her milk, but also cast infants into the rivers" ("καὶ ἴδον γυναῖκα κρεμαμένην, καὶ τέσσαρα θηρία θηλάζοντα τοὺς μαστοὺς αὐτῆς. καὶ εἶπόν μοι οἱ ἄγγελοι· αὕτη τὸ γάλα ἐφθόνησεν τοῦ δοῦναι, ἀλλὰ καὶ τὰ νήπια ἐν τοῖς ποταμοῖς ἔρριψεν," ed. Tischendorf 1866; trans. Stone 1992, 576).

The *Apocalypse of Peter* survives in Greek in fragmentary form (5th–late 6th/7th c. AD)[17] and in a fuller version preserved in Ethiopic (most probably translated from an Arabic translation of the original Greek which is to be dated in the 2nd c. AD).[18] The *Apocalypse of Peter* was popular in the early Christian centuries

---

13   Frankfurter 1993, 21–25; Alexander 1967, 39.
14   Much of the ambivalence towards milk in antiquity stems from the fact that breastmilk was considered to be transformed menstrual blood. For medical and ethical associations of the milk–blood connection, see Chapters 5 and 6 in this volume.
15   Frankfurter 1993, 24–25 on the relationship between the two texts.
16   Stone 1992, 563; Himmelfarb 1983, 25.
17   Van Minnen 2003.
18   Bauckham 1998, 162; Müller 1992, 625. On the date see Bauckham 1998, 160–258; Himmelfarb 1983, 8–9.

and was even regarded as canonical.[19] In this text, there is an inversion: it is not creatures that attack female breasts from the outside, but the other way around:

> women who procured abortions are up to their neck in a lake of excrement, the aborted children watching them (Ethiopic version: 'lightnings go forth from those children which pierce the eyes of those who, by fornication, have brought about their destruction'). And the milk of the mothers flows from their breasts and congeals and smells foul and from it come beasts that devour flesh. (Trans. Müller 1992, 629–630)

The final text that records punishments inflicted on women's breasts was also the most popular by far in the Byzantine world: the *Apocalypse of the Theotokos*. Written in Greek and dated between the ninth and eleventh centuries AD, it is preserved in more than fifty manuscripts (7th–17th c. AD), and it enjoyed a vivid afterlife in printed pamphlets.[20] Jane Baun, who produced the authoritative study of this textual genre, dubbed the thought-world of this text "village Christianity" and emphasized its focus on transgressions that disrupt social cohesion.[21]

The *Apocalypse of the Theotokos* includes both motifs encountered so far: the Mother of God in her tour of hell sees deaconesses who defiled their bodies in fornication hanging on a cliff, with two-headed beasts gnawing at their breasts. In a very late version (perhaps 17th c. AD) of the text produced in Crete and written in Latin letters but in the Cretan dialect, the Theotokos sees women hung up by the feet and fire coming out of their mouths. "And the Angel says to her: These are women with milk; these hated [their own children] and gave suck to children not their own" ("aftes ine en do gala aftes i misandes chie v (? u) chie visasan etera gnipia," ed. and trans. Dawkins 1929–1930, 301).[22]

The traditions connecting female breasts and afterlife punishments for transgressions are obviously the result of the intermingling of many different strands. There is no straightforward genealogy, in my mind – at least none that can be inferred from the surviving evidence, be it textual or visual. We have to bear in mind that many texts (for example, the Greek version of the *Apocalypse of Elijah*) and even more monuments that could have preserved images like the ones I have discussed above have been lost. At present, for example, most visual representations of the punishment for not nursing come from rural milieux. The textual traditions and the ways in which they were much later translated into images of mothers who were punished for not nursing, or not nursing the right infants, are the result of complex processes. The apocryphal texts that provided glimpses into the future and the afterlife were, more often than not, produced in communities that were outside

---

19 Jacab 2003.
20 Baun 2007, 18–20. While Delatte (1927, 272) wrote that he had found the text sold in the streets of Athens, it is now mostly diffused through the internet; see https://neataksi.blogspot.com/2010/02/blog-post_24.html. Accessed 30 May 2022.
21 Baun 2007, 323–325.
22 Baun 2007, 40.

mainstream Christianity.[23] Their reception was supported by the fact that they obviously filled a gap in the knowledge about the afterlife that Scripture had not covered.[24] Ideas from these texts about the punishment of female transgressions were translated into images. It seems that the earliest extant representations emerged in a monastic milieu – for example at Yılanlı and Tebtunis – and perhaps represent a kind of "monastic misogyny."[25] From there, they were gradually adopted in non-monastic churches, from where the later evidence has been gathered. Despite the many uncertainties in the processes of formation and dispersion I have outlined above, I think it is helpful to examine the material as a whole and reach some conclusions that can help contextualize the ideas behind it.

Conclusions

The earliest textual and visual traditions seem to have a strong Egyptian element in common. The episode in the Coptic *Apocalypse of Elijah* shows what David Frankfurter calls "the convergence of Egyptian and Christian worldviews."[26] In his astute analysis, he emphasizes the ancient Egyptian images and texts that connect serpents, breasts, milk, and blood and shows that the striking image of women nursing snakes has "a special symbolism indigenous to Egyptian culture."[27] The image of Cleopatra dying by suicide by nursing one snake (or two snakes) at her breast is powerful. There are ancient Egyptian ritual spells for the protection of breasts against demons and snakebites, and Frankfurter makes the case that "the forcible application of serpents to breasts would have constituted an unimaginable horror."[28]

The highly symbolic importance of both breastmilk and blood as magical substances could be used to denote the inversion or reversal that is characteristic of the end of times and the afterlife, as symbolized, for example, by the parable of the Rich Man and the Poor Lazarus (Luke 16:19–31), in which the merciless Rich Man finds himself suffering after his death while the long-suffering Lazarus enjoys comfort and bliss.[29] In our case, life-sustaining breastmilk is turned to blood and ultimately to poison in a complete reversal of human life experience. Frankfurter also brings to the discussion a passage from the Life of the Alexandrian pope Peter I (AD 300–311) in the *History of the Patriarchs of the Coptic Church* in which a mother cut her breast and used drops of her blood to perform an emergency baptism of her children because she believed that the ship they were travelling on would perish in a storm (ed. Evetts 1907, 122–123).[30] From these textual traditions

---

23 Sim 1996, 245; Frankfurter 1993, 296–298.
24 Stathakopoulos 2020, 22–25.
25 Walters 1989, 207; Thierry and Thierry 1960, 166.
26 This is part of the title of the second part of Frankfurter 1993, 159–240.
27 Frankfurter 1993, 207.
28 Frankfurter 1993, 209.
29 Stathakopoulos 2020, 24 with reference to bibliography.
30 Frankfurter 1993, 209–210. The text was "edited in the eleventh century" but was based on earlier material and includes later recensions designed to update the catalogue, a process of literary

connecting breasts, milk, blood, and serpents, it is not difficult to see the formation of the visual tradition of female sinners tormented by serpents on their breasts. The fact that some of the earlier extant images are linked to Egypt further corroborates this point. This connection is, naturally, evident in the image from Tebtunis, but the Cappadocian image from Yılanlı Kilise has also been linked by various scholars to Egyptian iconographic traditions.[31]

According to the inscriptions accompanying the relevant images, the transgression that is punished by the serpents biting female breasts in the afterlife can be divided into three categories that occasionally overlap: those who refuse to nurse, those who refuse to nurse others' infants, and those who nurse children who are not their own. The first category is phrased at times explicitly (those who do not nurse) but also less directly (those who turn themselves away from infants/turn infants away). In the latter case, although the images make a clear connection with breastfeeding, we can assume that another sin is (additionally) implied, that of abandoning or exposing infants. Such a reading agrees with the passage quoted above from the Greek *Apocalypse of Ezra*. Exposing infants was a widespread phenomenon, particularly among poorer strata or for children born out of wedlock.[32] Nursing an infant was obviously crucial for the survival of the child; the inability or, as implied in the cases mentioned above, unwillingness to nurse would most often lead to a child's death. This is indirectly corroborated by an *Euchologion* dated to the thirteenth century AD which records that if a newborn child is not nursing, it is a certain sign of imminent death and it should be baptized immediately (Athens, Nat. Lib. 662 (*Diktyon* 2598), *fr.* 79v).[33]

There is a variant attested in a few representations of punishment in the afterlife, as in the Church of Panagia in the village of Hagia Eirini, where the punished woman is identified as "She who does not breastfeed another's infant" ("ἡ μὴ θηλάζουσα ξένω βρέφος"). It is even more explicit in a scene found in the Church of the Archangel Michael in Ano Boularioi in Mani and dated to the late thirteenth century, where the woman (whose breasts are bitten by serpents) is labelled as "She who refuses to nurse orphans" ("ἡ μὴ θηλάζουσα τάρφανά").[34] Given that many mothers died in childbirth, it was obviously essential to nurse infants who had lost their mothers or risk their death.[35]

---

expansion that has extended even into the twentieth century; see Davis and Gabra 2004. There is an interesting inversion of the milk–blood binary recorded in the *Passion of Pistis, Elpis, and Agape*, daughters of Sophia, when Elpis has her breasts cut off and milk, rather than blood, flows from them; see Christodoulos Papavarnavas, *Cult of Saints, E06900*, http://csla.history.ox.ac.uk/record.php?recid=E06900. Accessed 30 May 2022. I am grateful to Christodoulos Papavarnavas for this reference. On the motif of milk emerging from female martyrs' breasts, see Constantinou 2024, in press. I would like to thank the author for providing me with an advance copy of the unpublished chapter.

31 Warland 2020, 245–252; much less explicitly Jolivet-Lévy 2006, 51 and 2001, 272.
32 Gasparis 2020, 100; Harris 1994.
33 I am grateful to Father Gregorios Ioannides for this reference.
34 Gerstel and Katsaphados 2020, 331–333.
35 Ariantzi 2012, 84–85. For high rates of mortality (of both infants and women) and their correlation to the spread of the phenomenon of wet nursing in antiquity and Byzantium, see Chapter 1 in this volume.

The third variant condemns women for the opposite of the previous sin, namely for nursing others' children, for being a wet nurse (as attested in Tebtunis and the 17th c. AD version of the *Apocalypse of the Theotokos*). This requires some unpacking. The immediate implication, since to be able to nurse meant that a woman must have given birth recently herself, is that the wet nurse would probably not be able to nurse her own children. In the particular context of Crete, there is also an additional dimension, the possibility that a woman could be employed as a wet nurse for an infant from a different ethno-religious background than her own. Evidence from Cretan notarial acts suggests that it was not uncommon for Greek women to be employed as wet nurses for Venetian infants.[36] Given that wet nurses ("βυζάστρες," *nutrices*) were well paid, seeking such employment must have been very tempting, especially for women from the lower socio-economic strata.[37]

The refusal to nurse an infant was considered a sin, as can be seen from its inclusion in a twelfth-century confession manual (penitentiary) as one of 94 sins that the priest should enquire about from those seeking confession: (Nr 39) "On women who turn away from nursing their own children" ("Περὶ ἀποστρεφηκῶν τοῦ μὴ βυζάνειν τὰ ἑαυτῶν παιδία," ed. Arranz 1993, 170).[38] It is worth highlighting that in similar penitential collections sins that are considered specifically female clearly highlight issues surrounding conception, abortion, and sexual behaviour.[39] The visual universe of sinners being punished after death displays similar emphases. In the majority of the wall paintings that include such scenes, women are punished for sins that disrupt the social cohesion of their communities and families: slandering, gossiping, eavesdropping, fornicating, and refusing to nurse.[40] We must assume that the function of the punishments shown in such images was to safeguard established norms and order, to curtail subversive behaviour – in short, to exercise social control.

The so-called *Strategikon* (now more accurately known as *Advice and Anecdotes*) by the eleventh-century author known as Kekaumenos, most probably a provincial military aristocrat, includes advice directed to his sons, among other things, and is clearly conversant with earlier collections of advice literature. In this work, there is a passage that is relevant to our discussion in a section dedicated to children's duty to honour and love their parents: "Remember your mother's

---

36 Maltezou 1984, 74. In a similar image from Epiros dated to the early nineteenth century, a woman is identified as "The woman who nurses Turkish children" ("Η γυνή όπου βυζάνη τα τουρκόπαιδα"), suggesting a similar transgression; see Tsiodoulos 2012, Figure 17, p. 37.

37 Evidence from the fourteenth century AD in Santschi 1969, 53, 60, 70. The average annual salary for wet nurses was 15.7 ducats, compared with, e.g., 12.4 for a smith and between 7.4 and 5 for a tailor.

38 On the date: the earliest manuscript is dated to the twelfth century AD, Vat. Gr. 1554 (*Diktyon* 68185), but the editor has not elaborated on the dating of the text apart from assigning it to the twelfth century; see Arranz 1993, 131.

39 Arranz 1993, 99, 181 (polluting men with their menses, performing abortions in various ways, taking herbs to avoid conception or produce abortions, killing infants once they have been born, masturbating).

40 Lymberopoulou 2020b, 143–148; Baun 2007, 324, 339–343.

labour-pains, and do not forget her breast" ("Μνήσθητι ὠδῖνος μητρός σου, θηλῆς δὲ αὐτῆς μὴ ἐπιλάθῃ," 63.1, ed. and trans. Roueché 2013).[41] While part of this passage alludes to Sirach 7:27 ("Do not forget the labour pains of your mother"), the mention of the mother's breast seems to be unique to Kekaumenos. It emphasizes the importance of nursing in a text that is chronologically close to the earliest depictions of the punishments meted out to women who did not nurse and, we can assume, is also closer to the thought-world of the audiences that were targeted by these images, the assumed "village Christianity." In such a world, refusing to nurse was such a grave transgression that it brought on dire punishment in the next world.

References

Texts: Editions and Translations

Alexander, P.J. ed. and trans. 1967. *The Oracle of Baalbek: The Tiburtine Sibyl in Greek Dress*. Washington, DC: Dumbarton Oaks Center for Byzantine Studies.

Arranz, M.S.J. ed. 1993. *I Pentitenziali Bizantini: Il Protokanonarion o Kanonarion Primitivo di Giovanni Monaco e Diacono e il Deuterokanonarion o "Secondo Kanonarion" di Basilio Monaco* (Kanonika 3). Rome: Pontificio Istituto Orientale.

Dawkins, R.M. ed. and trans. 1929–1930. "A Cretan Apocalypse of the Virgin," *Byzantinische Zeitschrift* 30: 300–304.

Delatte, A. 1927. *Anecdota atheniensia*. Vol. 1. Liège: H. Vaillant-Carmanne, 272–280.

Evetts, B. ed. and trans. 1907. *History of the Patriarchs of the Coptic Church of Alexandria: Arabic Text Edited, Annotated, and Translated by B. Evetts. Patrologia Orientalis* 1. Paris: Firmin-Didot, 99–214.

Frankfurter, D. ed. and trans. 1993. *Elijah in Upper Egypt: The Apocalypse of Elijah and Early Egyptian Christianity*. Minneapolis: Fortress Press.

Müller, C.D.G. trans. 1992. "Apocalypse of Peter," in W. Schneemelcher (ed.) *New Testament Apocrypha*, vol. 2: *Writings Relating to the Apostles, Apocalypses and Related Subjects*. Cambridge: James Clark and Co., 620–638.

Roueché, C. trans. 2013. *Kekaumenos, Consilia et Narrationes*. Sharing Ancient Wisdoms/ SAWS 2013, https://ancientwisdoms.ac.uk/mss/viewer.html?viewColumns=greekLit%3 Atlg3017.Syno298.sawsEng01. Accessed 30 May 2022.

Stone, M.E. trans. 1992. "Greek Apocalypse of Ezra (Second–Ninth Century A.D.)," in J.H. Charlesworth (ed.) *The Old Testament Pseudepigrapha*, vol. 1: *Apocalyptic Literature and Testaments*. New York: Doubleday and Co., 561–579.

Tischendorf, C. ed. 1866. *Apocalypses Apocryphae*. Leipzig: Mendelssohn.

Secondary Works

Ariantzi, D. 2012. *Kindheit in Byzanz: Emotionale, geistige und materielle Entwicklung im familiären Umfeld vom 6. bis zum 11. Jahrhundert*. Berlin and Boston: De Gruyter.

Bauckham, R. 1998. *The Fate of the Dead: Studies on the Jewish and Christian Apocalypses*. Leiden, Boston and Cologne: Brill.

Baun, J. 2007. *Tales from Another Byzantium: Celestial Journey and Local Community in the Medieval Greek Apocrypha*. Cambridge: Cambridge University Press.

41 Roueché 2013.

Constantinou, S. 2024. "The Martyr's Body: Sanctification through Blood, Milk, and Water," in P. Sarris (ed.) *Blood in Byzantium*. London and New York: Routledge, in press.

Constantinou, S., and A. Skouroumouni-Stavrinou. 2024. "The Other Mother: Ancient and Early Byzantine Approaches to Wet Nursing and Mothering," *Journal of Hellenic Studies* 145, in press.

Davis, S. J., and G. Gabra. 2004. "Editors' Introduction," in S.J. Davis (ed.) *The Popes of Egypt*, vol. 1: *The Early Coptic Papacy*. Cairo and New York: The American University in Cairo, ix–xi.

Gasparis, G. 2020. "Venetian Crete: The Historical Context," in Lymberopoulou 2020a, 60–116.

Gerstel, S.E.J., and P.S. Katsaphados. 2020. "Images of Hell and the Afterlife in the Churches of Laconia," in Lymberopoulou 2020a, 310–345.

Harris, W.V. 1994. "Child-Exposure in the Roman Empire," *Journal of Roman Studies* 84: 1–22.

Himmelfarb, M. 1983. *Tours of Hell: An Apocalyptic Form in Jewish and Christian Literature*. Philadelphia: University of Pennsylvania Press.

Jacab, A. 2003. "The Reception of the Apocalypse of Peter in Ancient Christianity," in J.N. Bremmer, and I. Czachesz (eds) *The Apocalypse of Peter*. Leuven: Peeters, 174–186.

Jolivet-Lévy, C. 1991. *Les églises byzantines de Cappadoce: Le programme iconographique de l'abside et de ses abords*. Paris: Editions du CNRS.

———. 2001. *La Cappadoce médiévale: Images et spiritualité*. Paris: Zodiaque.

———. 2006. "Prime rappresentazioni del Giudizio Universale nella Cappadocia bizantina," in V. Pace (ed.) *Alfa e omega: Il giudizio universale tra Oriente e Occidente*. Castel Bolognese: Itaca, 47–52.

Kalopissi-Verti, S. 2012. "The Murals of the Narthex: The Paintings of the Late Thirteenth and Fourteenth Centuries," in A. Weyl Carr, and A. Nicolaïdès (eds) *Asinou across Time: The Architecture and Murals of the Panagia Phorbiotissa, Cyprus*. Washington, DC: Dumbarton Oaks Research Library and Collection, 115–208.

Lymberopoulou, A. ed. 2020a. *Hell in the Byzantine World: A History of Art and Religion in Venetian Crete and the Eastern Mediterranean*, vol. 1: *Essays*. Cambridge: Cambridge University Press.

———. 2020b. "Hell on Crete," in Lymberopoulou and Duits 2020, 117–190.

Lymberopoulou, A., and R. Duits. eds. 2020. *Hell in the Byzantine World: A History of Art and Religion in Venetian Crete and the Eastern Mediterranean*, vol. 2: *A Catalogue of the Cretan Material*. Cambridge: Cambridge University Press.

Maltezou, C.A. 1984. "Η παρουσία της γυναίκας στις νοταριακές πράξεις της περιόδου της Βενετοκρατίας," *Κρητολογία* 16–19: 62–79.

Meyer, M. 2009. "Porneia: Quelques considerations sur la representation du péché de chair dans l'art byzantine," *Cahiers de civilisation médiévale* 52: 225–244.

Ousterhout, R.G. 2017. *Visualizing Community: Art, Material Culture, and Settlement in Byzantine Cappadocia*. Cambridge, MA: Harvard University Press.

Santschi, E. 1969. "Contrats de travail et d'apprentissage en Crète vénitienne au XIVᵉ siècle d'après quelques notaires," *Schweizerische Zeitschrift für Geschichte* 19: 34–74.

Sim, D.C. 1996. *Apocalyptic Eschatology in the Gospel of Matthew*. Cambridge: Cambridge University Press.

Stathakopoulos, D. 2020. "From Crete to Hell: The Textual Tradition on Punishments in the Afterlife and the Writings of Joseph Bryennios on Crete," in Lymberopoulou 2020a, 21–59.

Thierry, N., and M. Thierry. 1960. "L'église du jugement dernier à Ihlara (Yilanli Kilise)," *Anatolia* 5: 159–168.

Tsiodoulos, T. 2012. *Τιμωρία, η Σκοτεινή Όψη της Σεξουαλικότητας*. Athens: Futura.

Van Minnen, P. 2003. "The Greek Apocalypse of Peter," in J.N. Bremmer, and I. Czachesz (eds) *The Apocalypse of Peter*. Leuven: Peeters, 15–39.

Walters, C.C. 1989. "Christian Paintings from Tebtunis," *Journal of Egyptian Archaeology* 75: 191–208.

Warland, R. 2020. "'When the Visual Order was Established': The Last Judgement and Punishments in Hell in Byzantine Cappadocia," in Lymberopoulou 2020a, 237–280.

Zellmann-Rohrer, M. 2019. "The Woman Who Gave Her Breast for Hire: Notes on a Christian Wall-Painting from Tebtunis," *Journal of Egyptian Archaeology* 105: 297–303.

Part II
Medicine and Practice

4 Breastmilk as a Therapeutic Agent in Ancient and Early Byzantine Medical Literature*

Petros Bouras-Vallianatos

Introduction

The nutritive character of various kinds of milk and dairy products (for example, butter and cheese) was well known in antiquity, with medical authors making consistent use of them.[1] A decade ago when I was doing my PhD at King's College London, situated on the Strand, a nearby shop in Covent Garden was selling fresh ice cream made of breastmilk. At the time I was shocked since I had never thought about breastmilk being consumed by adults. The so-called "Baby Gaga"-flavour ice cream was regularly selling out, although it was extremely expensive compared to the usual ice cream. Breastmilk was pasteurized before being churned with Madagascan vanilla pods and lemon zest. It was selling for about £14 per serving compared to £4 for regular ice cream. The London-based ice cream company The Licktators re-launched the product in 2015 as "Royal Baby Gaga" at £19.99 per 500 ml in celebration of the birth of Princess Charlotte and to remind people of the benefits of breastfeeding.[2] All proceeds were donated to a breastfeeding charity. The product was advertised as natural, organic, "free-range," and highly nutritional.[3] Subsequently, I found out that several sites on the Internet, especially in the US and the UK, were functioning as platforms for lactating mothers who wanted to sell their excess milk for newborns or even adults for various scientifically unproven benefits, such as (allegedly) building muscle or beating cancer. These mothers usually emphasized their healthy and organic diet, and quite recently one could even find mothers who were on a gluten-free or vegan diet, eager to sell their breastmilk.[4]

* I would like to thank Stavroula Constantinou, Aspasia Skouroumouni-Stavrinou, and the anonymous referee for their helpful comments. I am also grateful to Anne Grons, Amber Jacob, and Nicola Reggiani for useful bibliographical suggestions. This study is dedicated to Tania Siahanidou, Professor of Pediatrics-Neonatology at the University of Athens, for taking care of Aristotelis in the first days of his life.

1 See the comprehensive survey by Rzeźnicka and Kokoszko 2020. All translations are mine, unless otherwise indicated.
2 Wikipedia. https://en.wikipedia.org/wiki/The_Licktators. Accessed 4 April 2022; Mail Online. 27 April 2015.https://www.dailymail.co.uk/femail/food/article-3057274/Breast-milk-ice-cream-released-time-royal-birth.html.
3 BBC News. 24 February 2011. https://www.bbc.com/news/uk-england-london-12569011.
4 E.g. Only the Breast. https://www.onlythebreast.com/. Accessed 4 April 2022. A mother has recently admitted that she made more than $20,000 by selling her breastmilk online to strangers: Mail

DOI: 10.4324/9781003265658-6

All this raises various ethical and moral concerns, which could be discussed at length. Nevertheless, the consumption of breastmilk, even by adults, is not just a modern fashion. For example, Galen's (AD 129–ca. 216/217) *Therapeutic Method* (*MM*) contains a passage involving a spectacular scene in which the Pergamene physician actively encouraged someone suffering from *phthisis*, a severe lung disease often identified by modern scholars as tuberculosis,[5] to drink milk by suckling a lactating mother or, if that was not possible, a female ass:

> I gave [him] ass's milk, after leading the ass to the room in which he lay sick. I was completely convinced that, if it was possible for the man himself to suckle the ass, he would have been cured in this way very quickly indeed … And, certainly, milk is best if someone draws it from the women themselves, as Euryphon and Herodicus did, for they had such a degree of confidence in this with regard to the restoration of bodies that they directed those who suffered wasting due to phthisis, when they had applied their mouths to the nipple of the woman's breast, to suck the milk. Since most people cannot bear to do this, it is better to transfer the warm milk from the breasts to the stomach of the patient as quickly as possible. Human [milk] is best because it is from the same species. However, since many are reluctant to use a woman's milk like infants, you must give them asses' milk, as if they were asses.[6]
>
> ἐδίδομεν ὄνειον γάλα τὴν ὄνον εἰς τὸν οἶκον εἰσάγοντες ἐν ᾧ κατέκειτο. ἐπεπείσμεθα γὰρ ὡς μάλιστα μὲν, εἰ αὐτὸν τὸν ἄνθρωπον οἷόν τε ἦν θηλάζειν τὴν ὄνον, οὕτως ἂν ἐθεραπεύθη τάχιστα … καὶ δὴ καὶ τὸ γάλα κάλλιστον μὲν εἰ ἐξ αὐτῶν τῶν θηλῶν ἐπισπῷτό τις, ὥσπερ Εὐρυφῶν καὶ Ἡρόδικος (Εὐρυφῶν καὶ Ἡρόδικος corr. Nutton in Johnston et Horsley: Εὐρυφῶν καὶ Ἡρόδοτος καὶ Πρόδικος Kühn) ἀξιοῦσιν· οἳ τοσοῦτον ἄρα τεθαρρήκεσαν αὐτῷ πρὸς ἀναθρέψιν σωμάτων ὥστε καὶ τοὺς ὑπὸ φθόης συντετηκότας ἐκέλευον ἐντιθεμένου τοῦ τιτθοῦ τῆς γυναικὸς τὴν θηλὴν βδάλλειν τὸ γάλα. τοῦτο δὲ οὐχ ὑπομενόντων ποιεῖν τῶν πλείστων ἄμεινόν ἐστιν ὅτι τάχιστα θερμὸν μεταφέρειν ἐκ τῶν τιτθῶν εἰς τὴν κοιλίαν τοῦ κάμνοντος αὐτό. τὸ μὲν οὖν ἀνθρώπειον ὡς ἂν ὁμόφυλον ἄριστον. ἐπεὶ δ᾽ ὑπομένουσιν οἱ πολλοὶ γάλα γυναικὸς προσφέρεσθαι δίκην παιδίων, ὡς ὄνοις αὐτοῖς δοτέον ὄνειον γάλα. (Gal. *MM* 2.6, 10.474.6–475.7K, ed. Kühn 1825; trans. Johnston and Horsley 2011, 262–264)

Having started with this analogy, which provides an introduction to ancient approaches to the use of breastmilk in medicine, it is worth pointing out that in antiquity medical authors actively encouraged the consumption of human milk for certain medical conditions, as we will see below. In this chapter, I would like to

---

Online. 16 October 2020. https://www.dailymail.co.uk/femail/article-8846853/Cash-strapped-mother-receives-backlash-making-close-20k-selling-breast-milk-strangers.html.

5 On *phthisis* in ancient medical texts, see Grmek 1989. Cf. Stamatu 2005.

6 For a discussion of this passage, see also Chapter 6 in this volume.

examine critically the role of breastmilk as a therapeutic agent in ancient and early Byzantine medical literature. I shall focus on both dietetics and pharmacology, although sometimes the boundaries between these two areas are not entirely clear in the medical texts under examination.[7] Particular attention will be paid to how an understanding of the curative role of breastmilk developed over the centuries.

The Classical Background

The first group of references to the use of breastmilk in ancient Greek medical literature are found in three gynaecological books in the Hippocratic corpus, the so-called *On Diseases of Women* (*Mul.*), which are dated to the late fifth/early fourth century BC.[8] Breastmilk is mentioned 18 times as an ingredient of a composite drug.[9] In most cases, it is used in combination with other ingredients in pessaries for uterine cleaning, and for drawing lochia and blood from the uterus. It can also be seen in three recipes for softening the cervix, two for promoting pregnancy, one for when the uterus does not retain the semen, one for a pessary if there is wind in the womb, and one in the form of an eye salve along with sap of black poplar for albugo, i.e. a white speck on the eye. All these composite medicaments consist mostly of two or three ingredients, including vegetal (for example, mandrake juice, peppercorn, and scammony), animal (for example, blister beetles, liver of sea turtle, marrow of goose, ox, or deer), and mineral ones (for example, lead and iron). Breastmilk is also used twice in pregnancy tests: in one it is given along with a plant called *boutyros* in the fasting state. If the woman burps, she is pregnant; if not, she is not. In the other, it is used to make bread; if it burns in fire, the child is a boy; if not, it is a girl.[10] In addition to the recipes mentioned above, we can find two more recipes for cleansing pessaries in *On the Nature of Woman* (*Nat. Mul.*), which are identical or quasi-identical to recipes in *On Diseases of Women*.[11] Lastly, there is one more mention in *On Diseases* (*Morb.*), where breastmilk is recommended as a simple drug for pain and pus in the ear.[12] So, apart from the last recipe, they are all clearly destined for women only.

Interestingly, in five cases in *On Diseases of Women* – one to promote pregnancy, one for a cleansing pessary, two for pessaries to soften the uterus, and one for a pregnancy test – the breastmilk is specified as milk produced for a male child

7 Cf. Totelin 2015.
8 The third book is also called *On Infertile Women*. For a brief introduction with references to relevant bibliography, see Craik 2015, 196–206.
9 [Hippoc.] *Mul.* 1.74, 8.156.8–11L; 1.74, 8.158.16–160.3L; 1.74, 8.160.12–13L; 1.75, 8.166.2–5L; 1.75, 8.166.7–12L; 1.78, 8.172.14–15L; 1.78, 8.176.14–16L; 1.78, 8.180.11–13L; 1.84, 8.206.12–14L; 1.84, 8.206.18–21L; 1.84, 8.208.7–14L; 1.105, 8.228.12–13L; 2.158, 8.336.7–10L; 2.162, 8.340.5–12L; 2.179, 8.362.8–15L; 2.205, 8.394.7–10L; 2.205, 8.396.3–6L; 3.243, 8.456.24–458.2L, ed. Littré 1853.
10 [Hippoc.] *Mul.* 3.214, 8.414.17–19L; 3.216, 8.416.21–23L.
11 [Hippoc.] *Nat. Mul.* 32, 7.352.13–14L, ed. Littré 1851 = 33.2–3, ed. Bourbon 2008 (identical with 8.176.14–16L); 109, 7.426.4–8L = 91.17–92.1 Bourbon (semi-identical with 8.336.8L).
12 [Hippoc.] *Morb.* 3.2, 7.120.8–9L = 72.1–3, ed. Potter 1980.

(*kourotrophos*).[13] This may be seen as reminiscent of influences from Egyptian medicine.[14] In fact, Tanja Pommerening has convincingly shown that the second Hippocratic pregnancy test could be considered a loan translation of a recipe surviving in the Egyptian Papyrus Berlin 3038 dated to 1250 BC.[15] The milk of a mother who has borne a male child is cited several times in Egyptian medical texts and has a ritualistic origin related to the goddess Isis and her infant son, Horus.[16] Although the original ritual significance might have been lost by the classical period, Julie Laskaris argues that the use of milk intended for a male child reflects the overall "fears regarding the breast and breast milk – and women's physical nature in general" in ancient Greece.[17] Still, we cannot exclude the independent development of some of these recipes in Egypt and Greece, as Laurence Totelin has pointed out.[18]

As well as from the references in the recipes of the Hippocratic corpus, we also learn about the use of breastmilk in classical medicine from a later source. In particular, Galen informs us three times about breastmilk being recommended for the treatment of *phthisis* by two late fifth-century BC physicians from Knidos, Euryphon (460–400 BC) and Herodikos (440–400 BC).[19] From the abovementioned passage of Galen's *Therapeutic Method*, we learn that the two physicians also insisted on using milk straight from the breast, lest it lose its nutritional value. In fact, they advocated adults suckling directly from the woman's breast. Interestingly, at least according to later sources, Euryphon was interested in gynaecology. For example, he is mentioned three times by the first-/early second-century AD Methodist author Soranos in his work *Gynaecology* (*Gyn.*), who informs us that he recommended the use of drugs for conception and for expelling the placenta[20]; for the latter, he also used a sort of ladder to shake women bound to it.[21] He also appears to have treated uterine prolapse by suspending women by their feet.[22]

---

13 [Hippoc.] *Mul.* 1.75, 8.166.2–5L; 1.84, 8.206.18–21L; 2.158, 8.336.7–10L; 2.162, 8.340.5–12L; 3.214, 8.414.17–19L.
14 See the evidence presented by Laskaris (2008, 460), who also states that the similarities between the recipes for unspecified milk and those from Egyptian papyri suggest that even the former were originally "kourotrophic" recipes. Cf. Dawson 1932, 12–15.
15 Pommerening 2010. Interestingly, the Greek word *boutyros* in this text does not signify "butter," but a plant of the gourd family. It seems to derive from the Egyptian *bdd*, the term for bottle gourd.
16 Pommerening 2015.
17 Laskaris 2008, 461.
18 Totelin (2009, 179–184) provides further bibliographical references on those who are for and those who are against the idea of Egyptian influence.
19 Apart from the passage cited above, there are two more references in the Galenic corpus, although these do not provide any further information. Gal. *On Good and Bad Humour* 4, 6.775.7–15K, ed. Kühn 1823 = 83.27–84.6, ed. Ieraci Bio 1987: εἰς τὰ φθινώδη πάθη; Gal. *On Withering* 9, 7.701.8–12K, ed. Kühn 1824: ἐπὶ τῶν φθινόντων. On Euryphon and Herodikos, see the entries by Manetti (2008a and 2008b).
20 Sor. *Gyn.* 1.11, 1.32.48–49 Burguière; 2.2, 2.11.17–21 Burguière, ed. Burguière 1988–2000.
21 Sor. *Gyn.* 2.2, 2.11.21–22 Burguière.
22 Sor. *Gyn.* 4.6, 4.25.66–70 Burguière. See also Gal. *On the Anatomy of the Uterus* 9, 2.900.15–16K, ed. Kühn 1821 = 48.23–24, ed. Nickel 1971, who refers to Euryphon's observations on the anatomy of the uterus.

This, together with the evidence presented above from the Hippocratic corpus, confirms that the early use of breastmilk in medicine must have originally been developed as an outcome of practical experience connected with the care of the female body. There is no other classical source confirming the use of adult breastfeeding for medical purposes. The next mention of the curative effects of breastmilk comes from the Roman Imperial period.

Evidence from the Roman Imperial Period

Both Greek and Latin authors made consistent use of breastmilk in their therapeutic recommendations, expanding its application to a wide variety of affections. However, some distinctions should be made in respect of the origins of evidence coming from a number of medical sources. For example, Dioskorides' work attempts to give an exhaustive list of all known simple drugs, although sometimes it is obvious that the author has little familiarity with some of them. Pliny's *Natural History* (*NH*) is clearly a work of an encyclopaedic nature. To some extent, the same could be said of the Galenic pharmacological works or the vast medical compendium by the sixth-century AD author Aetios of Amida, which were clearly not meant to serve everyday needs. On the other hand, the collection of recipes by the second-century AD medical author Aelius Promotus, or later the work of the sixth-century medical writer Alexander of Tralles, seems to be more closely connected with everyday practice. The same could be said to some extent of surviving recipes in scattered papyri, although in most cases a proper contextualization is not possible.

To start with evidence from Latin authors, Scribonius Largus (ca. AD 1–50) is the author of a collection of pharmacological recipes in Latin (*Prescriptions* (*Comp.*)) who makes four mentions of breastmilk: as an ingredient of composite drugs in two cases, namely for various eye conditions, including pustules, redness, and swelling, and for the treatment of gout.[23] In two more cases, Scribonius recommends the consumption of breastmilk in order to eliminate symptoms similar to those of *phthisis* and dropsy resulting from the bites of the sea hare and a kind of poisonous beetle (*bouprēstis*), respectively.[24] This recalls Euryphon's and Herodikos' corresponding advice for *phthisis*, although, unlike his predecessors, Scribonius does not specify how the patient should be given the breastmilk. Celsus lived in the reign of Tiberius (AD 14–37) and wrote the Latin work *On Medicine*, which is largely based on ancient Greek medical knowledge; he refers to the use of breastmilk four times.[25] These references are helpful in making some connections between the evidence from the classical period and that from later centuries. First, breastmilk mixed with the juice of squirting cucumber appears as an ingredient in a pessary for inducing

---

23 Scribonius Largus, *Comp.* 26, 114.15–18 Sconocchia; 158, 158.1–2 Sconocchia, ed. Sconocchia 2020.
24 Scribonius Largus, *Comp.* 186, 218.4–7 Sconocchia; 190, 220.20–222.2 Sconocchia.
25 On the use of milk in Celsus' work, see Kokoszko and Dybała 2016.

menstruation,[26] which recalls the above-mentioned Hippocratic recipes, where the squirting cucumber (*elatērion*) was used three times in combination with breast-milk in the *On Diseases of Women*: twice for a cleansing pessary and once together with pepper for a pessary to soften the uterus.[27] In the other three references by Celsus, breastmilk is recommended twice for inflammation of the eye and once for inflammation and pain in the ear.[28] In the former cases, it is recommended that eye salves be added when the inflammation is severe to make the application milder, while in the case of the ear remedy, it is used along with frankincense in combination with other medicines. The use of breastmilk for eye and ear conditions was very rare in the Hippocratic corpus, where we find only one reference to it for the treatment of albugo. However, from the first centuries AD onwards, it became by far the most common use of breastmilk cited in medical authors.

Pliny the Elder (AD 23/24–79) in his *Natural History* offers the most extensive account of human breastmilk. In the specific chapter devoted to it, he refers to the therapeutic effect of breastmilk in chronic fevers, lung affections, affections of the stomach and bowels, the so-called "gnawing sensation," gynaecological affections, such as pains in the uterus, gout, and as an emmenagogue and also for poisoning by the sea hare, a kind of poisonous beetle (*bouprēstis*) mentioned above, the plant dorycnium,[29] and henbane.[30] There is particular emphasis on eye and ear affections. In addition to details about the direct injection of breastmilk into the eye or its use along with honey and frankincense or with goose grease for earache, Pliny includes some information with superstitious connotations. For example, he notes that the use of milk from a mother and daughter can save an individual from any eye affection for the rest of their life. Interestingly, reference to the use of breastmilk from a mother who has given birth to a male child (*marem enixa*) recurs here with an additional note on the even greater effectiveness of the milk from a mother with male twins (*geminos maris*).[31] Furthermore, in Pliny, one finds the only explicit reference in the ancient corpus of Greek and Latin authors to the use of milk from a woman who has given birth to a female child, which was to be used only for the treatment of facial diseases.[32] The latter confirms that breastmilk from a woman with a male child was not always readily available, so the author provides a

26 Celsus, *On Medicine* 5.21.1b, 207.15–18, ed. Marx 1915. *Cucumis silvestre* in Latin and *elatērion* in Greek is usually identified with *Ecballium elaterium*. See André 1985, s.v. cucumis on p. 80.2, and elatērium on p. 93.1.
27 [Hippoc.] *Mul.* 1.84, 8.206.12L; 1.84, 8.208.9L; 2.205, 8.396.5L.
28 Celsus, *On Medicine* 6.6.8b, 263.12–13 Marx; 6.6.14, 266.24–7 Marx; 6.7.1e, 276.11–13 Marx.
29 *OLD*, s.v. dorycnion: "a kind of nightshade."
30 Pliny the Elder, *NH* 28.7.21, 4.169.2–33, ed. Mayhoff and Jan 1875–1906.
31 On multiple births in antiquity, see Dasen 1997.
32 Reference to the use of milk from a woman who has given birth to a female child (*gala gynaikeion thēlytrophou*) is also found in the pseudo-Galenic work *On Procurable Remedies* 3, 14.556.18–557.1K, ed. Kühn 1827, where it is recommended for anointing the head in cases of headache. This work is of uncertain date. It is worth noting that the third book contains recipes which clearly date to the later Byzantine period. On this, see Bouras-Vallianatos 2021, 1005, n. 215. A later reference in the Latin work by Marcellus is also attested; see n. 104 below.

recommendation for the use of milk from a woman with a female child (*feminam enixa*). No rational explanation can be offered for the specific connection of the latter with facial diseases, and it should be seen as recalling folk medicine, something which is often included in Pliny's accounts.[33]

In his long *On Medical Substances* (*Materia medica*), the Greek author Dioskorides (fl. 1st c. AD) devotes a specific chapter to breastmilk as a simple drug and mentions this substance another six times as an ingredient of a composite drug for a variety of diseases.[34] His account has some similarities with that of Pliny, especially as regards its use for gnawing stomach, fever, *phthisis*, gout, and being bitten by sea hares; there is also one reference to eye and another to ear affections. Moreover, it is here that one finds the first references to its beneficial effects in the treatment of headache, epilepsy, and spleen and liver diseases. In one case, the term *arrenotokou* is used rather than the most common word used in classical texts for the milk of a nursing mother with a male child: *kourotrophou*.[35] The former word resembles the one found in the sole surviving reference to the medical use of breastmilk (*arsenikou*) in a papyrus (P. CtYBR inv. 1443) dated to the late first– early second century AD. In this case, the breastmilk of a woman nursing a male child is mixed with juniper berries to make a vaginal pessary.[36]

I would now like to turn to the second-century AD, probably Alexandrian, physician Aelius Promotus, who is the author of a pharmacological manual, the so-called *Dynameron*.[37] This is not a huge work; it has just 130 chapters. Each chapter deals with a certain disease and consists of recipes for composite drugs, often mixed with advice on the use of simples. In his proem, the author appears to have practised medicine for many years and refers to his first-hand knowledge (*peira*) of drugs, which he was eager to write down and share with the new generation of physicians (*paides*).[38] In fact, Aelius Promotus repeatedly refers to his experience in his work in an attempt to show that he has tested and proven the effectiveness of a certain drug,[39] much as the practising physician and medical author Alexander of Tralles used *peira* and its cognates in the sixth century.[40] Thus, his work could be seen as representing the most commonly used drugs, by contrast, for example, with the two Galenic works on compound drugs, which are eight times longer and attest to Galen's attempt to include every known drug.

33 Stannard 1982.
34 Dioskorides, *Materia medica* 2.70, 1.145.12–23 Wellmann; 1.26, 1.31.1–2 Wellmann; 2.78.3, 1.160.5–6 Wellmann; 2.136, 1.208.9–10 Wellmann; 4.64.4, 2.220.4–5 Wellmann; 5.126.1, 3.94.6–7 Wellmann; 5.127.2, 3.95.14–15 Wellmann, ed. Wellmann 1907–1914.
35 Dioskorides, *Materia medica* 5.84.3, 3.56.12–13 Wellmann.
36 See the new edition of this Egyptian papyrus along with the corresponding commentary by Monte 2022, 88.10–12, 94–95.
37 On this author, his works and *floruit*, see Crismani 2002, 7–17; see also Mavroudis 2013, 244–259.
38 Aelius Promotus, *Dynameron* pr., 40.1–7, ed. Crismani 2002.
39 Among the numerous cases, see e.g. Aelius Promotus, *Dynameron* 3.13, 48.6 Crismani; 29.7, 102.2–3 Crismani; 59.14, 150.6 Crismani; 60.8, 152.4–5 Crismani; 126.1, 240.13–14 Crismani.
40 See n. 89, below.

In Aelius Promotus, there are in total eight references to breastmilk.[41] It is used three times for ear affections, including ringing in the ears and earache, and mixed with vegetal ingredients, such as centaury, myrrh, and opium.[42] In two further cases, it is recommended as a simple for washing out eyes or as a basis for the application of a collyrium for ulcers in the eyes.[43] In the third case related to eyes, it is part of a composite drug for cataract that includes animal (cock's marrow), vegetal (wild rue and fennel), and mineral ingredients (*chalkanthon*).[44] All these cases clearly confirm its popularity and potentially proven effectiveness in these kinds of ailments. In the last two cases, it is recommended as a simple drug in a nasal drench for cleaning the brain and as an ingredient in a soporific pessary along with opium, castoreum, and myrrh, which is administered rectally.[45]

Before I proceed to discuss evidence from Galen, I would like to add a few words on some aspects of modern research confirming the immunological efficacy of breastmilk, which may explain its extensive use for eye and ear affections in premodern medicine. The use of breastmilk for eye affections in newborns is recommended by experts even today with extremely good results. Over the last three decades, several studies have reported the inhibitory effect of breastmilk on tested neonatal pathogens, including *Staphylococcus aureus* (a common cause of eye infections), *Candida albicans* (a common cause of neonatal infections associated with significant mortality), and *Acinetobacter baumanii* (responsible for bloodstream and respiratory tract infections in neonates).[46] A more recent study by National Jewish Health and the University of Iowa published in 2019 gives milk even more credit as a substance with strong antibiotic characteristics. This study has identified that the presence of glycerol monolaurate (GML) in human breastmilk is 20 times greater than in cow's milk, while infant formula has been shown to have none.[47]

Colostrum is even more effective than mature breastmilk, and it has recently been suggested as an alternative prophylactic option to antibiotics for neonatal conjunctivitis (an infection of the conjunctive membrane in the eye), which can, in extreme cases, lead to blindness.[48] This is most probably connected with leukocytes and various kinds of immunoglobulins, immune cells, and antibodies that

41 One can also find a reference to the consumption of breastmilk in cases of poisoning with henbane in the work *On Venomous Animals and Poisonous Drugs* ascribed to Aelius Promotus 66, 73.6–7, ed. Ihm 1995.
42 Aelius Promotus, *Dynameron* 75.3, 166.15–17 Crismani; 78.4, 168.12 Crismani; 78.12, 168.25–26 Crismani.
43 Aelius Promotus, *Dynameron* 96.13, 190.8–14 Crismani; 96.26, 192.33–37 Crismani.
44 Aelius Promotus, *Dynameron* 101.9, 202.15–18 Crismani. *LSJ* gives "solution of blue vitriol (copper sulphate)" for "χάλκανθον."
45 Aelius Promotus, *Dynameron* 10.1, 58.16–18 Crismani; 90.1, 180.2–4 Crismani.
46 Among the various studies available, see the most recent ones by Aakhila and Feminamol 2021; and Ackerman et al. 2018.
47 Schlievert et al. 2019. Glycerol monolaurate (GML) is a monoglyceride well known for its antibacterial and antiviral activity *in vitro*.
48 Ghaemi et al. 2014. On colostrum, see also Chapter 5 in this volume.

are contained in the colostrum. Interestingly, ancient and early Byzantine authors do not make any reference to the use of colostrum (*pyar* or *prōton gala*) for therapeutic purposes.[49] In fact, medical authors did not recommend the consumption of colostrum by newborns, since it was considered too thick and hard to digest; newborns, they said, should be fed with honey or with a mixture of honey and water (*hydromeli*) or a mixture of honey with goat's milk during the first two to three days of their lives, and then with breastmilk.[50]

To return to the evidence from the Imperial period, I would like to briefly refer to the case of Aretaios of Cappadocia, a very little-studied author, whose exact dates are a matter of debate.[51] He was probably active in the first century AD, and although he gives importance to the role of *pneuma*, he does not seem to be formally affiliated with the so-called Pneumatist school, whose founder is considered to be Athenaios of Attalia (1st c. AD).[52] Aretaios refers to breastmilk only once, when he recommends its consumption from a mother who has recently given birth to a male child (*gynaikos neotokou kai kourotrophou*) for those suffering from syncope associated with fevers and inflammations, a heart disease related to sudden loss of strength and a term much wider in scope then than now.[53] In order to emphasize the importance of breastmilk in this case, Aretaios literally describes those patients as needing nursing like newborns (*hokōs artitokoi paides*),[54] although he does not explicitly refer to the act of suckling as in the classical case from Euryphon and Herodikos that we saw above. Aretaios is, however, the only post-classical source that retains the exact Hippocratic term, *kourotrophos*, to mean a woman who has given birth to a male child.

In his huge corpus, Galen makes numerous references to the use of breastmilk for various diseases, in line with his predecessors. He pays particular attention to its anti-inflammatory action, suggesting its use in composite drugs for eye and ear affections,[55] and even for inflammation of the anus.[56] Furthermore, Galen is the

---

49 There are cases referring to the "first milk" produced by an ass or a horse (Aet. *Tetrabiblos* (*Tetr.*) 11.18, 103.3–4, eds Daremberg and Ruelle 1879) or later on by a goat (e.g. *Hippiatrica Ludgunensia* 44.5, 2.285.4, eds Oder and Hoppe 1924–1927), and other cases where it is not clear whether the sources refer to human or animal colostrum (e.g. Aet. *Tetr.* 16.107, 142.18–19, ed. Zervos 1901). I have managed to identify only one reference to the use of human colostrum (*prōton gala gynaikeion*) for therapeutic purposes, in the Byzantine author Paul of Nicaea (ca. 9th/10th c. AD), *De re medica* 65, 145.15–16, ed. Ieraci Bio 1996, who recommends its consumption for the treatment of dysentery. Cf. Rzeźnicka and Kokoszko 2020, 141–147.

50 Sor. *Gyn.* 2.7, 2.26.48–57 and 2.27.77–84 Burguière; Orib. *Synopsis for Eustathios* (*Eust.*) 5.5, 3.155.16–18, ed. Raeder 1926; Aet. *Tetr.* 4.3, 1.360.22–25, ed. Olivieri 1935–1950.

51 Leven 2005, 80–81.

52 Nutton 2013, 210, 386, n. 19.

53 Aretaios, *On the Causes and Symptoms of Acute Diseases* 2.3, 21.27–23.12, ed. Hude 1958.

54 Aretaios, *Therapeutics of Acute Diseases* 2.3, 130.25–29 Hude.

55 E.g. Gal. *On the Composition of Drugs According to Places* (*Comp. Med. Loc.*) 3.1, 12.601.12K, 12.602.6K, 12.634.10–11K, 12.641.8K; 4.8, 12.750.1K, 12.751.18K, 12.795.2K, ed. Kühn 1826. See also Kokoszko 2016, 37–38, 45.

56 Gal. *Comp. Med. Loc.* 9.6, 13.309.13K, ed. Kühn 1827. For the therapeutic uses of breastmilk, see also Chapter 6 in this volume.

only author of the Roman Imperial period who actively recommends adult consumption of breastmilk by suckling for the treatment of *phthisis*, something he does three times in his corpus. In all cases, he gives the example of the aforementioned authors, Euryphon and Herodikos, in order to strengthen his argument.[57] He notes that in the case of those who are not willing to suck from a mother directly, breastmilk should be consumed as soon as possible, which aligns with modern recommendations on milk storage. For example, the Breastfeeding Network in Scotland suggests that the maximum time for the use of milk stored at normal room temperature is six hours.[58]

The adult consumption of human milk seems to have been socially acceptable under certain circumstances in ancient Rome. There are, for example, stories about aged, imprisoned parents who survived because they received breastmilk from a daughter.[59] The *columna lactaria*, the so-called "milk column" in ancient Rome where orphans and infants whose mother could not breastfeed them were given milk, suggests that there was a high demand for this commodity in the city.[60] Tara Mulder goes so far as to suggest that mothers could have provided breastmilk there even to adults for the treatment of certain diseases.[61] Although the latter cannot be excluded, one should take into consideration the overall concept of someone who is severely ill suckling from the mother of a baby. Any person with such a disease would have been considered a great threat to the woman, who would want to stay healthy in order to be able to feed her baby and not spoil her milk or – in the case of a wet nurse – to be able use her breastmilk as her main source of subsistence. In my view, the chances of finding a woman eager to give her milk directly to someone with *phthisis*, even for a considerable sum of money, would have been minimal. One, of course, could have received breastmilk indirectly from a mother who removed milk from her breast manually or using a breast pump, since archaeological evidence confirms that breast pumps were most probably in use, at least in the Roman era.[62] The other thing that we learn from Galen's accounts is that asses' milk could be substituted for human milk in the first instance. In fact, Galen reports that asses' milk is the best animal milk for this particular purpose, since it is very thin, does not curdle, and is distributed rapidly throughout the body.[63] Modern research has shown that ass's milk is particularly rich in minerals and vitamins, and it is also

57 See n. 19, above.
58 The Breastfeeding Network. https://www.breastfeedingnetwork.org.uk/wp-content/pdfs/BFN %20Expressing%20Leaflet%202019.pdf
59 See Mulder 2017, who examines critically the relevant sources. See also Chapter 9 in this volume.
60 On the *columna lactaria*, see Beagon 2005, 314.
61 Mulder 2017, 239.
62 Gourevitch 1990. Cf. Centlivres Challet 2016.
63 Gal. *MM* 2.6, 10.475.7–12K. On the various kinds of animal milk and their characteristics in Galen, see *On the Capacities of Foodstuffs* (*Alim. Fac.*) 3.15, 6.681.12–689.8K = 199.5–206.4, ed. Wilkins 2013, and *On the Capacities of Simple Drugs* (*SMT*) 10.2, 12.263.12–266.6K.

reported as a significant source of folic acid, including 0.83 μM, unlike human milk and cow's milk, which contain only 0.37 and 0.02 μM, respectively.[64]

The role of breastmilk as a dietary agent for preserving the health of infants was particularly important for premodern societies, especially in the absence of modern substitutes, such as formula milk. Galen emphasizes the nutritive quality of mother's milk in various parts of his corpus. For example, in the *On the Capacities of Simple Drugs* (*SMT*), he states that human milk is superior to that of various animals, especially if the woman has a good diet (*kalōs diaitōmenēs*) and her body is in good condition (*euektousēs*).[65] If the milk is not of good quality and is full of unhealthy humour as a result of her diet, it could infect the body of a newborn with ulcers[66]; harmful (*mochthēron*) milk could also be the cause of abscesses in infants.[67] The quality of milk could allegedly also be affected by sexual intercourse. Galen argues that it becomes less sweet, and harmful, and if a mother wants to get pregnant again, she should find a wet nurse whose milk is better in taste, appearance, and odour.[68]

The author who pays most attention to the production and quality of good milk is the late first-/early second-century AD Greek physician Soranos. He practised at Rome and followed the medical theoretical concept of Methodism, although he often pays more attention to the individual characteristics of patients.[69] He is mostly known for his long work *Gynaecology* in four books, which was particularly influential in the Middle Ages.[70] Book 2 focusses on the care of the newborn. Soranos devotes particular thematic units to "The selection of a wet nurse," "Testing the milk," "How to conduct the regimen of the nurse," and "What one should do if the milk stops, or becomes spoiled or thick or thin." As regards choosing a wet nurse, the focus is on how to ensure that the milk will be of good quality, judging this by factors ranging from the skin colour of the woman to the size of her breasts and nipples, her abstinence from sexual intercourse and drinking.[71] According to Soranos, the testing of milk is of primary importance, since low-quality milk does not protect the infant from potential diseases. Thus, he makes a direct reference to the role of milk as an agent for preserving infant health.[72] He then goes on to

---

64 Vincenzetti et al. 2021. A lack of folic acid is the main reason for babies developing megaloblastic anaemia shortly after birth. Goat's milk is also very low in folic acid. See Bourbou 2010, 165–166, who discusses the nutritive value of various kinds of milk in light of osteoarchaeological evidence from Byzantine Crete.

65 Gal. *SMT* 10.2, 12.265.6–8K.

66 Gal. *Alim. Fac.* 3.15, 6.686.2–5K = 203.7–10 Wilkins. According to Galen, breastmilk, like semen, was generated from perfectly concocted blood: *On the Function of the Parts of the Body* (*UP*) 16.10, 4.322.9–10K, ed. Kühn 1822 = 2.419.21–22, ed. Helmreich 1907–1909. On stories of milk that poisons children, see Gourevitch 2001, and Totelin 2019, 38–39.

67 Gal. *Comp. Med. Loc.* 6.9, 12.988.8–9K.

68 Gal. *Hygiene* 1.9, 6.46.15–47.10K = 22.19–29, ed. Koch 1923.

69 Hanson and Green 1994, 988–1005.

70 Hanson and Green 1994, 1042–1060.

71 Sor. *Gyn.* 2.8, 2.28.1–32.117 Burguière.

72 Sor. *Gyn.* 2.9, 2.32.6–33.16 Burguière.

discuss various kinds of tests related to the colour, smell, composition, density, and taste of the milk, and whether the milk becomes sour quickly when stored. For each characteristic, he gives a list of criteria. For example, the right colour and taste are medium white and sweet, respectively, and so on.[73] He also suggests that the milk of a wet nurse should be tested and its quality should remain the best.[74] In terms of regimen, he considers a wide variety of inputs, suggesting moderate exercise, consumption of foodstuffs that do not contain noxious humours (for example, bread, egg yolks, fish, and pork), and avoidance of vegetables, such as garlic and onion and all kinds of preserved meat.[75] Interestingly, he also recommends taking *oinomeli* (a mixture of honey and wine) 40 days after the start of breastfeeding, followed, later on, by some white wine.[76] Soranos' exciting account ends with some advice on how to rectify spoiled milk, for example, by massaging the breast, exercising, and bathing.[77] Finally, it should be noted that neither Galen nor Soranos refers anywhere in their surviving corpora to the allegedly better quality of milk produced by a mother who has given birth to a male child. The texts of these authors are generally free of superstitious connotations and this kind of cliché, although Galen is not always as rational as one might expect.[78] This designation is also absent in the corpus of the surviving papyri that have preserved contracts for wet nurses, which will be discussed below. This suggests that the option of using milk from a mother with a male child probably played very little role in reality, especially when good milk quality was not always easily procurable.

A last comment should be made about the significant number of surviving wet-nursing contracts recorded in late Roman and early Byzantine Greek papyri from Egypt. These are mainly dated to between the first century BC and the fourth century AD, while there is a single surviving papyrus dated to the third century BC. In this rich body of information, there are some stipulations that align with the relevant Galenic and Soranic advice. For example, there are several mentions of the fact that the quality of the wet nurse's milk should be pure and unadulterated (*katharō kai aphthorō*).[79] There is also a reference commonly found in many papyri to the need for the nurse to be careful not to spoil the milk (*mē phtheirousan to gala*), perhaps suggesting that she needs to follow a good regimen and not suffer from any diseases that may affect its quality, in addition to further specified provisions of not sleeping with a man (*mēd' androkoitousan*), becoming pregnant again (*mēd'*

---

73 Sor. *Gyn.* 2.9, 2.33.16–34.63 Burguière.
74 Sor. *Gyn.* 2.9, 2.34.64–35.78 Burguière. On this, see also Aboul Aly 1998.
75 Sor. *Gyn.* 2.10, 2.35.1–38.87 Burguière.
76 Sor. *Gyn.* 2.10, 2.38.88–39.100 Burguière. It is worth pointing out that in two of the surviving wet-nursing contracts wine is included among the supplies provided, i.e. P. Bour. Inv. 43, 140.15, ed. Manca Masciadri and Montevecchi 1984; and P. Ross. Georg. II 18, 148.313 Manca Masciadri and Montevecchi. Cf. Aboul Aly 1996, 90.
77 Sor. *Gyn.* 2.11, 2.40.1–42.58 Burguière.
78 Jouanna 2011.
79 *BGU* 4.1106, 61.11 Manca Masciadri and Montevecchi; *BGU* 4.1107, 65.7 Manca Masciadri and Montevecchi; *BGU* 4.1108, 81.6 Manca Masciadri and Montevecchi; *BGU* 4.1109, 87.6–7 Manca Masciadri and Montevecchi; P. Berol. Inv. 25416, 95.9–10 Manca Masciadri and Montevecchi.

epikyousan), or breastfeeding another child (*mēd' heteron/allo parathēlazousan paidion*).[80] Interestingly, in one case, we are explicitly informed that the wet nurse was needed because the milk of the mother was spoiled due to an illness (*en astheneia … diaphtharthai to tautēs gala*).[81] The latter confirms my observation above that breastfeeding mothers would have avoided coming into contact with adults who might transmit a serious illness to them, such as *phthisis*. Unfortunately, the papyri do not preserve any specific details about particular dietary recommendations for the wet nurse or any kind of process for testing the milk, and the rest of the information mainly focusses on payment, whether monetary or in kind, including *inter alia* clothes and various foodstuffs, the duration of the contract, and the breastfeeding.[82]

Early Byzantine Medical Literature

The surviving medical handbooks from the fourth century AD onwards consist mainly of quotations from earlier authors, in an attempt to summarize the best medical theories of antiquity. Each manual differs in content, the author's expertise, and selection of material. For example, Alexander of Tralles' *Therapeutics* (*Ther.*) does not include advice on invasive surgery. Furthermore, although the theories of Galen dominated rational medical approaches in this period, one can see a few independent voices, including, for example, the African author Caelius Aurelianus (5th c. AD), who writes in Latin and mainly bases himself on the Methodist Soranos, and the author of *Medicina Plinii* (ca. 4th c. AD) who provides an abridged version of the medical advice in Pliny's *Natural History*.[83] I shall start my examination by focussing on three Greek medical authors: Oribasios (fl. second half of the 4th c. AD), Aetios of Amida (fl. first half of the 6th c. AD), and Paul of Aegina (fl. first half of the 7th c. AD). They do not seem to show any sort of originality in their recommendations for the use of breastmilk but they give indicative examples of how ancient knowledge on breastmilk was received in early Byzantium.

All three authors devote three to four chapters exclusively to milk given to infants and make use of similar passages, mainly based on Soranos, most probably

80 *BGU* 4.1104, 58.29–31 Manca Masciadri and Montevecchi; *BGU* 4.1106, 62.28–31 Manca Masciadri and Montevecchi; *BGU* 4.1107, 66.12–14 Manca Masciadri and Montevecchi; *BGU* 4.1108, 81.14–15 Manca Masciadri and Montevecchi; *BGU* 4.1109, 87.18–19 Manca Masciadri and Montevecchi; P. Berol. Inv. 25416, 94.16–95.19 Manca Masciadri and Montevecchi; P. Bour. Inv. 43, 141.19–21 Manca Masciadri and Montevecchi; P. Ross. Georg. II 18, 145.74 Manca Masciadri and Montevecchi; P. Cair. Preis. 31, 148.316–149.317 Manca Masciadri and Montevecchi; P. Oxy. 78.5168, 16–17, not in Manca Masciadri and Montevecchi. Cf. P. Rein. Inv. 2111, 98.18–19, Manca Masciadri and Montevecchi; P. Ryl. II 342, 125.21–23 Manca Masciadri and Montevecchi. See also Tawfik 1997, 945–950.

81 *BGU* 4.1109, 86.11–12 Manca Masciadri and Montevecchi.

82 Strauss 2018; Ricciardetto and Gourevitch 2017; Parca 2017. It is worth noting that the vast majority of the contracts are for exposed infants, usually taken from rubbish pits (*apo koprias*) to be raised as slaves. For this type of nurslings, see also Chapter 1 in this volume.

83 On early Byzantine medical handbooks, see Bouras-Vallianatos 2019.

using passages from otherwise lost works for the rest. Paul, in particular, seems most likely to have based himself directly on Oribasios. On the same topics, Soranos' text extends to almost 11 printed pages, while in Aetios, it is four, and in Oribasios and Paul, just two and three printed pages, respectively. Among the various topics discussed, we can see chapter titles, such as "On the wet nurse," "On the milk of the wet nurse," "How to correct the bad qualities of milk," "On testing the milk," and "On the management of the infant."[84] Thus, great importance is given to the milk being of good quality, in line with the ancient accounts. There are various ways of testing milk, mainly in terms of its consistency, colour, smell, and taste, as we observed in Soranos. Oribasios and Paul also suggest mixing milk in a glass vessel with an equal quantity of rennet and observing whether the cheesy part is smaller than the serous; if it is, it is not of good quality, whereas, if it is the other way round, it will be difficult to digest. The best milk has each of these in more or less equal proportions.[85] From a terminological point of view, we can see an expansion in the variety of terms used for breastmilk of bad quality. Thus, apart from the adjectives used in Galen and Soranos, i.e. *mochthēron* and *phaulon*,[86] we notice the use of *ponēron*[87]; all of them can basically be rendered in English as "harmful." The selection of a wet nurse is a central topic in these accounts as well. Interestingly, according to Oribasios and Paul of Aegina, it was better to employ one who had given birth to a boy (*arren mallon*),[88] although there is no mention of this in Soranos' similar account or in the surviving contracts.

Perhaps the most original contribution is that by Alexander of Tralles on the treatment of an epileptic child. Alexander practised in the reign of Justinian I and, as a result of his own extensive clinical experience, he produced two major works, one *On Fevers* (*Febr.*) and a handbook known as the *Therapeutics*, which are both marked by his strong authorial presence and his persistent attempts to supplement pre-existing material with new elements.[89] Thus, compared to the works of the three

84 Orib. *Eust.* 5.2–5, 3.154.1–155.23 Raeder; Aet. *Tetr.* 4.3–6, 1.360.4–363.31 Olivieri; Paul Aegin. *Epitome of Medicine* (*Epitome*) 1.2–5, 1.9.10–11.6, ed. Heiberg 1921–1924. Cf. Orib. *Medical Collections Incerti* (*Med. Coll. Inc.*) 31, 2/2.121.25–124.26, ed. Raeder 1928–1933. On the sources of these passages, see the *apparatus critici* of the relevant editions.
85 Orib. *Eust.* 5.3, 3.154.20–24 Raeder; Orib. *Med. Coll. Inc.* 32, 2/2.125.23–32 Raeder; Paul Aegin. *Epitome* 1.3, 1.9.28–10.4 Heiberg. Cf. Aet. *Tetr.* 4.5, 1.361.26–362.7.
86 On *mochthēron*, see n. 67, above. On *phaulon*, see e.g. Sor. *Gyn.* 2.9, 2.35.70–77 Burguière. On milk terminology in ancient and early Byzantine medical literature, see the recent comprehensive study by Constantinou and Skouroumouni-Stavrinou 2022.
87 On this adjective, see e.g. Orib. *Eust.* 5.4, 3.155.11 Raeder.
88 Orib. *Eust.* 5.2, 3.154.7–8 Raeder; Paul Aegin. *Epitome* 1.2, 1.9.15–16 Heiberg. Oribasios refers explicitly one more time to the milk of a mother who has given birth to a male child by using the term *arrenotokou* (*Medical Collections* 13.Σ.4, 1/2.176.7 Raeder). The term is also found once in Book 3 of the pseudo-Galenic treatise *On Procurable Drugs* 3, 14.519.16–17K, which is clearly of late date. On this, see n. 32, above. Interestingly, the term *arrenotokos* is also found in early Byzantine alchemical recipes referring to breastmilk as an ingredient: Zosimos of Panopolis, *On Divine Water* 184.8, eds Berthelot and Ruelle 1988; Zosimos of Panopolis, *On Instruments and Furnace* 226.12 Berthelot and Ruelle; Pseudo-Iamblichos, *Tincture* 286.6 Berthelot and Ruelle.
89 Bouras-Vallianatos 2014.

authors mentioned above, Alexander's recommendations are more closely related to everyday medical practice. In his account of epilepsy, he devotes a special section to epilepsy in infants and children. He considers the quality of the milk of the wet nurse very significant, describing harmful milk as *mochthēron* ("harmful") and *pachy* ("thick").[90] He then goes on to discuss a number of foodstuffs that could improve its quality and make the milk thinner, such as fennel, anise, dill, rocket, rue, and leek, and also suggests some gentle exercise for the nurse.[91] Alexander's focus on the role of milk in epileptic infants is in line with modern research published in the *Journal of Paediatrics* showing that breastfeeding is linked to fewer seizures in infants after their first year. In particular, babies who had their mother's milk for more than nine months had a 60 per cent lower risk of epilepsy after the first year of life compared with children who were breastfed for less than a month.[92] Interestingly, in Alexander, we also find a piece of aetiological information that to the best of my knowledge is not found so explicitly in any other surviving ancient or early Byzantine medical work. Alexander connects the use of thick milk, in particular, with the onset of seizures (*spasmous*), explaining that it blocks the nerves (*emphrattein ta neura*).[93] The role of breastmilk in mitigating epileptic seizures in infants is also emphasized by Caelius Aurelianus, although his account is significantly shorter.[94]

So far, I have only referred to the consumption of milk by infants. We have already referred to Galen's advice about the adult consumption of breastmilk for *phthisis*, which goes back to the classical period. The only similar case is one in Book 4 of Alexander's *On Fevers*, which gives some interesting information.[95] Here, Alexander recommends the use of breastmilk in the diet of those affected by hectic fevers, a kind of fever that occurs at an advanced stage in an exhausting disease, such as *phthisis*:

> … and so the woman's milk is valued most and ass milk comes second. Since some people do not like to take the former, they have to be given ass's milk … It is clear that you have to take care of the animal and feed it at home with barley, myrtle, mastic tree and oak leaves. In this way the milk will not become harmful.
>
> … τὸ μὲν οὖν γυναικεῖον γάλα προτετίμηται καὶ δεύτερον πάλιν τὸ ὄνειον. ἀλλ' ἐπειδὴ δυσχερῶς ἓν ἐκ τούτων ἀνέχονται λαμβάνειν, τὸ ὄνειον αὐτοῖς δοτέον γάλα … δῆλον δὲ ὅτι καὶ φροντίζειν δεῖ τοῦ ζῴου τρέφοντα αὐτὸ ἐν οἴκῳ διὰ κριθῶν καὶ μυρσίνης καὶ σχίνου καὶ δρυὸς φύλλων. οὕτω γὰρ οὐκέτι φθαρτικὸν τὸ γάλα. (Alex. Tralles, *Febr.* 4, 1.365.5–10 Puschmann)

---

90 Alex. Tralles, *Ther.*1.15, 1.539.1, ed. Puschmann 1878–1879.

91 Alex. Tralles, *Ther.* 1.15, 1.539.2–7 Puschmann.

92 Sun et al. 2011.

93 Alex. Tralles, *Ther.* 1.15, 1.539.18–19 Puschmann.

94 Caelius Aurelianus, *Acute Diseases* 1.77–79, 474.18–476.4, ed. Bendz 1990.

95 Orib. *Eust.* 9.4, 3.276.27–28 Raeder, also suggests the use of milk for those suffering from *phthisis*, but he does not specify the origin of the milk. Furthermore, Aet. *Tetr.* 8.75, 2.542.16–17 Olivieri, recommends the use of ass's milk as the best for the treatment of *phthisis*.

Alexander accepts that it is hard to convince these patients to drink human milk, which is reminiscent of the difficulties described by Galen in his *Therapeutic Method* regarding getting patients to agree to suckle directly from a nursing mother. As an alternative, Alexander notes that it is easier to consume ass's milk, just as his predecessor had done. He recommends that the family of the patient should have this animal in their household, so they can regulate its diet to ensure it does not produce harmful (*phthartikon*) milk.[96]

The use of breastmilk for gynaecological purposes also continued in early Byzantium. The relevant texts preserve passages that recall the uses that I discussed with reference to the Hippocratic corpus above. For example, the author of the collection of gynaecological recipes ascribed to a certain Metrodora, which must have been written by the sixth century,[97] makes three references to its use in composite drugs in the form of pessaries, viz. for uterine inflammation, for flow of red and white menses, and for an accumulation of gluey humours in the uterus.[98] In the first case, it refers to the milk of a woman who has given birth to a male child (*gynaikos arrenotokou*), alluding to its use in the Hippocratic corpus, although the text retains the term that was used earlier by Dioskorides.[99] Similarly, Aetios of Amida in his gynaecological section, Book 16, refers to the use of breastmilk 12 times, showing that its use was not just confined to ear and eye affections but that it was in regular use for uterine affections too. This is confirmed by the references in the relevant chapters in Oribasios and Paul of Aegina (see Table 4.1).

Table 4.1 shows a list of mentions of the use of breastmilk in early Byzantine medical authors. In Oribasios' surviving corpus, we see 15 references to its use as a simple drug or as an ingredient of composite drugs. In Aetios, Alexander, and Paul, we can see 38, 10, and 13 pharmacological references, respectively. The greater number of references in Aetios is certainly connected with the length of the work, which is three times longer than, for example, that by Paul. By far, the most common use is for pains and inflammations in the eyes or ears, followed by other uses such as for the so-called gnawing stomach, as an ingredient in antidotes, and also for gynaecological affections. It is worth noting that in most cases where milk is found as an ingredient in composite drugs, these drugs are not complicated ones, but mostly consist of only two or three ingredients, such as egg white, poppy, and saffron. Egg white, in particular, is well known for its richness in antimicrobial proteins, including ovotransferrin and lysozyme.[100]

---

96 On the superiority of ass's milk compared to that of other animals in Alexander of Tralles' works, see also *Ther.* 5.6, 2.215.24–1217.15 Puschmann.

97 On this collection, with references to further bibliography, see Totelin 2017, 109–114. The sole surviving manuscript, Laurentianus Plut. 75.3, dates to the tenth/eleventh century AD. On the various opinions about the dating of Metrodora's work, see Totelin 2017, 110, n. 33.

98 Metrodora, *On Female Diseases* 4, 43.19–21, Del Guerra; 9, 46.18–22 Del Guerra; 18, 50.10–18 Del Guerra, ed. Del Guerra 1953. The last recipe is similar to one found in the Hippocratic corpus for a pessary to draw blood out of the uterus: [Hippoc.] *Mul.* 1.74, 8.160.12–13L.

99 See n. 35, above.

100 Guyot et al. 2016.

Table 4.1 Uses of breastmilk in the works of Oribasios, Aetios of Amida, Alexander of Tralles, and Paul of Aegina

Author	Use
Oribasios,[1] *Synopsis for Eustathios*	3.122, 3.99.14–19 Raeder (mixed with various other ingredients in a collyrium for eye epiphora)
	9.9, 3.279.2–3 Raeder (mixed with hemlock juice for inflammation of the breast)
	9.50, 3.307.19 Raeder (mixed with saffron for uterine ulcers)
	9.51, 3.308.9–11 Raeder (as a simple; also mixed with saffron, opium, and hyssop to form a pessary for uterine cancer)
Oribasios, *Books to Eunapios*	2.1, 3.357.12–15 Raeder (as a simple for an ulcerated uterus and any kind of inflammation)
	3.64, 3.431.1–6 Raeder (mixed with other ingredients in an antidote for deadly drugs)
	4.14, 3.445.6–7 Raeder (mixed with egg for eye inflammation)
	4.23, 3.447.5–7 Raeder (mixed with saffron and gum for eye ulcers)
	4.24, 3.447.20–22 Raeder (mixed with wild lettuce for blister on the eye)
	4.26, 3.448.15–18 Raeder (mixed with haematite stone for a burst blood vessel in the eye)
	4.36, 3.450.17–18 and 450.24–25 Raeder (mixed with egg white; mixed with egg white and poppy juice for earache)
	4.39, 3.452.20–21 Raeder (mixed with leek juice for tinnitus)
	4.82, 3.469.21–22 Raeder (mixed with hemlock juice for inflammation of the breast)
Aetios of Amida,[2] *Tetrabiblos*	1.165, 1.76.14–16 Olivieri (mixed with wild lettuce for blister on the eye)
	1.360, 1.131.21–22 Olivieri (mixed with squirting cucumber for headaches)
	2.157, 1.210.25–27 Olivieri (mixed with ash of goat's hooves for eye wounds)
	4.12, 1.365.18–20 Olivieri (mixed with egg white for inflammation in the ears)
	5.125, 2.100.25–26 Olivieri (mixed with egg white for earache)
	6.76, 2.222.8–9 Olivieri (mixed with egg white for earache)
	6.81, 2.226.16–18 Olivieri (mixed with egg white for earache)
	6.81, 2.226.22–24 Olivieri (mixed with egg white and opium for earache)
	7.24, 2.271.26 Olivieri (mixed with egg for deep wounds)
	7.33, 2.284.11–12 Olivieri (as a simple for washing out an eye ulcer)
	7.33, 2.284.20–21 Olivieri (mixed with quince and saffron for eye ulcer)
	7.34, 2.285.5–6 Olivieri (as a simple to wash out a malignant eye ulcer)
	7.34, 2.285.10–11 Olivieri (mixed with either washed lead slag or starch for malignant eye ulcer)

(*Continued*)

Table 4.1 (Continued)

Author	Use
	7.36, 2.287.25–27 Olivieri (mixed with nightshade juice for pain due to a defect in the cornea)
	7.41, 2.293.12–15 Olivieri (mixed with black pigment and honey for eye leucoma)
	7.45, 2.299.8–13 Olivieri (mixed with various other ingredients for eye rheums)
	7.48. 2.302.12–13 Olivieri (mixed with onion juice and honey for those suffering from day blindness)
	7.80, 2.328.16–18 Olivieri (mixed with several other ingredients for baldness in the eyelids)
	7.104, 2.364.17–365.3 Olivieri (mixed with several other ingredients for eye epiphora)
	7.105, 2.367.17–19 and 7.106, 2.372.6 Olivieri (to wash out the eye along with the administration of some kinds of eye collyria)
	7.117, 2.394.18 Olivieri (mixed with several other ingredients to form a collyrium for *myiokephala*, i.e. an eye affection where the uvea protrudes like the head of a fly)
	8.6, 2.410.1–6 Olivieri (mixed with other ingredients for cleaning the face)
	8.20, 2.431.6–7 Olivieri (as a simple for washing out a tubercle on the lips)
	8.35, 2.450.8–13 Olivieri (mixed with cumin, squirting cucumber, and myrrh for tooth decay and earache)
	9.37, 368.1 Zervos 1911 (mixed with black cumin for the treatment of helminths)
	16.45, 63.2 and 9–10 Zervos (as a simple or mixed with melilots after the removal of a uterine cancer)
	16.82, 128.25–27 and 129.13–15 Zervos (mixed with nightshade leaves for inflammation of the uterus)
	16.88, 136.17 Zervos (mixed with litharge for uterine abscess)
	16.101, 139.9 Zervos (mixed with saffron for ulceration of the uterus)
	16.105, 142.15–17 Zervos (mixed with white wax and rose oil for ulceration of the uterus)
	16.109, 143.32, 144.23, 144.13–14, 144.16–18 and 144.29 Zervos (mixed with nightshade leaves; mixed with mallow leaves; as a simple; mixed with saffron, opium, and hyssop, as a base for the application of other drugs for uterine cancer)
Alexander of Tralles, *On Fevers*	4, 1.365.5–10 Puschmann (as a simple/dietary agent for the treatment of hectic fevers)

Alexander of Tralles, *Therapeutics*	1.11, 1.477.7–8 Puschmann (mixed with various other ingredients for headache)
	2, 2.7.6–7 Puschmann (mixed with egg yolk and rose oil for eye inflammation)
	2, 2.9.3–10 Puschmann (mixed with several other ingredients for eye inflammation)
	3, 2.73.21–22 Puschmann (mixed with oregano and honey for earache and inflammation)
	3, 2.77.22–24 Puschmann (mixed with egg white for earache)
	3, 2.81.4–6 Puschmann (mixed with horned poppy juice and opium for earache and inflammation)
	3, 2.87.16–17 Puschmann (mixed with goose fat for ear inflammation)
	3, 2.87.18–19 Puschmann (mixed with saffron for ear inflammation)
	12, 2.575.12–17 Puschmann (mixed with opium and cerate for inflammation in a gout attack)
Paul of Aegina, *Epitome*	3.22, 1.174.18 Heiberg (a simple drug to be infused for a suffusion of blood in the eye)
	3.23, 1.187.22–23 Heiberg (mixed with a collyrium for earache)
	3.23, 1.188.7–8 Heiberg (mixed with oregano and honey for earache)
	3.23, 1.188.23–24 Heiberg (mixed with opium and castoreum for earache)
	3.23, 1.189.4 Heiberg (as a simple drug to be instilled into the ear for earache)
	3.50, 1.262.24–25 Heiberg (mixed with squirting cucumber for the treatment of jaundice)
	3.64, 1.281.10–11 Heiberg (mixed with poppy juice for uterine inflammation and pain)
	3.66, 1.283.11–12 Heiberg (mixed with saffron for ulceration of the uterus)
	3.67, 1.285.6 Heiberg (as a simple to be infused for pain in uterine cancer)
	3.67, 1.285.8–9 Heiberg (mixed with saffron, poppy juice, and hyssop for uterine cancer)
	5.33, 2.28.21 Heiberg (as a simple against the bite of the poisonous beetle, *bouprēstis*)
	7.3, 2.202.21–22 Heiberg (general description of the various kinds of milk in the list of simples; breastmilk as superior to all animal milks)
	7.24, 2.395.19–24 Heiberg (mixed with several other ingredients for inflammations and indurations)

1   For Oribasios, I am not including evidence from the *Collection of Remedies* (better known as *Eclogae medicamentorum*), since the authorship of this work is dubious. See Raeder 1933, 2/2.viii.

2   Note that a considerable part of Aetios' work (Books 10 and 14, and parts of Book 13) is still unedited.

Before I conclude, I would like to offer some remarks on a few Latin medical works dated between the fourth and fifth century AD. Generally speaking, these Latin compendia do not present too many references to the use of breastmilk. Cassius Felix (fl. first half of the 5th c. AD) and Theodore Priscianus (fl. late 4th/early 5th c. AD) do not mention breastmilk at all. Caelius Aurelianus reports one case of its use, which is found only in Paul of Aegina (see Table 4.1). To be specific, before the patient enters the bath for the treatment of jaundice, he recommends pouring a mixture of soapwort or the juice of squirting cucumber or cyclamen juice with either human or ass's milk into the nostrils of the patient so that the yellow bile may be carried out through the nose.[101] *Medicina Plinii* makes only three references to breastmilk as an ingredient in composite drugs for ear and eye affections, and for the treatment of ruptures and wrenches.[102] Lastly, Marcellus (fl. early 5th c. AD) in his *On Drugs* (*De Med.*), who mainly bases himself on Scribonius Largus, refers to the use of human milk three times. In the first case, breastmilk mixed with sulphur is recommended for earache.[103] In the second, there is a particular reference to the milk of a woman who has given birth to a female child being mixed with honey and oil for stains of burning,[104] which reminds us of Pliny's similar mention discussed above. The last case is related to the preparation of an ointment for lung diseases.[105] After having listed a large number of ingredients, Marcellus goes on to mention human milk:

Preparation of an ointment for the same lung disease … one *quartarius* human milk, a milk that can only be added at the time when the sick person is to be anointed and that cannot be warmed up together with the other ingredients, and, lying on the bed, it should be rubbed in adequately by hand.

Confectio unctionis ad ipsam pulmonis causam … lactis humani quartarium, quod lac sub hora, qua aeger ungendus est, mittatur nec calefaciat cum ceteris speciebus, et iacens in lecto unguatur lenta satis manu. (Marcellus, *De Med.* 16.105, 294.5–15 Niedermann and Liechtenhan)

Marcellus' remark states that the ointment must be added at the time when the sick person is to be anointed, and the fact that it should not be warmed up with the other ingredients confirms the fragile nature of human milk, also alluded to by Galen in the passage mentioned above from the *Therapeutic Method*.

Lastly, the popularity of breastmilk for certain eye conditions even saw it included in the treatise known as the *Kyranides*, a textbook of magico-medical

---

101 Caelius Aurelianus, *Acute Diseases* 3.72, 722.12–16 Bendz.
102 *Medicina Plinii* 1.6.11, 15.4–5 Önnerfors; 1.8.1, 16.14–15 Önnerfors; 3.30.10, 90.19–20 Önnerfors, ed. Önnerfors 1964.
103 Marcellus, *De Med.* 9.110, 186.23–24, ed. Niedermann and Liechtenhan 1968.
104 Marcellus, *De Med.* 19.37, 316.16–17 Niedermann and Liechtenhan. See n. 32, above.
105 It is worth noting that in Marcellus one also finds a rare reference to the use of the very first faeces, or the so-called meconium, of a male infant after a first drink of breastmilk (*stercus infantis, quod primum dimittit, statim ex lacte mulieris*), as an ingredient in a composite drug. See Marcellus, *De Med.* 8.136, 150.7–11 Niedermann and Liechtenhan.

remedies written in Greek, which was first put together at some point in the third/ fourth century AD. It is most famous for the large number of details it contains on gemstones and amulets, as well as its significant use of animal substances. Human milk is mentioned five times mixed with animal substances, such as deer's horn, the faeces of lizards, burnt nail of ass, the droppings of the turtledove, and the bile of a bogue (*bōps*), in line with the absurd medical ingredients commonly found in this text. In the cases of deer's horn and ass's nail, the milk of a woman who has given birth to a male child (*gynaikeiō arrenotokō*) is explicitly mentioned. As might be expected, in all cases, the resulting drugs are recommended for various eye conditions (trachoma, leucoma, amblyopia, and for the promotion of sharp-sightedness).[106]

Conclusions

By examining a large number of Greek and Latin medical sources from the fifth century BC to the seventh century AD, I have shown how the use of breastmilk for therapeutic purposes was developed over the centuries. The curative effects of breastmilk seem to have been originally related to the treatment of the female body, where it was used for a variety of gynaecological affections according to the surviving recipes in the Hippocratic corpus. At the same time, breastmilk was recommended as a sort of panacea for severe lung diseases, such as *phthisis*, even in adults. Moreover, we have noted how its use expanded to cover a large number of diseases by the first centuries AD, although the vast majority of these references continued to concentrate on its constantly reported efficacy for eye and ear infections. As we have seen, this is consistent with modern research emphasizing breastmilk's high content of immune cells and antibodies compared to animal and formula milk.

Another point that came up was the recurrent motif of the use of milk from a mother who has given birth to a male child (described as either *kourotrophos* or *arrenotokos*), which most probably reflects influence from Egypt. This superstitious connotation is first found in the Hippocratic corpus, but it is notably missing from the works of Galen and Soranos. It is then found again in early Byzantine medical compilations, which are often based on earlier sources, and quite predictably in the *Kyranides*, the medieval bestseller of magical healing. It remains uncertain whether this had any actual impact on daily medical practice. For example, the medical handbooks of Aelius Promotus and Alexander of Tralles, which seem to align more closely with everyday treatment of patients, do not mention this specification.

An equally significant outcome of this study was the paramount importance often given by medical authors to the good quality of breastmilk, along with special advice on the regimen of the wet nurse. In an era in which milk substitutes did not exist, the nutritive role of breastmilk remained central to the growth and

---

106 *Kyranides* 2.11, 135.22–23 Kaimakis; 2.29, 161.8–9 Kaimakis; 2.31, 163.13–14 Kaimakis; 3.43, 231.3–4 Kaimakis; 4.7, 247.4–5 Kaimakis, ed. Kaimakis 1976.

development of children, and also had a prophylactic role as regards infantile diseases, such as epilepsy. The latter is also confirmed by the number of references to the quality of milk and the various provisions, such as abstinence from sexual intercourse and not feeding other babies concurrently, included in the surviving corpus of wet-nursing contracts in papyri. Finally, I hope this chapter can play a part in encouraging breastfeeding nowadays by showing the beneficial effects of breastmilk for infants and, at the same time, emphasizing the need for expert advice and guidance for mothers on various issues, including daily regimen, from the early stages of breastfeeding.

References

Texts: Editions and Translations

Bendz, G. ed. 1990. *Caelii Aureliani Celerum passionum libri III, Tardarum passionum libri V.* Berlin: Akademie Verlag.

Berthelot, M., and C.E. Ruelle. eds. 1888. *Collection des anciens alchimistes grecs.* Vol. 2. Paris: Steinheil.

Bourbon, F. ed. 2008. *Hippocrate. Tome XII, 1re partie: Nature de la femme.* Paris: Les Belles Lettres.

Burguière, P. ed. 1988–2000. *Soranos d'Ephèse: Maladies des femmes I–IV.* 4 vols. Paris: Les Belles Lettres.

Crismani, D. ed. 2002. *Elio Promoto Alessandrino, Manuale della salute (Δυναμερόν).* Alessandria: Edizioni dell'Orso.

Daremberg, C., and C.E. Ruelle. eds. 1879. *Oeuvres de Rufus d'Ephèse.* Paris: Imprimé par l'autorisation du gouvernement à l'Imprimerie Nationale.

Del Guerra, G. ed. 1953. *Il Libro di Metrodora: Sulla malattie delle donne e il ricettario di cosmetica e terapia.* Milan: Ceschina.

Heiberg, J.L. ed. 1921–1924. *Paulus Aegineta.* 2 vols. Leipzig: Teubner.

Helmreich, G. 1907–1909. *Galeni De usu partium libri xvii.* 2 vols. Leipzig: Teubner.

Hude, C. ed. 1958. *Aretaeus.* Berlin: Akademie Verlag.

Ieraci Bio. A.M. ed. 1987. *Galeno. De bonis malisque sucis.* Naples: D'Auria.

———. ed. 1996. *Paolo di Nicea: Manuale medico.* Naples: Bibliopolis.

Ihm, S. ed. 1995. *Der Traktat περὶ τῶν ἰοβόλων θηρίων καὶ δηλητηρίων φαρμάκων des sog. Aelius Promotus: Erstedition mit textkritischem Kommentar.* Wiesbaden: Ludwig Reichert Verlag.

Johnston, I., and G.H.R. Horsley. ed and trans. 2011. *Galen: Method of Medicine,* vol. 1: *Books 1–4.* Loeb Classical Library 516. Cambridge, MA: Harvard University Press.

Kaimakis, D. ed. 1976. *Die Kyraniden.* Meisenheim am Glan: Hain.

Koch, K. ed. 1923. *De sanitate tuenda.* Leipzig and Berlin: Teubner.

Kühn, C.G. ed. 1821–1833. *Claudii Galeni opera omnia.* 20 vols in 22. Leipzig: Knobloch.

Littré, E. ed. 1839–1861. *Oeuvres complètes d'Hippocrate: Traduction nouvelle avec le texte grec en regard, collationné sur les manuscrits et toutes les éditions; accompagnée d'une introduction, de commentaires médicaux, de variantes et de notes philologiques; suivie d'une table générale des matières.* 10 vols. Paris: J.-B. Baillière.

Manca Masciadri, M., and O. Montevecchi. eds. 1984. *I contratti di baliatico.* Milan: Tipolitografia Tibiletti.

Marx, F. ed. 1915. *A. Cornelii Celsi.* Leipzig and Berlin: Teubner.

Mayhoff, K., and L. Jan. eds. 1875–1906. *C. Plinii Secundi Naturalis historiae libri XXXVII.* 5 vols. Leipzig: B.G. Teubner.

Nickel, D. ed. 1971. *Galeni De uteri dissectione.* Berlin: Akademie Verlag.

Niedermann, M., and E. Liechtenhan. eds. and J. Kollesch, and D. Nickel. trans. 1968. *Marcelli De medicamentis liber.* 2 vols. Berlin: Akademie Verlag.

Oder, E., and K. Hoppe. eds. 1924–1927. *Corpus Hippiatricorum Graecorum.* 2 vols. Leipzig: Teubner.

Olivieri, A. ed. 1935–1950. *Aetii Amideni Libri medicinales.* 2 vols. Leipzig: Teubner.

Önnerfors, A. ed. 1964. *Plinii Secundi Iunioris qui feruntur De medicina libri tres.* Berlin: Akademie Verlag.

Potter, P. ed. 1980. *Hippocratis: De morbis III.* Berlin: Akademie Verlag.

Puschmann, T. ed. 1878–1879. *Alexander von Tralles: Original-Text und Übersetzung nebst einer einleitenden Abhandlung. Ein Beitrag zur Geschichte der Medicin.* 2 vols. Vienna: W. Braumüller.

Raeder, H. ed. 1926. *Oribasii Synopsis ad Eustathium; Libri ad Eunapium.* Leipzig and Berlin: Teubner.

———. ed. 1928–1933. *Oribasii Collectionum medicarum reliquiae.* 2 vols in 4 pts. Leipzig and Berlin: Teubner.

Sconocchia, S. ed. 2020. *Scribonii Largi Compositiones.* Berlin: De Gruyter.

Wellmann, M. ed. 1907–1914. *Pedanii Dioscuridis Anazarbei De materia medica libri quinque.* 3 vols. Berlin: Weidmann.

Wilkins, J. ed. 2013. *Galien: Sur les facultés des aliments.* Paris: Les Belles Lettres.

Zervos, S. ed. 1901. *Aetii Sermo sextidecimus et ultimus.* Leipzig: A. Mangkos.

———. ed. 1911. "Ἀετίου Ἀμιδηνοῦ λόγος ἔνατος," *Ἀθηνᾶ* 23: 273–390.

Secondary Works

Aakhila, A., and V. M. Feminamol. 2021. "Antimicrobial Activity of Breast Milk against Neonatal Pathogens," *Acta Scientific Microbiology* 4 (4): 197–207.

Aboul Aly, A. 1996. "The Wet Nurse: A Study in Ancient Medicine and Greek Papyri," *Vesalius* 2 (2): 86–97.

———. 1998. "Testing Women's Milk," in G. Argoud, and J.-Y. Guillaumin (eds) *Sciences exactes et sciences appliquées à Alexandrie.* Saint-Etienne: Université de Saint-Etienne, 207–215.

Ackerman, D.L., K.M. Craft, R.S. Doster, J.-H. Weitkamp, D.M. Aronoff, J.A. Gaddy, and S.D. Townsend. 2018. "Antimicrobial and Antibiofilm Activity of Human Milk Oligosaccharides against *Streptococcus agalactiae*, *Staphylococcus aureus*, and *Acinetobacter baumannii*," *ACS Infectious Diseases* 4 (3): 315–324.

André, J. 1985. *Les noms de plantes dans la Rome antique.* Vol. 1. Paris: Les Belles Lettres.

Beagon, M. 2005. *The Elder Pliny on the Human Animal: Natural History Book 7.* Oxford: Oxford University Press.

Bouras-Vallianatos, P. 2014. "Clinical Experience in Late Antiquity: Alexander of Tralles and the Therapy of Epilepsy," *Medical History* 58: 337–353.

———. 2019. "Galen in Late Antique Medical Handbooks," in P. Bouras-Vallianatos and B. Zipser (eds) *Brill's Companion to the Reception of Galen.* Leiden: Brill, 38–61.

———. 2021. "Cross-Cultural Transfer of Medical Knowledge in the Medieval Mediterranean: The Introduction and Dissemination of Sugar-Based Potions from the Islamic World to Byzantium," *Speculum* 96 (4): 963–1008.

Bourbou, C. 2010. *Health and Disease in Byzantine Crete (7th–12th centuries AD)*. Farnham: Ashgate.

Centlivres Challet, C.-E. 2016. "Tire-lait ou biberons romains?" *L'Antiquité Classique* 85: 157–180.

Constantinou, S., and A. Skouroumouni-Stavrinou. 2022. "Premodern 'Galaktology': Reading Milk in Ancient and Early Byzantine Medical Treatises," *Journal of Late Antique, Islamic and Byzantine Studies* 1: 1–40.

Craik, E. 2015. *The 'Hippocratic' Corpus: Content and Context*. Abingdon: Routledge.

Dasen, V. 1997. "Multiple Births in Graeco-Roman Antiquity," *Oxford Journal of Archaeology* 16 (1): 49–63.

Dawson, W.R. 1932. "Adversaria Aegyptiaca," *Aegyptus* 12: 9–16.

Ghaemi, S., P. Navaei, S. Rahimirad, M. Behjati, and R. Kelishadi. 2014. "Evaluation of Preventive Effects of Colostrum against Neonatal Conjunctivitis: A Randomized Clinical Trial," *Journal of Education and Health Promotion* 3: 63.

Gourevitch, D. 1990. "Les tire-lait antiques et la consommation médicale de lait humain," *Histoire des sciences médicales* 24: 93–98.

———. 2001. "Le nourrisson et sa nourrice: Étude de quelques cas pédiatriques chez Galien," *Revue de philosophie ancienne* 19 (2): 63–76.

Grmek, M. 1989. *Diseases in the Ancient Greek World*. Baltimore: Johns Hopkins University Press.

Guyot, N., V. Labas, G. Harichaux, M. Chessé, J.-C. Poirier, Y. Nys, and S. Réhault-Godbert. 2016. "Proteomic Analysis of Egg White Heparin-Binding Proteins: Towards the Identification of Natural Antibacterial Molecules," *Scientific Reports* 6: 27974.

Hanson, A.E., and M.H. Green. 1994. "Soranus of Ephesus: *Methodicorum princeps*," *Aufstieg und Niedergang der römischen Welt* 37 (2): 968–1075.

Jouanna, J. 2011. "Médecine rationnelle et magie: Le statut des amulettes et des incantations chez Galien," *Revue des études grecques* 124: 47–77.

Kokoszko, M. 2016. "Galen's Therapeutic Galactology (γαλακτολογία ἰατρική) in *De simplicium medicamentorum temperamentis ac facultatibus*," in I. Anagnostakis, and A. Pelletieri (eds) *Latte e latticini: Aspetti della produzione e del consumo nelle società mediterranee del'Antichità e del Medioevo*. Lagonegro: Grafica Zaccara, 33–48.

Kokoszko, M., and J. Dybała. 2016. "Medical Science of Milk Included in Celsus' Treatise *De medicina*," *Studia Ceranea* 6: 323–353.

Laskaris, J. 2008. "Nursing Mothers in Greek and Roman Medicine," *American Journal of Archaeology* 112: 459–464.

Leven, K.-H. 2005. "Aretaios v. Kapapdokien," in K.-H. Leven (ed.) *Antike Medizin: Ein Lexikon*. Munich: Beck, 80–81.

Manetti, D. 2008a. "Euruphōn of Knidos," in P.T. Keyser, and G.L. Irby-Massie (eds) *The Encyclopedia of Ancient Natural Scientists*. London: Routledge, 321–322.

———. 2008b. "Hērodikos of Knidos," in P.T. Keyser, and G.L. Irby-Massie (eds) *The Encyclopedia of Ancient Natural Scientists*. London: Routledge, 381.

Mavroudis, A. 2013. *Τὰ ἰοβόλα ζῷα καὶ τὰ δηλητήρια φάρμακα στὴν ἀρχαία ἑλληνικὴ ἰατρική*. Athens: Academy of Athens.

Mulder, T. 2017. "Adult Breastfeeding in Ancient Rome," *Illinois Classical Studies* 42: 227–243.

Monte, A. 2022. "Medical Recipes for All Occasions: A *receptarium* from Tebtunis? (P.CtYBR inv. 1443)," *Greek, Roman, and Byzantine Studies* 62: 77–109.

Nutton, V. 2013. *Ancient Medicine*. 2nd ed. Abingdon: Routledge.

Parca, M. 2017. "The Wet Nurses of Ptolemaic and Roman Egypt," *Illinois Classical Studies* 42 (1): 203–226.

Pommerening, T. 2010. "βούτυρος, '*Flaschenkürbis*' und κουροτόκος im Corpus Hippocraticum, *De sterilibus* 214: Entlehnung und Lehnübersetzung aus dem Ägyptischen," *Glotta* 86: 40–54.

———. 2015. "Milch einer Frau, die einen Knaben geboren hat," in P. Kousoulis and N. Lazaridis (eds) *Proceedings of the Tenth International Congress of Egyptologists: University of the Aegean, Rhodes, 22–29 May 2008*. Vol. 2. Leuven: Peeters, 2083–2095.

Ricciardetto, A., and D. Gourevitch. 2017. "Entre Rome et l'Egypte romaine: Pour une étude de la nourrice entre littérature médicale et contrats de travail," in M.-H. Marganne, and A. Ricciardetto (eds) *En marge du Serment hippocratique: Contrats et serments dans le monde gréco-romain*. Liège: Presses Universitaires de Liège: 67–117.

Rzeźnicka, Z., and M. Kokoszko. 2020. *Milk and Dairy Products in the Medicine and Culinary Art of Antiquity and Early Byzantium (1st–7th Centuries AD)*. Lódź and Kraków: Lódź University Press and Jagiellonian University Press.

Schlievert, P.M., S.H. Kilgore, K.S. Seo, and D.Y.M. Leung. 2019. "Glycerol Monolaurate Contributes to the Antimicrobial and Anti-inflammatory Activity of Human Milk," *Scientific Reports* 9: 14550.

Stamatu, M. 2005. "Phthisis," in K.-H. Leven (ed.) *Antike Medizin: Ein Lexikon*. Munich: Beck, 701–702.

Stannard, J. 1982. "Medicinal Plants and Folk Remedies in Pliny, *Historia naturalis*," *History and Philosophy of the Life Sciences* 4 (1): 3–23.

Strauss, J.A. 2018. "Les contrats et les reçus de salaire de nourrice relatifs à des esclaves dans la documentation papyrologique grecque de l'Egypte romaine," *Papyrologica Lupiensia* 27: 69–94.

Sun, Y., M. Vestergaard, J. Christensen, and J. Olsen. 2011. "Breastfeeding and Risk of Epilepsy in Childhood: A Birth Cohort Study," *Journal of Pediatrics* 158 (6): 924–929.

Tawfik, Z. 1997. "Wet-Nursing Stipulations in Greek Papyri and Arabic Sources," *Archiv für Papyrusforschung, Beiheft* 3: 939–953.

Totelin, L. 2009. *Hippocratic Recipes: Oral and Written Transmission of Pharmacological Knowledge in Fifth- and Fourth-Century Greece*. Leiden: Brill.

———. 2015. "When Foods Become Remedies in Ancient Greece: The Curious Case of Garlic and Other Substances," *Journal of Ethnopharmacology* 167: 30–37.

———. 2017. "The Third Way: Galen, Pseudo-Galen, Metrodora, Cleopatra and the Gynaecological Pharmacology of Byzantium," in L. Lehmhaus and M. Martelli (eds) *Collecting Recipes: Byzantine and Jewish Pharmacology in Dialogue*. Berlin: De Gruyter, 103–122.

———. 2019. "Sweet Honey and Hare's Brains: Ancient Pharmacology for Children's Diseases," in C. Lamburgo (ed.) *Una favola breve: Archeologia e antropologia per la storia del'infanzia*. Florence: Edizioni All'Insegna del Giglio, 37–42.

Vincenzetti, S., G. Santini, V. Polzonetti, S. Pucciarelli, Y. Klimanova, and P. Polidori. 2021. "Vitamins in Human and Donkey Milk: Functional and Nutritional Role," *Nutrients* 13 (5): 1509.

5 Weaning and Lactation Cessation in Late Antiquity and the Early Byzantine Period

Medical Advice in Context

Laurence Totelin

Introduction

I open this chapter with a story that is very evocative of the pains associated with lactation cessation: that of the martyrdom of Perpetua and Felicity, as told in the *Passion of Perpetua and Felicity* (*PPF*), a text that exists both in Latin and in Greek. As the Latin version is likely to be the primary one, it is the one I will use.[1]

In AD 203, under the rule of Septimius Severus, near Carthage, a group of Christians were put to death in the arena, where they had to fight against wild beasts. The crowds, we are told, were particularly shocked at the appearance of two women in the group, Perpetua and Felicity:

> Thus, stripped naked and covered with nets, they were brought forward. The crowd shuddered when it gazed upon them: one a tender girl [Perpetua], the other [Felicity] with her breasts dripping [milk], as she had recently given birth.
>
> Itaque dispoliatae et reticulis indutae producebantur. Horruit populus alteram respiciens puellam delicatam, alteram a partu recentem stillantibus mammis. (*PPF* 20.2, eds Farrell and Williams 2012)

This scene is, as scholars have noted, implausible, as well as being erotically charged. It would not have been possible for the spectators, perhaps even those nearest to the women, to discern the milk dripping from Felicity's breasts.[2] Yet, this far-fetched scene played an important role in the *PPF*'s narrative; in the words of Alicia Myers, it "reinforce[d] the physicality of the miracles provided by God."[3] For the bodies of Felicity and Perpetua, each representing a different stage in the

---

1 There is much scholarship on the *PPF*. See e.g. Cobb and Jacobs 2021; Gold 2018; Heffernan 2012; Bremmer and Formisano 2012b. For the primacy of the Latin, see Bremmer and Formisano 2012a, 2. For the *PPF*, with a focus on the Greek text, see Chapter 1 in this volume. Unless stated otherwise, all translations from the Latin and Greek are mine.

2 See e.g. Bremmer 2012; Heffernan 2012, 340; Frankfurter 2009, 221–224.

3 Myers 2017, 144.

DOI: 10.4324/9781003265658-7

lactation cycle had been transformed by the grace of God. Felicity, upon praying to God for deliverance, had given birth to a girl in the famously dangerous eighth month, a few days before the games; her milk was flowing on the arena, perhaps for the first time.[4] Perpetua, for her part, had recently ceased to breastfeed her son and therefore to lactate. We are told the story of this lactation cessation in Perpetua's own first-person narrative, a rare record of an ancient woman's voice, if it is indeed authentic.

In her account, Perpetua referred on several occasions to the breastfeeding of her son, whose age is not specified. Translator and commentator Thomas Heffernan gives this age as 18 months but there is very little to substantiate this claim in Perpetua's narrative.[5] All we can tell is that the child was not a very small infant when his mother was arrested. Perpetua described in detail the pain she felt upon being separated from her son when she and her companions were arrested and put in prison. She was "distressed by anxiety for [her] baby" (*PPF* 3.6), an anxiety which, as argued by Stamatia Dova, might have been both mental and physical, as Perpetua's breasts became engorged when they were not drained of milk.[6] The Christian group, however, was later moved to another part of the prison, where visitors were allowed. Perpetua then breastfed her son whom she found "weakened because of the lack of food" (*PPF* 3.8). After a few days, mother and son were allowed to stay in prison together, an event which had a very positive effect on Perpetua: "immediately I regained strength, as I was relieved from pain and anxiety for my baby" (*PPF* 3.9). The child stayed with his mother, "receiving the breast," until, at a hearing, the Christians were condemned to death in the arena (*PPF* 6.7). Perpetua's father removed the child, refusing him a last feed, and condemning Perpetua to painful torments. She was, however, saved by God:

> But this was God's will, not only did the child no longer long for my breasts, but also they did not cause me fever, so that I may not be distressed by anxiety for my baby and pain in my breasts.
>
> Et quomodo Deus voluit, neque ille amplius mammas desideravit neque mihi fervorem fecerunt ne sollicitudine infantis et dolore mammarum macerarer. (*PPF* 6.8)

Dova interpreted the mention of a *fervor* (fever), *phlegmonē* (inflammation) in the Greek version, as one of "weaning fever," which can accompany sudden lactation cessation.[7] This touching and detailed description of lactation cessation is unique for antiquity. It is particularly noteworthy for its acknowledgement of the pain, both physical and psychological, that sudden weaning can cause to both mother

---

4 The description of the birth is at *PPF* 15. See Totelin 2021a, 247–249.

5 Heffernan 2012, 151.

6 See Dova 2017, 254.

7 Dova 2017, 257–258. Heffernan (2012, 207) takes the references to engorgement as a sign that "male authorship [is] less probable."

and child. By contrast, Felicity's pain at being separated from her daughter while her milk was coming in is glossed over in the *PPF*. This silence, perhaps, better reflects the situation in the ancient literature, where women's and children's experiences of breastfeeding, its initiation and cessation, and its emotional impact on the breastfeeding dyad (whether it is constituted of biological mother and child, or nurse and child) are to be read between the lines, teased out from often dispassionate texts, such as the writings of ancient physicians.

In this chapter, I focus on the descriptions of two linked processes, lactation cessation (in a lactating woman) and weaning (in a child), in the works of the Byzantine medical authors, Oribasios of Pergamon (doctor and friend of the emperor Julian the Apostate in the 4th c. AD), Aetios of Amida (active in the 6th c. AD, and perhaps associated with the court of Justinian), and Paul of Aegina (active in the 7th c. AD).[8] As these authors are known to have abbreviated earlier medical authors, I will at times mention those, and in particular Soranos (1st–early 2nd c. AD), Dioskorides (fl. 1st c. AD), and Galen (AD 129–ca. 216/217). I also refer to texts that are very difficult to date but which fall roughly within our chronological span: Metrodora's gynaecological text, and pseudo-Galen's second book *On Procurable Remedies* (*Rem. Parab.*).[9] Finally, where relevant, I call upon a few non-medical texts, as well as bioarchaeological evidence.

Weaning

Byzantine medical authors made occasional reference to weaning, *apogalaktismos*, or the act of weaning, *apogalaktizō*.[10] As these words make clear, the ancients considered weaning as the act of taking away (*apo*) the breastmilk (*gala*) that infants consumed. The advice that they gave, however, indicated that they considered this "taking away from the breast" as the end of a long process, taking place over several months during which infants were slowly accustomed to taking some semi-solid and then solid foods, as well as other drinks. In what follows, I will refer to the starting point of this process as "initiation of weaning," when after a period of exclusive breastfeeding, infants are introduced to supplementary foods. I will refer to the end point of the process as "cessation of breastfeeding" or "completion of

---

8 Information on all the ancient medical authors mentioned in this chapter can be found in Keyser and Irby-Massie 2008. Several of the texts studied here are also examined in Gourevitch 1995 and in Lascaratos and Poulakou-Rebelakou 2003. On these and other medical texts, see also Chapters 2, 4, and 6 in this volume.

9 Calà and Chesi (2022) suggest a date in the first century AD and discuss other dates, which range between the first and the sixth centuries AD. On the pseudo-Galenic *Rem. Parab.*, see Totelin 2021b.

10 *Apogalaktismos*: Orib. *Medical Collections Incerti* (*Med. Coll. Inc.*) 39.1 (CMG 6.2.2, 138.22–23), ed. Raeder 1933; Aet. *Tetrabiblos* (*Tetr.*) 4.29 (CMG 8.1, 370.27), ed. Olivieri 1935. *Apogalaktizō*: Aet. *Tetr.* 4.28 (CMG 8.1, 370.26). The phrase "*apo tou galaktos*" also appears in, e.g., Orib. *Med. Coll. Inc.* 39.1 (CMG 6.2.2, 138.19).

weaning."[11] The process of weaning was – and still is – one that could be risky for the child, who became more prone to illnesses. It also marked an important change in the relation between an infant and its breastfeeder, whether its biological mother or a nurse, and therefore was a turning point in the development of an infant's personhood.[12]

Oribasios is the Byzantine medical author who provided the most advice about the weaning process. In his *Medical Collections* (*Med. Coll.* or *Med. Coll. Inc.*), he presented various summarized passages on the matter which he had extracted from earlier authors (Galen, Rufus of Ephesos, Mnesitheos, and Athenaios), not seeking to resolve differences between them. It is therefore very difficult to determine what exactly Oribasios' views on weaning were. The first author whom Oribasios summarized on the topic of weaning was quite naturally Galen, who had described the weaning process in his *Hygiene* (*San. Tu.*):

> From Galen's works, on the rearing of the nursling (*paidiou*) until the age of fourteen. At first, one must feed the nursling (*paidion*) with milk alone. But when **its front teeth have grown**, one must already accustom it in some way to bear some thicker food, as indeed women do, taught by experience, when they pre-chew food and then put it in nurslings' (*paidiōn*) mouths: first a little bread, and next pulses, meats, and other similar things.
>
> Ἐκ τῶν Γαληνοῦ. Περὶ τροφῆς παιδίου ἄχρι ἐτῶν ιδ. Τρέφειν δὲ τὸ παιδίον τὰ μὲν πρῶτα γάλακτι μόνῳ· **ἐπειδὰν δὲ φύῃ τοὺς πρόσθεν ὀδόντας**, ἐθίζειν ἤδη πως αὐτὸ καὶ τῆς παχυτέρας ἀνέχεσθαι τροφῆς, ὥσπερ οὖν καὶ τοῦτο αὐτὸ πείρᾳ διδαχθεῖσαι ποιοῦσιν αἱ γυναῖκες, ἄρτου μέν τι πρῶτον, ἐφεξῆς δ' ὀσπρίων τε καὶ κρεῶν [καὶ] ὅσα τ' ἄλλα τοιαῦτα προμασώμεναι κἄπειτα ἐντιθεῖσαι τοῖς στόμασι τῶν παιδίων. (Orib. *Med. Coll. Inc.* 35 (CMG 6.2.2, 129.21–27))[13]

Galen had identified the cutting of the front teeth as a turning point in an infant's growth. This was by no means a fixed time since, if we assume that teething patterns have not changed much since antiquity, some infants can start teething before four months (some can even be born with teeth), while others will only acquire their first teeth after 12 months. Most infants, however, start teething around six months.[14] Galen acknowledged women's experience in preparing foods for infants

---

11 In his important review of the anthropological evolution of infant feeding, Daniel W. Sellen defined weaning as "The termination of suckling. Weaning is a uniquely mammalian life history marker that may or may not be preceded by a period of feeding on other foods in addition to mother's milk" (Sellen 2007, 126). The language I employ is closer to that used in Fulminante 2015.

12 See Marklein and Fox 2020, 574 for further references.

13 The corresponding passage in Galen is *San. Tu.* 1.10.1 (CMG 5.4.2, 23.4–9), ed. Koch 1923; an English translation of *Hygiene* is available: Johnston 2018. The vocabulary referring to young children is not always precise. Here, I adopt the translation suggested by Golden 2015, 11.

14 See https://www.nhs.uk/conditions/baby/babys-development/teething/baby-teething-symptoms/. Accessed April 2022.

by pre-chewing them, a practice still witnessed in some parts of the world.[15] Not all ancient authors, however, approved of pre-chewing. Mnesitheos (4th c. BC), whose views on weaning were also preserved by Oribasios, noted that "one must not give [the infant] any pre-chewed food, but one must give boiled wheaten flour, cereal meal, or triturated millet. All these must be boiled well and for a long time" (Orib. *Med. Coll. Inc.* 37.4–5 (CMG 6.2.2, 135.25–28)). Despite what is sometimes mentioned in the modern scholarship, neither Galen nor Oribasios in his summary gave a timeline for the completion of weaning and the cessation of breastfeeding at three years of age.[16] Galen, followed by Oribasios, had indicated that until the third year of a child's life (that is, from its second to its third birthday), its nurse should take precautions so that the *krasis* of her milk remains good (Gal. *San. Tu.* 1.9.1 (CMG 5.4.2, 21.34–22.4)).[17] These medical authors did not, however, give a fixed point for breastfeeding cessation, perhaps allowing for flexibility in response to individual circumstances.

Oribasios also preserved Rufus of Ephesos' (1st c. AD) advice on infant feeding, which differed from that of Galen:

From the works of Rufus, on the care of the nursling (*paidiou*) … Until a certain time, then, one must maintain [the child] on milk alone, and not give it any other food; but when **it itself is eager to take some other food** and gives us the hope that it will be able to digest it, then give crumbs of bread in watery wine. One must above all avoid giving meat, because the belly is not yet ready to digest it … One must also avoid thick soups and porridges, because nothing thick is appropriate for a child since, even without that, it tends by nature to produce phlegm … **It is sufficient to feed the child with milk for two years**, and then to change onto [solid] foods.

Ἐκ τῶν Ῥούφου. Περὶ κομιδῆς παιδίου … μέχρι μὲν οὖν τινος ἐπὶ μόνου τοῦ γάλακτος φυλάσσειν, σιτίον δ' ἄλλο μηδὲν προσφέρειν· ὅταν δ' **αὐτό τε πρόθυμον ᾖ λαμβάνειν** καὶ ἐλπίδα παρέχῃ ἐκπέψειν, τηνικαῦτα ἤδη <καὶ> σιτίον διδόναι, ἄρτον εἰς ὑδαρῆ οἶνον καταθρύψαντας. τὰς δὲ τῶν κρεῶν προσφορὰς πεφυλάχθαι παντὸς μάλιστα· οὐ γάρ πω ἱκαναὶ αἱ γαστέρες καταπέσσειν … πεφυλάχθαι δὲ καὶ τὰ ἔτνη καὶ τὰ ῥοφήματα· παχὺ γὰρ οὐδὲν παιδίῳ συμφέρει διὰ τὸ καὶ ἄλλως τὴν φύσιν πρὸς τὸ φλεγματῶδες ῥέπειν … **ἀρκεῖ δ' ἔτη δύο τρέφειν τῷ γάλακτι**, τὸ δ' ἐντεῦθεν μεταβάλλειν πρὸς σιτία. (Orib. *Med. Coll. Inc.* 38.13–23 (CMG 6.2.2, 137.12–138.3))

Like Galen, Rufus did not give a fixed time for the initiation of weaning, stating that one should take cues from the child itself, a practice that recalls modern

15 Danielle Gourevitch (1995, 286) reported having witnessed this "répugnante habitude" ("disgusting habit") in France in her childhood.
16 Valerie Fildes stated that "the child should be weaned completely from the breast at the age of three, according to Galen" (Fildes 1986, 35). This is often repeated in the literature on ancient weaning.
17 Cf. Orib. *Med. Coll. Inc.* 30.1 (CMG 6.2.2, 121.10–14).

"baby-led weaning."[18] Rufus did, however, display a certain anxiety towards supplementary foods, especially those that were "too thick." Rufus also mentioned that
it was sufficient to feed an infant on milk for two years. This is a rather ambivalent
statement, which can be interpreted either as a recommendation to stop breastfeeding once the infant has reached 24 months or as an acknowledgement that the
infant can be exclusively breastfed for two years, even though it might wish to take
some food earlier.[19] The former interpretation (breastfeeding to end at 24 months)
is perhaps more likely but the recommendation does not amount to a prohibition of
breastfeeding beyond two years.

In his shorter works, the *Synopsis for Eustathios* (*Eust.*) and the *Books to Eunapios* (*Eun.*), Oribasios gave advice that was similar to that found in Rufus, perhaps
indicating his own preference:

> *Synopsis for Eustathios*: Care of the nursling (*paidiou*) … When it itself is
> eager to take it and gives us hopes that it will be able to digest it, then give
> it food, **avoiding surfeit**. If by mistake the child is overfilled, it will imme-
> diately become sleepier and sluggish, there will be swelling in the belly and
> flatulence, and the urine will be more watery. When this is recognized, one
> must not give the child anything until the food has been consumed. **It is suf-
> ficient to feed the child with milk for two years**, and then to change onto
> [solid] foods.
>
> Κομιδὴ παιδίου … ὅταν δ' αὐτό τε πρόθυμον ᾖ λαμβάνειν καὶ ἐλπίδας
> παρέχῃ εἰς πέψιν, τηνικαῦτα ἤδη καὶ σιτίον διδόναι **μὴ ἐμπιπλᾶσαν**. εἰ δέ που
> λαθόντα πληρωθείη, ὑπνωδέστερά τε εὐθὺς γίνεται καὶ νωθρότερα, καὶ ὄγκος
> ἐν γαστρὶ ἔνεστι καὶ φῦσα, καὶ οὐρεῖ ὑδατωδέστερα, οἷς χρὴ τεκμαιρομένην
> μηδὲν διδόναι, ἔστ' ἂν καταναλώσῃ. **ἀρκεῖ δ' ἔτη δύο τρέφειν τῷ γάλακτι**,
> τὸ δ' ἐντεῦθεν μεταβάλλειν πρὸς σιτία. (Orib. *Eust.* 5.5 (CMG 6.3, 155.15–
> 23), ed. Raeder 1926)
>
> *Books to Eunapios*: When the nursling (*paidiou*) is able to use other foods
> [than milk], there should be no obstacle to its efforts, for it is by nature that
> it reaches for exercises and foods. For **there won't be surfeit**, since much
> blood is consumed by growth.
>
> τοῦ δὲ παιδίου καὶ τῶν ἄλλων τροφῶν οἵου τε ὄντος ἤδη προσφέρεσθαι,
> μηδαμῶς ταῖς προθυμίαις ἐμποδὼν γίνεσθαι, φυσικῶς ὁρμῶντος ἐπὶ τὰ
> γυμνάσια καὶ τροφάς· **οὐ γὰρ ἔσται πλησμονὴ** πλείονος τοῦ αἵματος εἰς
> τὴν αὔξησιν ἀπαναλισκομένου. (Orib. *Eun.* 1.1.8 (CMG 6.3, 320.23–27), ed.
> Raeder 1926)

18 See https://www.nhs.uk/conditions/baby/weaning-and-feeding/babys-first-solid-foods/. Accessed
 29 June 2022.

19 For the second interpretation, see Gourevitch and Chamay (1992, 79), who note that some unspecified breastfeeding contracts stipulate a two-year period of exclusive breastfeeding. Children usually
 reach for food earlier, when they can stay in a sitting position and when their hand–eye coordination
 allows them to bring food to their mouth. See https://www.nhs.uk/conditions/baby/weaning-and-
 feeding/babys-first-solid-foods/. Accessed 29 June 2022.

The *Synopsis for Eustathios* passage is particularly close to that of Rufus. It expresses anxiety about surfeit in the infant who is being weaned. That anxiety is not found in the *Books to Eunapios* passage, which emphatically states that surfeit will not occur at this time of growth. This unease around surfeit is also found in a passage of Athenaios (1st c. AD) excerpted by Oribasios, which seems to focus on slightly older children, who have recently completed weaning:

> From the works of Athenaios, on healthy regimen. One must allow infants (*nēpious*) who have been taken off milk [i.e. weaned] to live in a relaxed way and in play ... One must give them light foods and in moderate amounts. For those who, during weaning, fill them with foods and try to give them foods that are rather nourishing lead them to poor nutrition and prevent their healthy growth because of the weakness of their nature. Many of these infants, because of frequent indigestion and the downward motions of the belly, suffer from ulcerations and inflammations of the intestines, from prolapses of the anus, and from severe diseases.
>
> Ἐκ τῶν Ἀθηναίου. Περὶ ὑγιεινῆς διαίτης. Τοὺς νηπίους καὶ ἀπὸ τοῦ γάλακτος γεγονότας ἐν ἀνέσει τε ἐᾶν καὶ παιδιᾷ ... καὶ τροφὰς αὐτοῖς προσφέρειν ἐλαφροτάτας καὶ τῷ πλήθει συμμέτρους· οἱ γὰρ διὰ τὸν ἀπογαλακτισμὸν ἐμφοροῦντες αὐτοῖς τὰς τροφὰς καὶ ταύτας πειρώμενοι πολυτροφωτέρας διδόναι εἰς κακοτροφίαν καὶ ἀναύξειαν αὐτοὺς περιτρέπουσι διὰ τὴν τῆς φύσεως ἀσθένειαν. πολλοῖς δ' αὐτῶν διὰ τὰς συνεχεῖς ἀπεψίας καὶ τὰς καταφορὰς τῆς κοιλίας ἑλκώσεις τε καὶ φλεγμοναὶ τῶν ἐντέρων καὶ προπτώσεις τῆς ἕδρας καὶ νόσοι χαλεπαὶ συμβαίνουσιν. (Orib. *Med. Coll. Inc.* 39.1–2 (CMG 6.2.2, 138.18–28))

These precautions around the introduction of new foods were legitimate. Demographic studies indicate a correlation between weaning and infant mortality in antiquity, as weaning exposed children to new bacteria and parasites, and could lead to "weanling diarrhoea."[20]

Oribasios, then, transmitted several different sets of advice on weaning, not really trying to reconcile them. One of his medical predecessors whose weaning recommendation he did not include was Soranos, whose *Gynaecology* (*Gyn.*) was, by contrast, Aetios' source on the topic of weaning. Here is Aetios' summary on the topic:

> When to wean (*apogalaktisteon*) infants (*nēpia*). Until the infant (*nēpion*) has become **firm**, it should be fed milk only. When its body has already strengthened, give some soft morsels in hydromel, honey-wine, sweet wine, or milk; and later eggs that can be sipped ... As a drink, give mixed wine.

20 See e.g. Parkin 2013, 55; Garnsey 1998, 267; Sallares 1991, 231. On the diseases which ancient medical thinking associated with weaning, see Bertier 1996, 2182–2184. On infant mortality more generally and its high rates in antiquity, see also Chapters 1 and 3 in this volume.

As soon as the newborn/small baby (brephous) can confidently take cereal food, which in the majority of cases occurs around the twentieth month, then stealthily and little by little wean from the breast (*aposunēthizein*). If the child becomes ill while being weaned (*apogalaktisthen*), one must again change to milk, and when the disease has stopped, and the little body has recovered, only then wean (*apogalaktizein*)

Πότε ἀπογαλακτιστέον τὰ νήπια. Μέχρις ἂν οὖν **παγῇ** τὸ νήπιον, γάλακτι τρεφέσθω. ἐστερεωμένου δὲ ἤδη τοῦ σώματος τροφὴν δίδου ψίχας τρυφερὰς ἐξ ὑδρομέλιτος ἢ οἰνομέλιτος ἢ γλυκέος οἴνου ἢ γάλακτος, εἶτα καὶ ὠὰ ῥοφητά· ... ποτὸν δὲ διδόναι οἶνον κεκραμένον· **ἤδη δὲ τοῦ βρέφους λαμβάνοντος ἀδεῶς τὴν σιτώδη τροφήν, ὅπερ ὡς ἐπὶ τὸ πολὺ γίγνεται περὶ τὸν κ μῆνα, τότε λεληθότως καὶ κατ᾽ ὀλίγον ἀποσυνηθίζειν αὐτὸ τοῦ μαστοῦ**· εἰ δ᾽ ἀπογαλακτισθὲν νόσῳ περιπέσοι, πάλιν αὐτὸ δεῖ μεταγαγεῖν ἐπὶ τὸ γάλα. καὶ μετὰ τὸ παύσασθαι τὴν νόσον ἀναλαβεῖν τὸ σωμάτιον καὶ οὕτως ἀπογαλακτίζειν. (Aet. *Tetr.* 4.28 (CMG 8.1, 370.17–26))[21]

Soranos and Aetios recommended initiating the weaning process when the baby's body became firm, a notion that does not really resonate with modern milestones (unless perhaps the ability to sit counts as "firmness") but is linked to ancient concepts of moulding the malleable body of an infant, which was like wax.[22] Soranos had specified that the firmness stage was unlikely to occur before the age of six months (Sor. *Gyn.* 2.46.3 (CMG 4, 86.9)), but Aetios omitted that information.[23] The importance of the "firmness" stage is signalled by the change of vocabulary to designate the infant: before it is firm, the infant is a *brephos* (newborn), then it becomes a *nēpios* (infant). Neither Soranos nor Aetios prescribed an end point for breastfeeding. Instead, they recommended slowly and stealthily withdrawing breastmilk: Soranos suggested doing so from the "third or fourth half-year of the infant's life" (Sor. *Gyn.* 2.47.1 (CMG 4, 86.26–27)), that is, from 12 months to 24 months, linking this stage to the growth of the teeth that enable mastication (molars), while Aetios indicated the 20th month. They also allowed for a return to exclusive breastfeeding if a child became ill during the weaning process.

The final main Byzantine medical encyclopaedist, Paul of Aegina, gave brief instructions on weaning, which are verbatim repetitions from two sections he found in Oribasios: Athenaios' advice on healthy infant diet and Oribasios' summary in his *Synopsis for Eustathios* 5.5 (CMG 6.3, 155.15–23).[24]

---

21 See Sor. *Gyn.* 2.46.3–47.1 (CMG 4, 86.7–31), ed. Ilberg 1927; for an English translation of Soranos' treatise, see Temkin 1956.

22 On infant-rearing as moulding wax, see Holman 1997.

23 Soranos recorded that Mnesitheos and Aristanax recommended weaning girls six months later than boys because they were weaker, a practice he rejected (*Gyn.* 2.48.2 (CMG 4, 87.9–13)). Soranos also indicated that some women attempted to give cereal foods from 40 days (*Gyn.* 2.46.2 (CMG 4, 86.2)).

24 Paul Aegin. *Epitome of Medicine* (*Epitome*) 1.5 (CMG 9.1, 10.27–11.6) and 1.14 (CMG 9.1, 13.15–14.3), ed. Heiberg 1921.

In sum, the Byzantine medical authors, and the predecessors from whom they borrowed, were more prescriptive about the beginning of weaning, which should not happen before certain milestones are reached (even if those milestones could be reached at different times by different babies), than about the end of the weaning process, on which they showed much flexibility, because they knew that the weaning period could be beset with dangers and bring with it risks of morbidity and mortality. In any case, they favoured relatively long-term breastfeeding, and never suggested completing weaning before the child had reached 24 months. It is difficult to determine who exactly would have followed this medical advice, but it can be assumed that the medical authors had as their main audience wealthy families, who could often afford wet nurses. As Tracy Prowse et alii rightly noted, these medical texts were "prescriptive rather than descriptive;" they depicted what their authors considered to be good practice and might bear little relation with the lived reality of infants and those who breastfed them.[25] Nevertheless, other types of ancient sources ("biographies," documents, and bioarchaeological data) do testify to the breastfeeding of toddlers.

Thus, we find references to children aged two and beyond being breastfed in several saints' Lives dating to the early Byzantine period.[26] For instance, in the *Miracles of Thekla* (2.24, ed. Dagron 1978), we read about a little child "who has just been weaned" (*apotitthon arti gegonos*), who risked losing his sight because he was crying so much as a result of his weaning. His nurse (*tithē*) therefore took him to the church of Thekla in Seleucia. While the exact age of the child is not given, we hear that he was able to walk, run, and play, which would suggest he was around 18 months. Further, in the *Life of Symeon Stylites the Younger* (5–6, ed. Van den Ven 1962), we read that the saint, after being baptized at age two, refused to take his mother's breast whenever she ate meat.

Documentary evidence from Ptolemaic and Roman Egypt, while a little early for the purpose of this chapter, also attests to long-term breastfeeding. Thus, in a letter preserved on a papyrus dating to the first century AD, a mother, Hikane, berates her son, Isidoros, for not writing to her, who had "carried [him] for ten months and nursed [him] for three years" (O. Ber. 2.129 = Trismegistos 89155). Wet-nursing contracts preserved on papyrus, for their part, specify a length of service for the wet nurse varying from 16 months to three years, with two years being the most commonly given period.[27]

Bioarchaeological data from the late antique and Byzantine period also testify to long-term breastfeeding. Indeed, isotopic investigations (the study of nitrogen and carbon isotopes) of the protein found in bone collagen or tooth dentin make it possible to discern breastfeeding and weaning patterns.[28] While there are geographical variations, sometimes significant, in these patterns, the bioarchaeological evidence

---

25 Prowse et al. 2008, 297. See also Powell et al. 2014, 91.
26 See e.g. Bourbou and Garvie-Lock 2015, 175–176; Rey 2004, 368; Beaucamp 1982, 552.
27 Parca 2017, 215.
28 See Marklein and Fox 2020 for introduction.

points to an onset of weaning in the second half of an infant's first year (that is, after six months) and a termination of breastfeeding between two and five years. I have summarized some of the findings of bioarchaeological studies in Table 5.1. My criteria for inclusion in Table 5.1 were those studies that made mention of medical writings (usually Soranos, Galen, but sometimes also Oribasios) in their discussion of the archaeological evidence. Some archaeologists have tentatively suggested that ancient populations read the medical texts that have come down to us.[29] It is probably safer, however, to assume that the concordance between medical texts and bioarchaeological data is coincidental, or rather that the concordance reflects the fact that breastfeeding and weaning advice circulated orally among populations, especially among women, mothers, midwives, and wet nurses.[30] The different types of sources, then, would reflect – in different ways – this oral knowledge, and its flexibility. It should be noted that studies of non-industrial populations have shown that five to six months is a common age for the initiation of weaning, that weaning is a process that can take several years, and that the cessation of breastfeeding generally occurs between two and five years.[31] In other words, it would be possible to find a correspondence between the vague recommendations preserved in ancient Greek medical texts and the weaning and breastfeeding practices in regions of the world where those texts could not have been read.

If breastfeeding anthropologically tends to last between two and five years, it is because it is a source of great comfort to children. That fact was acknowledged in the story of the child distraught by his weaning experience in the *Miracles of Thekla* and quietly hinted at in Soranos' and Aetios' recommendations to return to exclusive breastfeeding if a child became ill during the weaning process. Long-term breastfeeding does require investment, both in terms of time and emotions, from the breastfeeder, who could feel ambivalent towards the act, whether they were the infant's biological mother or a hired or enslaved nurse. Ancient breast-feeders at times used means to speed up the process. Thus, Soranos noted that some women anointed their nipples with bitter substances, a practice he opposed:

> For thus [if the advice on weaning is followed] the infant will be weaned without harm, getting away little by little from the first habit. At the same time, the milk of the child's nurse will simply dry up because of the gradual elimination of suckling. For it is harmful to anoint the nipple with some bitter and ill-smelling things and thus wean the infant suddenly, because the sudden change has an injurious effect and because sometimes the infant becomes ill when the stomach is damaged by drugs.
>
> οὕτω γὰρ ἂν μᾶλλον τὸ βρέφος ἀποσυνεθισθήσεται ἀλύπως κατὰ βραχὺ τῆς πρώτης ἀποχωροῦν συνηθείας, ἅμα δὲ ἀπεριέργως σβεσθήσεται τὸ γάλα

---

29 See e.g. Cocozza et al. 2021, 435; Fulminante 2015, 41; Powell et al. 2014, 106 (who reject the idea; see the next note).
30 On oral tradition, see Powell et al. 2014, 106–107.
31 See Dettwyler 2017; see also Centlivres Challet 2017, 897.

Table 5.1 Bioarchaeological studies of weaning pattern that mention ancient medical authors, alphabetically by modern country

Site(s)	Date of evidence	Type of evidence	Initiation of weaning	Completion of weaning	Ancient author(s) mentioned	Author(s) of study(/-ies)
Dakhleh Oasis, modern Egypt	ca. AD 250	Isotopic data from 49 bone samples and dentin of 102 individuals	Around 6 months	By 3 years	Soranos, Galen	(Dupras et al. 2001) (Dupras and Tocheri 2007)
Various sites in modern Greece (including Crete)	6th–15th c. AD	Isotopic data from bones of 61 individuals	Around 6 months	Between 3 and 4 years	Oribasios, Aetios, Paul, and other Byzantine sources	(Bourbou 2020; Bourbou and Garvie-Lock 2015; Bourbou et al. 2013; Bourbou and Garvie-Lock 2009)
Isola Sacra, Rome, Italy	1st–3rd c. AD	Isotopic data from 37 bone samples	End of first year	2–2.5 years	Soranos, Galen, Oribasios, wet-nursing contracts	(Prowse et al. 2008)
Avenches, modern Switzerland	1st–3rd c. AD	Isotopic data from bones of 30 individuals	Not specified	Around 3 years	Soranos	(Bourbou et al. 2019)
Leptiminus, modern Tunisia	2nd–5th c. AD	Isotopic data from bones of 99 individuals	Before 2 years	By 3 years	Soranos, Galen	(Keenleyside et al. 2009)
Queenford Farm, Oxfordshire, modern UK	4th–mid 6th c. AD	Isotopic data from 87 bone samples	Not possible to establish but before 1.5 years	2–4 years	Soranos, Galen, Oribasios	(Fuller et al. 2006)
London, modern UK	1st–5th c. AD	Isotopic data from bones of 58 individuals	Around 6 months	By 4 years	Soranos, Galen	(Redfern et al. 2018; Powell et al. 2014)
Bainesse, modern UK	1st–5th c. AD	Isotopic measurement on tooth increments from five individuals	Around 6 months	Between 2 and 5 years	Soranos, Galen, Oribasios	(Cocozza et al. 2021)

τῆς τιτθευούσης τὸ νήπιον τῇ κατὰ μικρὸν ὑφαιρέσει τῆς ἐκμυζήσεως. τὸ γὰρ πικροῖς τισι καὶ δυσώδεσι περιχρίειν τὰς θηλὰς καὶ ἀθρόως ἀπογαλακτίζειν αὐτὸ βλαβερὸν διὰ τὸ τὸν ἐν τῇ ἀθρόᾳ μεταβολῇ ξενισμὸν ἐμποιεῖν καὶ διὰ τὸ κακούμενον ὑπὸ τῶν φαρμάκων τὸν στόμαχόν ποτε πάσχειν. (Sor. *Gyn.* 2.47.2 (CMG 4, 86.30–87.4))

One of the bitter substances used for this purpose of weaning might have been worm-wood, which is used in this way in Shakespeare's *Romeo and Juliet*.[32] Interestingly, none of the Byzantine medical authors referred to the practice of anointing the nip-ples with bitter drugs. We do, however, find allusions to this practice in religious and philosophical texts of the period. Thus, John Chrysostom (AD 340/350–407) alluded to the practice in an analogy he drew between a mother trying to wean her child off the breast and God trying to wean his devotees off Jerusalem:

A tender mother who has breastfed (*hupomazein*) her child but wants to lead it away from milk-nourishment and lead it towards other forms of food, when she sees that it is unwilling and vexed, and seeks for the breast, and insinuates itself into her motherly bosom, smears gall or some other bitter juice around the nipple of her breast, and thus forces it, unwillingly, to turn away from the source of milk.

Καὶ καθάπερ μήτηρ φιλόστοργος ὑπομάζιον ἔχουσα παῖδα, εἶτα αὐτὸν ἀπαγαγεῖν τῆς γαλακτοτροφίας σπουδάζουσα καὶ πρὸς ἑτέραν ἀγαγεῖν τροφήν· ἐπειδὰν ἴδη μὴ βουλόμενον καὶ δυσανασχετοῦντα καὶ τὸν μαζὸν ἐπιζητοῦντα καὶ πρὸς τὸν κόλπον καταδυόμενον τὸν μητρικόν, αὐτὴν τοῦ μαζοῦ τὴν θηλὴν κύκλῳ χολὴν περιχρίσασα ἢ καὶ ἑτέρῳ τινὶ πικροτάτῳ χυμῷ, καὶ ἄκοντα ἀναγκάζει τοῦ γάλακτος ἀποστραφῆναι λοιπὸν τὴν πηγήν. (John Chrys. *Homily against the Jews* 2, eds and trans. Pradels, Brändle, and Heimgartner 2000, 42–44)

And the Neoplatonist philosopher Simplikios (6th c. AD), in a discussion on pleas-ure and pain (*On Epictetus* (*In Epict.*)), referred to physicians and mothers who apply bitter drugs:

Accordingly, the good physician, by applying unpleasant [things], causes them [the souls] to turn away from what they lean towards, just as women who wish to wean infants anoint their nipples with something bitter.

Ὁ τοίνυν ἀγαθὸς ἰατρός, ἀνιαρὰ ταῦτα εἰς ἃ νένευκεν αὐτῇ προσφέρων, ἀποστρέφεσθαι ποιεῖ αὐτά, ὥσπερ αἱ τὰ παιδία ἀπογαλακτίζειν βουλόμεναι πικρῷ τινι τὰς θηλὰς ὑπαλείφουσι. (Simpl. *In Epict.* 14, ed. Hadot 1996)

Both John Chrysostom and Simplikios described the practice of anointing the breasts with a bitter drug in neutral to positive terms, unlike Soranos, who had seen

---

32 Shakespeare, *Romeo and Juliet* Act 1, Scene 3, v. 28, ed. Levenson 2000.

it as injurious to the child. These authors implicitly acknowledged that a breast-feeder might at times have wished to wean an infant off the breast, although they did not give explanations as to why she might have wanted to do so, beyond her wish to give the child some other forms of nourishment.

Weaning in the Byzantine period, in sum, was a process that ideally was gradual. Byzantine medical authors did not mention the physical effects this weaning would have on mothers and nurses, presumably because they expected it to lead to painless lactation cessation – if that effect was the one wished for. Indeed, we must not forget that some women might have had other children to breastfeed. Neither did the Byzantine medical authors describe the psychological effects that weaning might have on the nursing woman; the ambivalence she might have felt towards the process is passed over entirely in silence.

Extinguishing the Milk

Byzantine medical authors, then, did not describe in any detail the gradual lactation cessation that accompanies weaning in the second year of a child's life. They did, however, mention several drugs that could induce a quick lactation cessation when needed. I now turn to these drugs and the contexts in which they would have been used. In the same way as the ancients knew of drugs that could promote lactation, they knew of drugs that could stop it.[33] These fell into two categories: simple drugs (single ingredients) and compound ones (recipes involving several ingredients). The references to simple drugs are found in treatises, or sections of treatises, devoted to simples, that is, lists of natural products, often organized alphabetically; the references to compound drugs are found in treatises, or sections of treatises, devoted to women's health.

Byzantine medical authors listed three simples as having the power to extinguish the milk: sweat, the faba bean, and wine lees (see Table 5.2). The Greek expressions used to refer to the powers of these ingredients are *gala sbennusi* or *gala sbennutai*, which have strong connotations of drying out the milk, of extinguishing it in the breasts. Oribasios also gave a general statement regarding the drugs that promoted the production of milk, and those that stopped it, indicating that thick substances could extinguish the milk – opposites (a thick substance) for opposites (fluid milk):

> In order to promote the production of milk, a substance must therefore be moderately warming and not at all thick, hence why such substances [that display this quality of being thick] extinguish the milk rather than promote it.
> δεῖται δὲ δήπου συμμέτρως εἶναι θερμὸν καὶ οὐδαμῶς παχὺ πρὸς τὴν τοῦ γάλακτος γένεσιν, ὅθεν ὅσα μὲν τοιαῦτα σβέννυσι μᾶλλον ἢ γεννᾷ τὸ γάλα.
> (Orib. *Med. Coll.* 14.63.6 (CMG 6.1.2, 234.4–6), ed. Raeder 1929)

33 See Chapter 4 in this volume.

Table 5.2 Simple remedies that are said to extinguish the milk in Byzantine medical works

Hidrōs, sweat	Aet. *Tetr.* 2.107 (CMG 8.1, 191.15–16): "This remedy, when used as an ointment, extinguishes the milk (*sbennusi gala*) accumulated in the breasts very well" ("τοῦτο τὸ φάρμακον ἐπιχριόμενον σβέννυσι γάλα πληθύνον ἐν τοῖς τιτθοῖς ἱκανῶς.").[1]
Kuamos, faba bean	Orib. *Eun.* 2.1k96 (CMG 6.3, 368.37): "It extinguishes milk (*gala sbennutai*) in a cataplasm" ("καὶ τὸ γάλα σβέννυται πρὸς τοῦ τοιούτου καταπλάσματος").
	Aet. *Tetr.* 1.233 (CMG 8.1, 98.11): "And it extinguishes the milk (*gala sbennutai*) in a cataplasm" ("καὶ γὰρ καὶ τὸ γάλα σβέννυται πρὸς τοῦ καταπλάσματος").
	Paul Aegin. *Epitome* 7.3.10 (CMG 9.2, 232.13): "In a cataplasm, it cures inflammation and swellings and extinguishes the milk in the breasts (*gala sbennusin*)" ("καταπλασσόμενος δὲ φλεγμονάς τε καὶ ὄγκους ἰᾶται καὶ γάλα σβέννυσιν ἐπὶ τῶν τιτθῶν").[2]
Trux oinou, wine lees	Paul Aegin. *Epitome* 7.3.19 (CMG 9.2, 267.22–23): "It extinguishes milk (*gala sbennusin*) in over-distended breasts" ("καὶ μαστῶν σπαργώντων τὸ γάλα σβέννυσιν").

[1] See also Gal. *On the Capacities of Simple Drugs (SMT)* 10.1.14, 12.284K, ed. Kühn 1826.
[2] See also Diosk. *Materia medica* 2.105.1; Gal. *SMT* 7.10.59, 12.50K.

Surprisingly, the Byzantine authors did not list hemlock among the simples that extinguished milk. That plant had been noted for this power by Dioskorides, who had stated that the plant could dry up both milk and semen:

> The herb and foliage [of hemlock], crushed and applied as a poultice to the testicles, help those who emit semen during their sleep; applied as a poultice, they relax the genitals, they dry up the milk, they prevent breasts from growing in young girls, and they make the testicles of boys atrophied.
>
> ἡ δὲ πόα καὶ ἡ κόμη λεῖα καταπλασσόμενα <ἐπὶ> τῶν διδύμων ὀνειρώττουσι βοηθεῖ· παρίησι δὲ καὶ αἰδοῖα καταπλασθέντα καὶ γάλα σβέννυσι, μαστούς τε ἐν παρθενίᾳ κωλύει αὔξεσθαι καὶ διδύμους ἀτρόφους ποιεῖ ἐπὶ παίδων. (Diosk. *On Medical Substances (Materia medica)* 4.78.2, ed. Wellmann 1907–1914)[34]

Both semen and milk were considered to be transformed blood, and it was therefore to be expected that a drug that would dry up one of those bodily fluids would dry up the other.[35]

The Byzantine descriptions of substances that dry up the milk posit a link between the wish to extinguish the milk and breast inflammation (see Table 5.2). They do not mention, however, that such inflammation can be very painful and lead to fevers, as Perpetua had feared. This inflammation, called mastitis, is today one of the reasons why mothers choose to stop breastfeeding; but, conversely, ending breastfeeding suddenly and early can lead to mastitis, as today's public health

34 An English translation of the full text of Dioskorides is available in Beck 2020.
35 See Pedrucci 2013.

messages make clear to women.[36] Yet, we should be wary of over-comparing our modern situation with that of the ancients: neonatal death was much more prevalent in the ancient world than it is today, at least in the Western world, and it must have been one of the main reasons why women needed to extinguish their milk. In their descriptions of simple drugs drying up the milk, however, Byzantine medical authors mentioned neither neonatal death nor any other context in which women developed breast inflammation and wished to stop lactating.[37]

We can gain some insights into these contexts from Byzantine treatises, or sections of treatises, devoted to women's health, in which medical authors described compound recipes to dry out the milk. For instance, Aetios gave the following recipe to extinguish the milk in his sixteenth medical book, the gynaecological book, in a chapter on "the curdling of milk in the breast":

> To prevent the curdling (*thrombousthai*) of the milk in the breasts … Another very good prescription: Asian stone and wax, of each two ounces; rose oil or kiki-oil, eight ounces. Mix together and use, changing twice a day. For it extinguishes the milk (*sbennuei gala*) and stops inflammations (*phlegmonas*).
>
> Πρὸς δὲ τὸ μὴ θρομβοῦσθαι τὸ γάλα ἐν μαστοῖς … Ἄλλο κάλλιστον. Λίθου ἀσίου, κηροῦ ἀνὰ γοβ´. ἤτοι οὐγ. β´. ἐλαίου ῥοδίνου ἢ κηκίνου γοη´. ἤτοι οὐγ. η´. ἀναλαβὼν χρῶ δὶς τῆς ἡμέρας ἀλλάσσων, σβεννύει γὰρ τὸ γάλα καὶ τὰς φλεγμονὰς παύει. (Aet. *Tetr.* 16.38, 51.28–52.1, ed. Zervos 1901)

And Oribasios gave a recipe for a similar purpose in the gynaecological sections of his *Synopsis for Eustathios* and *Books to Eunapios*:

> Oil scrapings [from palaestrae] are a very effective remedy when applied to inflamed (*phlegmainontōn*) breasts. If it appears to you to be too dry, soften it with henna oil or rose oil. And this remedy is also very useful to extinguish the milk (*sbesai to gala*) which has transformed into cheese (*turōthen*) in the breasts after childbirth (*ek toketōn*).
>
> Πάτος φλεγμαινόντων τιτθῶν βοήθημά ἐστι δραστικώτατον ἐπιτιθέμενον· ἐὰν δὲ ξηρότερόν σοι φαίνηται, κυπρίνῳ μάλαττε ἢ ῥοδίνῳ. καὶ πρὸς τὸ ἐκ τοκετῶν δὲ σβέσαι τὸ γάλα τυρωθὲν κατὰ τοὺς μαστοὺς χρήσιμον ἱκανῶς ἐστιν. (*Eust.* 9.9.1–2 (CMG 6.3, 278.12–15))[38]

Curdling of the milk in the breast is not a recognized condition in modern medicine but it was one that preoccupied physicians in antiquity and beyond. Like any process of milk curdling, the curdling in the breast turned the milk cheesy, as Oribasios made clear in the recipe above. The thick and cheesy breastmilk was allegedly very

---

36 See Gianni et al. 2019.

37 There is a reference to mothers with "full breasts" (*uberibus plenis*) dripping milk upon infants' funeral pyres in Statius' *Silvae* 5.5.15–17 (1st c. AD), ed. and trans. Shackleton Bailey 2003, 361.

38 The same recipe also appears at *Eun.* 4.82.1 (CMG 6.2.3, 469.7–8).

difficult to digest for the infant; worse, according to Soranos, it could lead to "clogging up" in a baby's body (*Gyn.* 2.18.1–3 (CMG 4, 64.21–65.13)). Ancient authors associated the curdling/thickening of the milk mainly with the onset of lactation, a time when, as I have argued elsewhere, the milk risked becoming tainted through contact with lochial blood.[39] Lochial blood is the blood that is shed in the days after childbirth; it flows at its heaviest in the first three to five days, that is, during the days when the body produces a thick, yellowish milk, which we now call the colostrum and consider as an extremely beneficial substance, but one which the ancients considered to be cheesy and dangerous for newborn babies, who would fare better if they were given some honey or were fed by other women until their mothers' "proper" milk came in (Sor. *Gyn.* 2.17–18.3 (CMG 4, 64.1–65.13); Orib. *Med. Coll. Inc.* 31.28 (CMG 6.2.2, 124.3–8); *Eust.* 5.5 (CMG 6.3, 155.16–18)).

The ancient anxiety about the curdling of the milk in the breast must not be dismissed. Some women and their physicians must have felt extreme fear of killing infants with bad milk, and this might have encouraged them to use rather unpleasant remedies to extinguish their milk.[40] We should not forget, however, that medicine can be a way for physicians to exert power over bodies, and in particular, over women's bodies.[41] Instilling fear of their bad milk in women might at times have been a way to dissuade them from breastfeeding, for a variety of reasons. One of these reasons might have been social perceptions, especially in wealthier families that could afford wet nurses, and where it might therefore have been considered unsightly for the mother to breastfeed – a physically demanding task.[42] Another reason to dissuade a woman from breastfeeding would have been to make her body available again for sexual intercourse. Indeed, there appears to have been a taboo against sexual intercourse while breastfeeding in antiquity, as it allegedly soured the milk, brought back the menses, and risked depriving the nursling from nourishment by redirecting it to the foetus.[43] Finally, as noted by Claude-Emmanuelle

---

39 Totelin 2021a.

40 Some of the remedies to extinguish the milk include some unpleasant ingredients. See for instance: Aet. *Tetr.* 16.41 (54.15, 56.5–6 Zervos): "Against inflammations of the breasts, according to Philoumenos … Or crush earthworms with quinces; or river crabs with egg. And this extinguishes the milk" ("Πρὸς τὰς τῶν μαστῶν φλεγμονὰς, Φιλουμένου … ἢ γῆς ἔντερα λειώσας μετὰ κυδωνίων ἢ καρκίνους ποταμίους μετὰ ᾠοῦ· τοῦτο καὶ τὸ γάλα σβεννύει").

41 The gender and social biases of medical writings are traceable in their language and style as well; see Constantinou and Skouroumouni-Stavrinou 2024, in press and 2022; see also Chapter 6 in this volume.

42 There were debates on maternal breastfeeding in antiquity, perhaps best exemplified by Favorinus' defence of maternal breastfeeding, preserved in Aulus Gellius' *Attic Nights* 12.1, ed. and trans. Rolfe 1927. One can also note a papyrus letter from the third century AD where a young mother's parent writes to their son-in-law, stating "I heard that you are compelling her to breastfeed. If she wants, let the baby have a nurse, for I do not want my daughter to breastfeed" (P. Lond. 3.951v = Trismegistos 31964, ll. 2–5). On the exhausting effects of breastfeeding, see also Sor. *Gyn.* 2.18.5 (CMG 4, 65.20–27).

43 See for instance Sor. *Gyn.* 2.19.11 (CMG 4, 67.28–68.2); Gal. *San Tu.* 1.9.4 (CMG 5.4.2, 22.10–13); Orib. *Med. Coll. Inc.* 30.3 and 31.19 (CMG 6.2.2, 121.17–20 and 123.18–20). Instructions to avoid sexual intercourse are also found in wet-nursing contracts on papyri from Ptolemaic and Roman Egypt; for references, see Ricciardetto and Gourevitch 2020, 54; Parca 2017, 211.

Centlivres Challet, avoiding breastfeeding, and placing that responsibility on someone else, might also have served as a mechanism, whether conscious or not, to protect families from emotional involvement with their infant in a world where infant mortality rates were high.[44]

It is also possible that women themselves exploited the rhetoric of curdled milk in order not to breastfeed, and to regain control – or perceived control – over their bodies.[45] They could have done so for all the reasons outlined above (wishing to resume sexual intercourse; social anxiety; fear of high emotional involvement), as well as for cosmetic reasons, to avoid the perceived effects that breastfeeding had on the body. In this context, one can note that sections on the care of the breasts in ancient medical treatises sometimes included recipes of a cosmetic nature alongside ones to prevent inflammation. For instance, Paul of Aegina's *Epitome of Medicine* 3.35, devoted to afflictions of the breasts, opens with advice on how to deal with inflammations when the milk has turned cheesy in the breast after childbirth, then turns to remedies against spreading ulcers in the breasts (extracted from Archigenes), and closes with recipes for "preservatives for the breasts." While one of these preservative recipes is clearly marked as being for virgin girls, the other is not, and might have been used by women at any life stage, including women concerned about the alleged sagging of their breasts while breastfeeding (Paul Aegin. *Epitome* 3.35 (CMG 9.1, 221.4–222.22)). Similarly, in Metrodora's gynaecological treatise, the section on the breasts mixes recipes against pains in the breasts, recipes to promote or check milk production, and recipes to keep the breasts small and dainty.[46] Finally, Chapter 15 of Pseudo-Galen's second book of *On Procurable Remedies* also includes recipes to maintain the beauty of the breasts, recipes to dry out milk, recipes against inflammations, and recipes to bring out the milk.[47]

Conclusions

I started this chapter with the story of the Christian martyr Perpetua's lactation cessation; I ended it with cosmetic recipes to keep the breasts dainty. It might seem callous to put these two things alongside each other but considerations of a cosmetic nature are not absent from Perpetua's story. The *PPF*'s narrator stressed that the martyr's body appeared beautiful and youthful in the arena. In her own account,

44 Centlivres Challet 2017, 898.
45 For refusal to breastfeed conceived as a punishable sin in religious contexts, see Chapter 3 in this volume.
46 Metrodora Chapters: 40–44 (remedies against afflictions in the breasts); 44–46 (recipes to make the milk come); 47 (recipes to dry out the milk); 48 (recipes to keep the breasts small); 49 (recipe to straighten drooping breasts); 50 (recipes to keep the breasts small and pert); 51 (recipes to make the breasts shiny and beautiful), ed. Del Guerra 1953.
47 Ps.-Gal. *Rem. Parab.* 2.15, 14.446–449K, ed. Kühn 1827: 15.1 (recipe to straighten drooping breasts); 15.2 (recipe so that the breasts remain dainty); 15.3 (recipe so that the breasts do not become large); 15.4 (recipe to dry out the milk); 15.5 (recipes against inflammation of the breasts); 15.6 (recipes to draw out the milk); 15.7 (recipe to prevent the flow of milk); 15.8 (preservatives of the breasts).

Perpetua stated that in a vision she saw herself during the preparations for the arena: she "became a man," whom assistants rubbed down with oil, as they would before an athletic contest – she became an athlete of God (*PPF* 10.7). In the arena, her firm body was contrasted to the dripping, leaking body of Felicity. Women in antiquity did at times feel anxiety about the appearance of their breasts while – and after – breastfeeding. In doing so, they might have internalized patriarchal views of the male body, supposedly firmer and stronger, as the norm from which the female body deviates, especially when it is put under the strains of childbirth and lactation. That is not, however, to diminish that anxiety, which compounded fears over breast inflammations and over the breastfeeder's ability to nourish a child and make it thrive.

Ancient medical sources relating to weaning and lactation cessation, whether sudden or gradual, when read in a sensitive manner, do much to reveal the ambivalence of women, of their physicians, and of society at large, towards lactating breasts, their power to impart nutrition, and their physical appearance. These sources also talk, even if very quietly, of the pain, both physical and psychological, that accompanies the separation of a nursing woman from her own child or charge, whether that separation be temporary or permanent.

References

Texts: Editions and translations

Beck, L.Y. trans. 2020. *Pedanius Dioscorides of Anazarbus: De materia medica.* Translated by L.Y. Beck. 4th enlarged ed. Hildesheim: Olms and Weidmann.

Dagron, G. ed. and trans. 1978. *Vie et miracles de Sainte Thècle.* Subsidia Hagiographica 62. Brussels: Société des Bollandistes.

Del Guerra, G. ed. and trans. 1953. *Il Libro di Metrodora: Sulla malattie delle donne e il ricettario di cosmetica e terapia.* Milan: Ceschina.

Farrell, J., and C. Williams. eds. 2012. "Passio Sanctarum Perpetuae et Felicitatis," in J.N. Bremmer, and M. Formisano (eds) *Perpetua's Passions: Multidisciplinary Approaches to the Passio Perpetuae et Felicitatis.* Oxford: Oxford University Press, 24–32.

Hadot, I. ed. 1996. *Simplicius: Commentaire sur le Manuel d'Epictète.* Leiden: Brill.

Heiberg, J.L. ed. 1921. *Paulus Aegineta, Libri I–IV, edidit J.L. Heiberg.* Corpus Medicorum Graecorum 9.1. Leipzig and Berlin: Teubner.

Ilberg, J. ed. 1927. *Sorani Gynaeciorum libri IV, De signis fracturarum, De fasciis, Vita Hippocratis secundum Soranum, edidit J. Ilberg.* Corpus Medicorum Graecorum 4. Leipzig and Berlin: Teubner.

Johnston, I. ed. and trans. 2018. *Galen: Hygiene. Books 1–4.* Loeb Classical Library 535. Cambridge, MA: Harvard University Press.

Koch, K., G. Helmreich, C. Kalbfleisch, and O. Hartlich. eds. 1923. *Galeni De sanitate tuenda libri IV, edidit K. Koch. De alimentorum facultatibus libri III, edidit G. Helmreich. De bonis malisque sucis liber, edidit idem. De victu attenuante liber, edidit C. Kalbfleisch. De ptisana liber, edidit O. Hartlich.* Corpus Medicorum Graecorum 5.4.2. Leipzig and Berlin: Teubner.

Kühn, K.G. ed. 1826. *Claudii Galeni opera omnia.* Vol. 12. Leipzig: Car. Cnoblochius.

———. ed. 1827. *Claudii Galeni opera omnia.* Vol. 14. Leipzig: Car. Cnoblochius.

Levenson, J.L. ed. 2000. *Romeo and Juliet.* Oxford: Oxford University Press.

Olivieri, A. ed. 1935. *Aetii Amideni Libri medicinales I–IV, edidit A. Olivieri.* Corpus Medicorum Graecorum 8.1. Leipzig and Berlin: Teubner.

Pradels, W., R. Brändle, and M. Heimgartner. eds. and trans. 2000. "Das bisher vermisste Textstück in Johannes Chrysostomus, *Adversus Judaeos*, Oratio 2," *Zeitschrift für Antikes Christentum/Journal of Ancient Christianity* 5: 23–49.

Raeder, J. ed. 1926. *Oribasii Synopsis ad Eustathium, Libri ad Eunapium, edidit J. Raeder.* Corpus Medicorum Graecorum 6.3. Leipzig and Berlin: Teubner.

———. ed. 1929. *Oribasii Collectionum medicarum reliquiae, libri IX–XVI.* Corpus Medicorum Graecorum 6.1.2. Leizpig and Berlin: Teubner.

———. ed. 1933. *Oribasii Collectionum medicarum reliquiae, libri XLIX–L, libri incerti, eclogae medicamentorum, edidit J. Raeder.* Corpus Medicorum Graecorum 6.2.2. Leipzig and Berlin: Teubner.

Rolfe, J.C. ed. and trans. 1927. *Gellius: Attic Nights. Volume 2: Books 6–13.* Loeb Classical Library 200. Cambridge, MA: Harvard University Press.

Shackleton Bailey, D.R. ed. and trans. 2003. *Statius: Silvae.* Loeb Classical Library 206. Cambridge, MA: Harvard University Press.

Temkin, O. trans. 1956. *Soranus' Gynecology.* Baltimore, MD: John Hopkins University Press.

Ven, P. van den. ed. 1962. *La vie ancienne de S. Syméon Stylite le jeune (521–592).* Subsidia Hagiographica 32. Brussels: Société des Bollandistes.

Wellmann, M. ed. 1907–1914. *Pedanii Dioscuridis Anazarbei De materia medica libri quinque.* 3 vols. Berlin: Teubner.

Zervos, S. ed. 1901. *Gynaekologie des Aëtios.* Leipzig: Fock.

Secondary Works

Beaucamp, J. 1982. "L'allaitement: Mère ou nourrice?," *Jahrbuch der Österreichischen Byzantinistik* 32 (2): 549–558.

Bertier, J. 1996. "La médecine des enfants à l'époque impériale," in W. Haase (ed.) *Aufstieg und Niedergang der römischen Welt. Band 37/3: Teilband Philosophie, Wissenschaften, Technik. Wissenschaften (Medizin und Biologie [Forts.]).* Berlin: De Gruyter, 2147–2227.

Bourbou, C. 2020. "Health and Disease at the Marshes: Deciphering the Human–Environment Interaction at Roman Aventicum, Switzerland (1st–3rd c. AD)," in G. Robbins Schug (ed.) *Routledge Handbook of the Bioarchaeology of Environmental Change.* London: Routledge, 141–155.

Bourbou, C., and S. Garvie-Lock. 2009. "Breast-Feeding and Weaning Patterns in Byzantine Times: Evidence from Human Remains and Written Sources," in A. Papaconstantinou, and A.-M. Talbot (eds) *Becoming Byzantine: Children and Childhood in Byzantium.* Washington, DC: Dumbarton Oaks Research Library and Collection, 65–83.

Bourbou, C., and S. Garvie-Lock. 2015. "Bread, Oil, Wine, and Milk: Feeding Infants and Adults in Byzantine Greece," *Hesperia Supplements* 49: 171–194.

Bourbou, C., B.T. Fuller, S.J. Garvie-Lock, and M.P. Richards. 2013. "Nursing Mothers and Feeding Bottles: Reconstructing Breastfeeding and Weaning Patterns in Greek Byzantine Populations (6th–15th centuries AD) Using Carbon and Nitrogen Stable Isotope Ratios," *Journal of Archaeological Science* 40: 3903–3913.

Bourbou, C., G. Arenz, V. Dasen, and S. Lösch. 2019. "Babes, Bones, and Isotopes: A Stable Isotope Investigation on Nonadults from Aventicum, Roman Switzerland (First–Third century CE)," *International Journal of Osteoarchaeology* 29: 974–985.

Bremmer, J.N. 2012. "Felicitas: The Martyrdom of a Young African Woman," in Bremmer and Formisano 2012b, 35–53.

Bremmer, J.N., and M. Formisano. 2012a. "Perpetua's Passions: A Brief Introduction," in Bremmer and Formisano 2012b, 1–13.

———. eds. 2012b. *Perpetua's Passions: Multidisciplinary Approaches to the Passio Pepetuae et Felicitatis*. Oxford: Oxford University Press.

Calà, I., and G. Chesi. 2022. "Alcune considerazioni sul trattaro attribuito a Metrodora: Le ricette cosmetiche," *Eugesta: Journal of Gender Studies in Antiquity* 12: 41–56.

Centlivres Challet, C.-E. 2017. "Feeding the Roman Nursling: Maternal Milk, Its Substitutes, and Their Limitations," *Latomus: Revue d'études latines* 76: 895–909.

Cobb, S., and A.S. Jacobs. 2021. *The Passion of Perpetua and Felicitas in Late Antiquity*. Berkeley, CA: University of California Press.

Cocozza, C., R. Fernandes, A. Ughi, M. Groß, and M.M. Alexander. 2021. "Investigating Infant Feeding Strategies at Roman Bainesse through Bayesian Modelling of Incremental Dentine Isotopic Data," *International Journal of Osteoarchaeology* 31: 429–439.

Constantinou, S., and A. Skouroumouni-Stavrinou. 2022. "Premodern 'Galaktology': Reading Milk in Ancient and Early Byzantine Medical Treatises," *Journal of Late Antique, Islamic and Byzantine Studies* 1: 1–40.

———. 2024. "The Other Mother: Ancient and Early Byzantine Approaches to Wet Nursing and Mothering," *Journal of Hellenic Studies* 145, in press.

Dettwyler, K.A. 2017. "A Time to Wean: The Hominid Blueprint for the Natural Age of Weaning," in P. Stuard-Macadam, and K.A. Dettwyler (eds) *Breastfeeding: Biocultural Perspectives*. London: Routledge, 39–74.

Dova, S. 2017. "Lactation Cessation and the Realities of Martyrdom in *The Passion of Saint Perpetua*," *Illinois Classical Studies* 42: 245–265.

Dupras, T.L., H.P. Schwarcz, and S.I. Fairgrieve. 2001. "Infant Feeding and Weaning Practices in Roman Egypt," *American Journal of Physical Anthropology* 115: 204–212.

Dupras, T.L., and M.W. Tocheri. 2007. "Reconstructing Infant Weaning Histories at Roman Period Kellis, Egypt Using Stable Isotope Analysis of Dentition," *American Journal of Physical Anthropology* 134: 63–74.

Fildes, V. 1986. *Breasts, Bottles and Babies: A History of Infant Feeding*. Edinburgh: Edinburgh University Press.

Frankfurter, D. 2009. "Martyrology and the Prurient Gaze," *Journal of Early Christian Studies* 17: 215–245.

Fuller, B.T., T.I. Molleson, D.A. Harris, L.T. Gilmour, and R.E.M. Hedges. 2006. "Isotopic Evidence for Breastfeeding and Possible Adult Dietary Differences from Late/Sub-Roman Britain," *American Journal of Physical Anthropology* 129: 45–54.

Fulminante, F. 2015. "Infant Feeding Practices in Europe and the Mediterranean from Prehistory to the Middle Ages: A Comparison between the Historical Sources and Bioarchaeology," *Childhood in the Past* 8: 24–47.

Garnsey, P. 1998. "Child Rearing in Ancient Italy," in P. Garnsey (ed.) *Cities, Peasants and Food in Classical Antiquity: Essays in Social and Economic History*. Cambridge: Cambridge University Press, 253–271.

Gianni, M.L., M.E. Bettinelli, P. Manfra, G. Sorrentino, E. Bezze, L. Plevani, G. Cavallaro, G. Raffaeli, B.L. Crippa, and L. Colombo. 2019. "Breastfeeding Difficulties and Risk for Early Breastfeeding Cessation," *Nutrients* 11: 1–10.

Gold, B.K. 2018. *Perpetua: Athlete of God*. Oxford: Oxford University Press.

Golden, M. 2015. *Children and Childhood in Classical Athens*. Baltimore: John Hopkins University Press.

Gourevitch, D. 1995. "L'alimentation animale de la femme enceinte, de la nourrice et du bébé sevré," in *Homme et animal dans l'Antiquité romaine: Actes du colloque de Nantes 1991*. Tours: Centre de Recherches A. Piganiol, 283–293.

Gourevitch, D., and J. Chamay. 1992. "Femme nourrissant son enfant au biberon," *Antike Kunst* 35: 78–81.

Heffernan, T.J. 2012. *The Passion of Perpetua and Felicity*. Oxford: Oxford University Press.

Holman, S.R. 1997. "Molded as Wax: Formation and Feeding of the Ancient Newborn," *Helios* 24: 77–95.

Keenleyside, A., H. Schwarcz, L. Stirling, and N.B. Lazreg. 2009. "Stable Isotopic Evidence for Diet in a Roman and Late Roman Population from Leptiminus, Tunisia," *Journal of Archaeological Science* 36: 51–63.

Keyser, P.T., and G.L. Irby-Massie. eds. 2008. *The Encyclopedia of Ancient Natural Scientists: The Greek Tradition and Its Many Heirs*. London: Routledge.

Lascaratos, J., and E. Poulakou-Rebelakou. 2003. "Oribasius (Fourth Century) and Early Byzantine Perinatal Nutrition," *Journal of Pediatric Gastroenterology and Nutrition* 36: 186–189.

Marklein, K.E., and S.C. Fox. 2020. "The Bioarchaeology of Children in Greco-Roman Antiquity," in L.A. Beaumont, M. Dillon, and N. Harrington (eds) *Children in Antiquity*. London: Routledge, 567–580.

Myers, A.D. 2017. *Blessed among Women? Mothers and Motherhood in the New Testament*. Oxford: Oxford University Press.

Parca, M. 2017. "The Wet Nurses of Ptolemaic and Roman Egypt," *Illinois Classical Studies* 42: 203–226.

Parkin, T. 2013. "The Demography of Infancy and Early Childhood," in J.E. Grubbs, T. Parkin, and R. Bell (eds) *The Oxford Handbook of Childhood and Education in the Classical World*. Oxford: Oxford University Press, 40–61.

Pedrucci, G. 2013. "Sangue mestruale e latte materno: Riflessioni e nuove proposte. Intorno all'allattamento nella Grecia antica," *Gesnerus* 70: 260–291.

Powell, L.A., R.C. Redfern, A.R. Millard, and D.R. Gröcke. 2014. "Infant Feeding Practices in Roman London: Evidence from Isotopic Analyses," in E.-J. Graham, and M. Carroll (eds) *Infant Health and Death in Roman Italy and Beyond*. Supplementary Series 96. Portsmouth, RI: *Journal of Roman Archaeology*, 89–110.

Prowse, T.L., S.R. Saunders, H.P. Schwarcz, P. Garnsey, R. Macchiarelli, and L. Bondioli. 2008. "Isotopic and Dental Evidence for Infant and Young Child Feeding Practices in an Imperial Roman Skeletal Sample," *American Journal of Physical Anthropology* 137: 294–308.

Redfern, R., R. Gowland, A. Millard, L. Powell, and D. Gröcke. 2018. "'From the Mouths of Babes': A Subadult Dietary Stable Isotope Perspective on Roman London (Londinium)," *Journal of Archaeological Science: Reports* 19: 1030–1040.

Rey, A.-L. 2004. "Autour des nourrissons byzantins et de leur régime," in V. Dasen (ed.) *Naissance et petite enfance dans l'Antiquité: Actes du colloque de Fribourg, 28 novembre–1er décembre 2001*. Fribourg: Academic Press, 363–375.

Ricciardetto, A., and D. Gourevitch. 2020. "The Cost of a Baby: How Much Did It Cost to Hire a Wet-Nurse in Roman Egypt?," in L. Totelin, and R. Flemming (eds) *Medicine and Markets in the Graeco-Roman World and Beyond: Essays on Ancient Medicine in Honour of Vivian Nutton*. Swansea: Classical Press of Wales, 41–69.

Sallares, R. 1991. *The Ecology of the Ancient Greek World*. Ithaca, NY: Cornell University Press.

Sellen, D.W. 2007. "Evolution of Infant and Young Child Feeding: Implications for Contemporary Public Health," *Annual Review of Nutrition* 27: 123–148.

Totelin, L. 2021a. "Breastmilk in the Cave and on the Arena: Early Christian Stories of Lactation in Context," in M. Bradley, V. Leonard, and L. Totelin (eds) *Bodily Fluids in Antiquity*. London: Routledge, 240–255.

———. 2021b. "Easy Remedies – Difficult Texts: The Pseudo-Galenic *Euporista*," in C. Petit, S. Swain, and K.-D. Fischer (eds) *Pseudo-Galenica: The Formation of the Galenic Corpus from Antiquity to the Renaissance*. London: Warburg Institute Colloquia, 31–46.

6 "Galaktology" and Genre

Simple Literary Forms on Milk and Breastfeeding in Ancient and Early Byzantine Medical Treatises*

Stavroula Constantinou and
Aspasia Skouroumouni-Stavrinou

Introduction

The diction (the choice of words and stylistic techniques), separate from the content (the choice of arguments), of ancient and early Byzantine medical debates constitutes a strategic means for communicating views on the science of milk – what we term "galaktology."[1] At the same time, diction flags the respective roles of milk producer, milk consumer, and milky product, which are crucial factors in understanding galaktology's mechanisms. This chapter aims to explore the literary profile of galaktology's diction by focussing on simple literary forms. In the examined texts, simple literary forms are relatively short, ranging from a short phrase to one or two pages of printed text, and they mostly fall into three categories: saying, anecdote, and ethnography. Although there are different degrees of complexity and elaboration also on the level of stylistics, content, and structure (for example, an anecdote is more complex than a saying), these forms are designated as "simple" to mark their status both as freestanding texts, also circulating orally, and as units embedded in extensive texts. In labelling them thus, we adopt André Jolles' terminology and generic system, in which simple forms are abstract pre-existing structures that take shape as actualized forms.[2] The former are collective creations, produced by language users in their attempt to decode and systematize their world ("mental dispositions"), while the latter (the actualizations) are individual and ar-

* The research for this chapter was co-funded by the European Regional Development Fund and the Republic of Cyprus through the Foundation of Research and Innovation (Project: EXCELLENCE/1216/0020), as well as by the University of Cyprus within the framework of an internal research project. Some of the ideas that inform the article's arguments were developed within the framework of the project "Network for Medieval Arts and Rituals" (NetMAR) which received funding from the European Union's Horizon 2020 research and innovation programme under grant agreement nr 951875. The opinions expressed in this document reflect only the authors' views, and in no way reflect the European Commission's opinions. The European Commission is not responsible for any use that may be made of the information it contains.

1 For galaktology in ancient and early Byzantine medical treatises, see Constantinou and Skouroumouni-Stavrinou 2022.
2 Jolles' investigation (1930, *Einfache Formen*; Eng. trans. as *Simple Forms* 2017) into the universal structures of narrative genres remains influential.

DOI: 10.4324/9781003265658-8

tificial creations modified by literary norms. Jolles distinguishes nine archetypical "verbal gestures" ("legend," "saga," "myth," "riddle," "saying," "case," "memorabile," "fairy tale," and "joke").

Following Jolles, we are trying to detect the ways in which medical authors resort to literary forms to decode the social and epistemic purposes influencing the use of these forms. Yet, our debts to Jolles do not extend to an adoption of all aspects of his systematic conception of the simple forms' genealogies or typologies. More specifically, although we acknowledge the heuristic value of Jolles' idea that simple forms derive from specific mental dispositions and are realized according to cultural codes and social conditions, we consider these forms both "simple" and "literary," not only at the level of their actualization as textual units but also as creative modes used to organize medical material and to present it in appealing ways.

The three simple literary forms discussed here – saying, anecdote, and ethnography – recur in medical discussions concerning the biology and mechanics of milk production and consumption, including the bodily organs and processes involved, the physiology and conduct of the human and animal milk producer, the texture and qualities of milk, and the more general condition of the infant and adult milk consumer. Like the milk terms and figurative tropes which are prominent in galaktology passages, simple literary forms are not restricted within their limits alone, but are found also in other parts of medical treatises dealing with other issues, such as embryology, obstetrics, and geriatrics.[3] They remain, however, common and recurrent techniques for elaborating and sustaining sections on galaktology in one or more medical authors. Their more widespread use within our ancient and early Byzantine medical corpus (1st–7th c. AD) further testifies to their value as efficient techniques of medical writing and as powerful means of explicating and promoting the examined authors' theories and ideas more generally. The content, aesthetics and function of each simple literary form are here set under scrutiny in a double way: within the immediate textual surroundings of a simple form's occurrence in galaktology sections of a given medical treatise; and, where applicable, within the wider intertextual context of re-formulations and alternative treatments of themes and simple narrative structures in the galaktology sections of different medical texts.

Our analysis is based on those Greek medical treatises in which galaktology sections figure most prominently. These are the works of Soranos (1st–early 2nd c. AD), Galen (AD 129–ca. 216/217), Oribasios (fl. 4th c. AD), and Aetios (fl. ca.

3 See e.g. Sor. *Gynaecology (Gyn.)* 1.39.1–2 (CMG 4, 27.28–38), ed. Ilberg 1927: the paradigm of the misshapen tyrant of the Cyprians used to exemplify the impact of the state of the soul on the moulding of the foetus; Sor. *Gyn.* 1.42.2.3–4 (CMG 4, 29.22–23): a saying of general wisdom in Soranos' discussion on conception as a healthful or unhealthful state for the woman ("As a matter of fact if a thing is useful it is not in every case healthful as well"; "οὐ πάντως γε μὴν εἴ τι ὠφέλιμόν ἐστιν, τοῦτο καὶ ὑγιεινόν"; trans. Temkin 1956, 41); Gal. *Hygiene (San. Tu.)* 5.4.9–15 (CMG 5.4.2, 143.17–144.15), ed. Koch 1923: the anecdote on the long-lived Antiochos' regimen of bodily care and nutrition. Several examples of the usage of a literary form in areas outside galaktology are also mentioned, where deemed relevant, in the following discussion.

530–560), with Alexander of Tralles (fl. 6th c. AD) and Paul of Aegina (fl. early 7th c. AD) occasionally providing parallels. These medical authors follow each other not only in terms of chronological sequence. Since Oribasios, Aetios, Alexander of Tralles, and Paul of Aegina repeat and re-elaborate earlier medical knowledge, including that of the authors under study (Galen and to a lesser extent Soranos, with Oribasios himself being a source for Aetios and so forth), these texts are also interlinked through the process of rewriting.[4] The analysis of the spread, thematic distribution and stylistic modulation (morphology and function) of the short literary forms most frequently employed in the examined medical treatises' galaktology sections is variously illuminating: for unravelling how the same themes take on different shapes and meanings through each author's use of literary forms, and for detecting how the usage and function of each literary form changes or remains the same through time.

Shedding light on medical rewriting in terms of its literary transformations is essential for a fuller understanding of ancient and early Byzantine galaktology and its evolution. Among other things, such an approach brings to light different aspects of galaktology that have remained hidden in previous studies that concentrate exclusively on the iteration of medical content.[5] Through the following analysis, the broader scientific, social, and cultural practices within which galaktology takes shape are significantly elucidated. Indeed, the attempt to reconstruct the interplay between the content and diction of galaktology by focusing on literary categories comes with an additional benefit: a contribution towards the unravelling of the evolution of ancient and Byzantine short literary forms and their rarely studied uses in scientific texts, such as medical treatises.[6]

Anecdote

Personal experience or knowledge of written and oral traditions on milk epistemology and praxis are the main reservoirs from which our medical authors draw to produce the anecdotes they include in their texts. In general, these anecdotes are short narratives referring to a medical author's practical experiences (for example, a personal encounter with a certain patient) or to the experiences of another physician, which the medical author incorporates in his text(s). Not, perhaps,

---

4 For the concept of rewriting as particularly appropriate for conceptualizing the interrelation of the examined medical texts, see Constantinou and Skouroumouni-Stavrinou 2022.

5 The argument that a highly developed medical milk theory existed already from the early first century BC, if not earlier, is variously made in studies focusing on the processes of selection (character and type of sources prioritized) and organization (citation and abbreviation techniques) of earlier medical material (primarily of the Galenic canonical material). See e.g. Rzeźnicka and Kokoszko 2020; Kokoszko et al. 2018, 985 (Sextius Niger and Dioskorides seen in relation to Galen and later authors); Kokoszko and Dybała 2016, 342, 346, 348 (comparative study of Celsus and Oribasios); Rzeźnicka 2016, 58, 63–64, 71 (Galen seen in relation to Rufus of Ephesos and later authors up to the 7th c. AD).

6 To our knowledge, no sustained study on the subject exists.

incidentally, Galen is the medical author of anecdotes *par excellence*.[7] Galenic anecdotes concerning his interaction with various patients recur in the context of his discussions on milk as pharmaceutical or dietetic substance. These anecdotes, which are inserted at strategic points of his galaktology discussions, invariably function as vehicles carrying forceful lessons about the quality and therapeutic uses of human and animal milk, as well as means of commenting on the ways in which the doctor's stature and the patient's stances mutually play a crucial role in matters concerning illness and its treatment.

A rich assortment of multiple anecdotes is found in *Therapeutic Method* (*MM*), in the context of Galen's discussion of ulcer treatment in the rough arteries (trachea and bronchial tree) through milk consumption. Galen flags the importance of this method emphatically, stating the novelty of his technique, which he executed with unfailing success during the Antonine plague of AD 165–180, the first pandemic affecting the Roman Empire (Gal. *MM* 5.12, 10.360.13–361.1K, ed. Kühn 1825).[8] Excellent-quality Tabian animal milk, consumed as fresh as possible, was the means that secured Galen's cure of those severe ulcers. The cases of two young men with ulcers in the rough arteries serve as illustrative examples of Galen's method (*MM* 5.12, 10.361.1–367.1K).

His acute diagnosis of the placement of the ulcer within each man's body is the first step towards the correct treatment and ultimate cure of the ulcer. Contrary to the doctors previously examining the first young man's mouth and not detecting the ulcer in his throat, Galen manages to reach a clearer diagnosis by providing a potion that is a mixture of vinegar and mustard which allows the patient to control his coughing (*MM* 5.12, 10.361.10–15K). As a result, Galen is able to see the ulcer that is responsible for the man's suffering. A treatment via drying and moist medications is applied before the patient's departure to Tabia for treatment with the high-quality regional milk.[9] In the case of the second young man, who suffers from catarrh, Galen again makes the right observations leading to the correct diagnosis and subsequent milk therapy in Tabia (*MM* 5.12, 10.366.16–18K; 10.367.1–2K). Galen also sends to Tabia a third young man, whose coughing is provoked by the cooling of his respiratory organs, as well as a number of other patients having similar symptoms (*MM* 5.13–14, 10.372.17–373.2K).

The way in which adult patients' stances and taboos may facilitate or hinder the doctor's work figure flagrantly in another anecdote, recounting Galen's treatment of a man suffering from dryness of blood in his arteries and veins (*MM* 7.6, 10.471–485K). Galen's goal is to moisten the man's stomach and whole body, which are dried up by the false therapies of previous doctors, who have administered astringent food, drinks, and medications. Galen's prescribed treatment

---

7 For Galen as a successful storyteller, see Xenophontos 2023, in press.

8 The Antonine plague was raging in the East by mid- to late AD 165 and could easily have reached Rome before the return of the army in mid AD 166, the traditional catalyst for its outbreak in Rome; see Gourevitch 2013.

9 Environmental factors defining the excellent quality of Tabian milk are described in Gal. *MM* 5.12, 10.363–366K; see also below under "Ethnography."

includes bathing followed by bodily rubbing with oil and consumption of donkey milk (*MM* 7.6, 10.472–473K, 10.479K). Although, as also remarked by previous medical authorities, Galen sees human milk directly suckled from a lactating woman's teats as the ideal medicament,[10] fresh donkey milk is prescribed in this case because the patient finds the direct consumption of human milk disgusting (*MM* 7.6, 10.475.1–3K). Galen criticizes the patient's approach leading to the rejection of the much more efficient treatment, by reducing him to the position of an ass that takes its share of the milk produced by a mother of its species (*MM* 7.6, 10.475.5–6K). This is a rare instance where animalistic imagery is directly applied to the milk consumer. In our corpus, it is mostly the human milk producer – biological mother or wet nurse – that is paralleled to animals or plants.[11]

That good knowledge of human physiology is crucial in understanding illness and configuring the right treatment is another emphatic message Galen aims to bring across by using anecdotes. A case in point is a discussion in his work *Affected Places* (*Loc. Aff.*) about the causes of diseases related to malfunctions of the human uterus or penis, where he uses an anecdote which also involves animals (goats), whose bodies figure prominently. This anecdote concerns the conduct and nutritional habits of an untimely delivered goat foetus which he discovers when dissecting a pregnant goat. After he has separated the premature animal from the mother's body and placed various bowls in front of it, each bowl containing a liquid such as wine, honey, oil, and milk, it is astonishingly observed

> that this premature animal walked from the start with its feet as if it had learned that it had feet for walking; secondly it shook off the moisture which covered it in the uterus; thirdly, it scratched its ribs with one foot. Then we saw that it sniffed at each one of the things laid out in the house. After it had smelled all of them, it drank the milk. At this moment we all exclaimed loudly.
>
> τὸ ἔμβρυον ἐκεῖνο πρῶτον μὲν βαδίζον τοῖς ποσὶν, ὥσπερ ἀκηκοὸς ἕνεκα βαδίσεως ἔχειν τὰ σκέλη· δεύτερον δ' ἀποσειόμενον τὴν ἐκ τῆς μήτρας ὑγρότητα· καὶ τρίτον ἐπὶ τούτῳ κνησάμενον ἑνὶ τῶν ποδῶν τὴν πλευράν· εἶτ' ὀσμώμενον εἴδομεν αὐτὸ τῶν κειμένων κατὰ τὸν οἶκον ἑκάστου· ὡς δὲ πάντων ὠσμᾶτο, τοῦ γάλακτος ἀπερρόφησεν, ἐν ᾧ καὶ ἀνεκεκράγαμεν ἅπαντες. (Gal. *Loc. Aff.* 6.6, 8.443.9–16K, ed. Kühn 1824; trans. Siegel 1976, 194)

Likewise, in two months' time, the baby goat instinctively aligns its nutritional habits to those of other goats of its age, turning "to the food to which adult goats are accustomed" (soft shoots of shrubs and leaves provided in Galen's bowls) and

---

10 This is a comment also made in passing in Galen's discussion about Tabian milk treatments (*MM* 5.12, 10.366.1–6K). For other instances of Galenic insistence on the freshness of milk, see Constantinou and Skouroumouni-Stavrinou 2022, 30, n. 100. For Galen's insistence on direct suckling from a woman's or an animal's teat, see also the discussion under "Ethnography", below.

11 *MM* 7.6, 10.475.5–6K. For the marked satirical irony of the passage, carried through animalistic imagery and other rhetorical means, see below, under "Ethnography"; see also Constantinou and Skouroumouni-Stavrinou 2022, 29–31.

ruminating them in the same manner (*Loc. Aff.* 6.6, 8.444.4–7K, 10K; trans. Siegel 1976, 194). Amazement over the natural faculties of animals and the workings of nature is again the spontaneous response (*Loc. Aff.* 6.6, 8.444.10–12K). Here and elsewhere in Galen's experimental anecdotes, his emphasis on the wondrous and awe-inspiring workings of nature, wisely crafting and providing for the reflexive predilection of the infant for milk, serves brilliantly to strengthen his fundamental doctrine on the unfailing and remarkable untaught nature of all bodily organs.[12] The anecdote of the goat inserted into Galen's discussion of the functions and malfunctions of genital organs not only provides an easier explanation of complex diseases but also presents in a more approachable and acceptable way issues related to bodily organs whose activities are traditionally categorized as taboo.

Galen's observational and deductive skills, leading to accurate *diagnoses* and inferences when curing patients, experimenting with dissection, and so on, effectively establish his authorial persona as an outstanding medical thinker and practitioner.[13] To put it differently, Galen's usage of anecdotes drawn from his practical experience aligns perfectly with his otherwise strong rhetoric of self-promotion.[14] That impression is further enhanced by the exceptionality of his extensive (both in terms of the quantity of examples and of the narrative length of each example) use of this literary form, which is unparalleled in his contemporary Soranos or later medical authors, such as Oribasios and Aetios.

In the context of his own discussion of infant nutrition and the ways of testing the quality of breastmilk, Soranos in his *Gynaecology*, for example, does not resort to anecdote, but to figures of speech and particularly to simile.[15] In order to raise a caveat on how the state of the infant should also be taken into consideration in evaluating the quality of a wet nurse's milk, he writes the following:

> For it is possible that the milk is suitable, but the child is prevented by some disease from being well nourished. For adults too who are sick become ill-nourished though they partake of the best food, the body spoiling what might be nourishing, just as vessels for vinegar spoil the wine that is poured into them, even if it is the best.

12 Cf. e.g. *Loc. Aff.* 6.6, 8.442.16–18K; 6.6, 8.444.18–19K; 6.6, 8.446.4–11K.
13 The strategies that showcase Galen's deductive skills in the narration of his case studies of patients have variously attracted comment. See e.g. Thumiger 2018, commenting on the "detective narrative" (p. 51) that shapes Galen's presentation of cases of cures, and differentiating them from Hippocratic case studies of patients in the *Epidemics*; Kim 2017, examining the rhetoric of Galenic stories of patient treatments with Calasiris' narratives in Heliodoros' *Ethiopics*. For studies turning attention to the usage of Galenic stories in general, see e.g. Kazantzidis and Tsoumpra 2018, 281–284, in the context of their examination of laughter as a response to disease from Hippocrates onwards.
14 For Galen's sustained and multiply promoted "rhetoric of success," see e.g. Nutton 2020, especially. 101–110; Petit 2018 (an extensive study on Galen's rhetorical skill and art); Lloyd 2008.
15 Soranos' similes are the most frequent and most expounded in their configuration (the lengthiest and the richest in complicated word images) in comparison to those of the other medical authors under study.

καὶ γὰρ τῶν τελείων οἱ νοσοῦντες ἀτροφοῦσιν καὶ τῆς ἀρίστης τροφῆς
μεταλαμβάνοντες, τοῦ σώματος φθείροντος τὸ θρέψαι δυνάμενον, καθάπερ
καὶ τὰ ὀξηρὰ τῶν ἀγγείων ἀφανίζει [καὶ] τὸν ἐγχεόμενον οἶνον εἰς αὐτά, κἂν
ἄριστος ᾖ. (Sor. *Gyn.* 2.21.2.7–10 (CMG 4, 69.15–18); trans. Temkin 1956, 95)

Although it is a hint that the milk is suitable if the child fed on it is in good physical
condition, it does not follow, on the other hand, that an ill-developed child is proof
of worthless milk. Soranos, imagining the body as a defective vessel, comments on
the sickly state of the consumer (whether infant or adult) as an important factor in
conceiving and determining the results of milk consumption.

Galen makes a similar point in the context of a different discussion, concerning
the appropriate foodstuff for old age. In his *Hygiene*, for instance, he at one point
considers the role of wine in the nutrition of aged people. This topic is taken on after
Galen's anecdote involving an eponymous man, the long-lived Telephos, grammarian of Pergamum (2nd c. AD). Telephos' longevity is the result of consistently receiving proper massage and his bathing habits, along with the careful consumption of
high-quality food in suitable quantities. As Galen explicates in the previous chapter,
these are important models for achieving good health in old age (*San. Tu.* 5.4 (CMG
5.4.2, 142.19–144.12), ed. Koch 1923). Telephos' habit of having for dinner bread
that has been soaked in mixed wine offers Galen the opportunity to introduce his
exposition on wine's potency as determined through its different types and modes of
consumption by old people (*San. Tu.* 5.5–5.6 (CMG 5.4.2, 144.13–147.26)).

Another anecdote in the same text, which refers to five milk-drinking men, aims
at further explicating Galen's theory about the strong interrelation between food – in
this case, the nature and potency of milk – and the bodily situation of the consumer:

Anyway, I knew a certain old man, a farmer, who had lived on the land for
more than a hundred years. His main nutriment was goat's milk … But someone who imitated this man, thinking the milk was the reason for his longevity,
was continually harmed, regardless of how it was taken. For the opening of
the stomach was weighed down by this, and afterward the right hypocondrium
was distended. And someone else, who similarly tried to use the milk, found
fault with none of the other things … But on the seventh day after he began,
he said he was clearly aware of a heaviness of the liver … Furthermore, I
know another person who formed a stone in the kidneys through using milk
for a long time, and someone else who lost all his teeth. This has also occurred
in many others who used a milk diet over a long period. And yet others have
used milk continually without trouble and with very great benefit, just like the
man who lived for more than a hundred years in the country, as I said. **For
when its quality has nothing inimical in nature to its use, and the passages
through the wide vessels of the internal organs are favorable, these people enjoy the benefits [of milk] and experience nothing bad.**

γέροντα γοῦν τινα γεωργικὸν ἔγνωμεν, ἔτη πλείω τῶν ἑκατὸν βιώσαντα
κατ᾽ ἀγρόν, ᾧ τὸ πλεῖον τῆς τροφῆς αἴγειον ἦν γάλα … ἀλλὰ τοῦτόν γέ
τις μιμησάμενος (ᾤετο γὰρ αἴτιον αὐτῷ τὸ γάλα τῆς πολυχρονίου ζωῆς

γεγονέναι) διὰ παντὸς ἐβλάβη καὶ κατὰ πάντα τρόπον προσφορᾶς. ἐβαρύνετο γὰρ αὐτῷ τὸ στόμα τῆς γαστρὸς καὶ μετὰ ταῦτα τὸ δεξιὸν ὑποχόνδριον ἐτείνετο. καί τις ἕτερος, ὁμοίως ἐπιχειρήσας χρήσασθαι τῷ γάλακτι, τῶν μὲν ἄλλων οὐδὲν ἐμέμφετο … ἑβδόμῃ δ᾿ ἡμέρᾳ μετὰ τὴν ἀρχὴν ἐναργῶς ἔφη τοῦ ἥπατος αἰσθάνεσθαι βαρυνομένου· … καὶ μὲν δὴ καὶ ἄλλον ἐπὶ γάλακτος χρήσει πολυχρονίῳ λίθον γεννήσαντα κατὰ τοὺς νεφροὺς οἶδα, καί τινα ἕτερον ἀπολέσαντα πάντας τοὺς ὀδόντας. τοῦτο μὲν οὖν καὶ ἄλλοις ἐγένετο πολλοῖς τῶν ἐπὶ γάλακτι μακρῶς διαιτηθέντων. ἀλύπως δ᾿ ἕτεροι διὰ παντὸς ἐχρήσαντο τῷ γάλακτι καὶ μετ᾿ ὠφελείας μεγίστης, ἄλλοι δὲ παραπλησίως τῷ κατ᾿ ἀγρὸν βιώσαντι πλείω τῶν ἑκατὸν ἐτῶν, ὡς ἔφην. **ὅταν γὰρ ἥ τε ποιότης αὐτοῦ τῇ τοῦ χρωμένου φύσει μηδὲν ὑπεναντίον ἔχῃ, τῶν τε σπλάγχνων εὐπετεῖς αἱ διέξοδοι διὰ τὴν τῶν ἀγγείων εὐρύτητα ὦσι, τῶν μὲν ὠφελίμων ἐκ γάλακτος ἀπολαύουσιν οὗτοι, μοχθηροῦ δ᾿ οὐδενὸς πειρῶνται.** (Gal. *San. Tu.* 5.7.10–15 (CMG 5.4.2, 148.21–149.11); trans. Johnston 2018b, 47–49; emphasis added)

On the one hand, we have those benefitting from the properties of milk in various ways, including longevity: the old farmer who uses goat's milk as his main nutriment and others that consume milk regularly without any trouble. On the other hand, we get those inflicted by various diseases, such as distention of the right hypochondrium, formation of stones in the liver or the kidneys, and loss of teeth. Galen's anecdote is not meant to deny the good properties of milk, already and rightly widely asserted by previous medical authors.[16] Caution should, however, be raised about their dependence on the condition of the consumer's organism, as well as on other influential factors related to the health and regimen of the milk producer (*San. Tu.* 5.7.17–20 (CMG 5.4.2, 149.15–25)) and the mode of milk consumption – for example, the combination of ass' and goat's milk is preferable (*San. Tu.* 5.7.21 (CMG 5.4.2, 149.27–30)).

In his *Tetrabiblos* (*Tetr.*), Aetios absorbs Galen's lessons concerning the ambiguous and conditional nature of milk. In fact, he acknowledges Galen, along with Rufus, as his key source (*Tetr.* 2.86 (CMG 8.1, 180.5), ed. Olivieri 1935). The phrasing and structure of his discussion of the role of the consumer's nature in determining the impact of milk consumption point to the Galenic hypotext in marked ways (as in the previous passage, we indicate in bold Galen's phraseology which is repeated in the Aetian passage):[17]

Those for whom milk is appropriate. Milk is the best of almost all we offer, being good-juiced and nutritious, and consisting of differing substances and

---

16 "The good aspects of milk have also been spoken of by many previous doctors – moderate downward evacuation of the stomach, euchymia and nourishment" ("τὰ δ᾿ ἐκ τοῦ γάλακτος ἀγαθὰ λέλεκται καὶ τοῖς ἔμπροσθεν ἰατροῖς, ὑπαγωγὴ μετρία γαστρὸς εὐχυμία τε καὶ θρέψις …" *San. Tu.* 5.7.16 (CMG 5.4.2, 149.11–14); trans. Johnston 2018b, 49).

17 We are employing the Genettean terms "hypertext" and "hypotext" to define the intertextual relationships of the examined texts, i.e. the role of Galen and Soranos as key sources of material

powers ... and **when its quality has nothing inimical in nature to its use, and the passages through the wide vessels of the internal organs are favourable, these people enjoy the benefits of milk and experience nothing malicious. The good aspects of milk have also been mentioned by many previous doctors – moderate downward evacuation of the stomach, the healthy state of the humours, and nourishment.**

Τίσι τὸ γάλα ἁρμόδιον. Εὐχυμότατον καὶ τροφιμώτατον πᾶν τὸ ἄριστον γάλα σχεδὸν ἁπάντων ὅσα προσφερόμεθα, συγκείμενον ἐξ ἐναντίων οὐσιῶν τε καὶ δυνάμεων ... καὶ ὅταν ἥ τε ποιότης αὐτοῦ τῇ τοῦ χρωμένου φύσει μηδὲν ὑπεναντίον ἔχῃ, τῶν τε σπλάγχνων εὐπετεῖς ὦσιν αἱ διέξοδοι διὰ τὴν τῶν ἀγγείων εὐρύτητα· τῶν μὲν οὖν ὠφελίμων ἐκ γάλακτος ἀπολαύουσιν οἱ τοιοῦτοι, μοχθηροῦ δὲ οὐδενὸς πειρῶνται. τὰ δὲ ἀγαθὰ τοῦ γάλακτος λέλεκται καὶ τοῖς ἔμπροσθεν ἰατροῖς, ὑπαγωγὴ μετρία γαστρὸς εὐχυμία τε καὶ θρέψις. (Aet. *Tetr.* 2.92.1–9 (CMG 8.1, 181.26–182.5))[18]

Aetios distils the epistemological arguments deduced in the Galenic anecdote of the five milk-drinking men, while excluding the anecdote from his own text.

In the following example, Aetios adopts a different method, as he rewrites a Galenic anecdote in the form of a summary. This time the Galenic anecdote revolves around infant care and the role of the wet nurse in the infant's upbringing. It concerns a nameless wet nurse whom Galen considers inexperienced in her mothering role:

At all events, on one occasion, when a baby was crying, restive and turning itself about in a violent and disorderly fashion for a whole day, and the nurse was at a loss, I myself discovered what was distressing it. ... I saw that his bed and its coverings, as well as his clothes, were rather soiled, and the baby himself was dirty and unwashed. I directed her to wash and clean him thoroughly, change the bed, and make all the clothing cleaner. Once these things had happened, he immediately stopped the excessive movements and straightway fell into a very sweet and very prolonged sleep. In properly evaluating all the things that distress a young child, not only is there need of wisdom but also of a long-continuing experience in nursing itself.

ἐγὼ γοῦν ποτε δι' ὅλης ἡμέρας παιδίου κλαίοντός τε καὶ θυμουμένου καὶ σφοδρῶς καὶ ἀτάκτως ἑαυτὸ μεταβάλλοντος ἐξεῦρον τὸ λυποῦν ἀπορουμένης τῆς τροφοῦ· ... ἐθεασάμην δ' ἐγὼ τὴν στρωμνὴν αὐτοῦ καὶ τὰ περιβλήματά τε καὶ ἀμφιέσματα ῥυπαρώτερα καὶ αὐτὸ τὸ παιδίον ἤδη ῥυπῶν τε καὶ ἄλουτον, ἐκέλευσα λοῦσαί τε καὶ ἀπορρύψαι καὶ τὴν στρωμνὴν ὑπαλλάξαι, καὶ πᾶσαν τὴν ἐσθῆτα καθαρωτέραν ἐργάσασθαι· καὶ τούτων γενομένων, αὐτίκα μὲν ἐπαύσατο τῶν ἀμέτρων κινήσεων, αὐτίκα δὲ καθύπνωσεν ἥδιστόν τε καὶ μακρότατον ὕπνον. εἰς δὲ τὸ καλῶς ἐστοχάσθαι πάντων τῶν

(both in terms of content and stylistics) for the later medical authors. For Genette's rewriting theory discussed in the context of approaching Byzantine rewriting and as a useful and apt exemplar for a better understanding of premodern rewriting in general, see Constantinou 2020, 10–62.

18   Unless otherwise indicated, translations are our own.

ἀνιώντων τὸ παιδίον οὐκ ἀγχινοίας μόνον, ἀλλὰ καὶ τῆς περὶ τὸ τρεφόμενον αὐτὸ συνεχοῦς ἐμπειρίας ἐστὶ χρεία. (Gal. *San. Tu.* 1.8.30–32 (CMG 5.4.2, 21.20–33); trans. Johnston 2018a, 65)

The three common remedies for an infant's distress, mentioned earlier in the same Galenic text – offering of the nipple, moderate movement, and a certain modulation in the nurse's voice – fail in the case of this infant boy (Gal. *San. Tu.* 1.7.22–24 (CMG 5.4.2, 18.7–18)).[19] With the nurse at a loss, it is Galen's acute observational and deductive skill, forcefully denoted via his use of first-person verbs accompanied by emphatic particles, which leads to the disclosure of the true reason for the infant's anguish: filthiness. Accordingly, he orders the baby's thorough washing and the changing of both the dirty bed coverings and the baby's soiled clothes. Galen's anecdote of his interaction with this nurse and infant is inserted into his discussion about how health is preserved in individuals with the best bodily situation from infancy to adult life. His emphasis on neatness and the nurse's role in sustaining a clean environment for the infant functions as a prompt for his detailed consideration of the good wet nurse's general profile. Apart from being wise and experienced, the wet nurse should have a certain diet and physical exercise, create sleep routines, and avoid sexual activity to secure the best milk quality and to provide the most suitable care for the nursing infant.[20]

Galen's anecdote reappears in Olivieri's edition of Aetios' *Tetrabiblos*.[21] At the end of a chapter entitled "On the selection of a wet nurse," we read the following:

The wet nurse should be such: *sōphrōn*, sober, not ill-tempered, clean, in good condition and not suffering from epilepsy. [I myself once, reports Galen, when a baby was in agitation and crying for a whole day, as I saw that its bed, coverings, and the baby itself were dirty, ordered for it to be washed and the bed and clothing to be changed. As soon as this was done, he stopped crying and being distressed, and he fell asleep.]

πρὸς τούτοις δὲ εἶναι χρὴ τὴν τιτθὴν σώφρονα ἀμέθυσον ἀόργητον καθάριον εὔχυμον καὶ μὴ ἐπίληπτον. [ἔγωγ' οὖν ποτε, φησὶν ὁ Γαληνός, παιδίου κλαίοντος δι' ὅλης τῆς ἡμέρας καὶ θυμουμένου, ἐπειδὴ ἐθεασάμην τήν τε στρωμνὴν αὐτοῦ καὶ τὰ ἱμάτια ῥυποῦντα καὶ αὐτὸ τὸ παιδίον ῥυπαρὸν ἐκέλευσα αὐτό τε λοῦσαι καὶ τὴν στρωμνὴν αὐτοῦ καὶ τὰ ἱμάτια ὑπαλλάξαι καὶ τούτου γενομένου τοῦ τε κλαυθμοῦ καὶ τῆς ὀργῆς ἐπαύσατο καὶ καθύπνωσεν.] (Aet. *Tetr.* 4.4.16–23 (CMG 8.1, 361.18–25))

Here Aetios' demand for a *katharios* (clean) wet nurse is substantiated through rewriting Galen's authorial experience with the nurse who failed to keep a clean

19 For this passage, see also the discussion under "Saying."
20 Gal. *San. Tu.* 1.8.32 (CMG 5.4.2, 21.31–33) and 1.9.1–6 (CMG 5.4.2, 22.1–21). For medical authors' treatment of the wet nurse, see also Chapter 2 in this volume; Constantinou and Skouroumouni 2024, in press.
21 The passage, which Olivieri retains in brackets, is omitted in some codices that transmit the text.

environment for her nursling. Aetios' rewriting of the Galenic anecdote repeats the latter's diction and main content, yet it is considerably shorter – Galen's narrative comprises 15 printed lines in Konrand Koch's edition, whereas Aetios' sentence takes up six lines in Olivieri's edition – and it has a different sequence and structure. Furthermore, while in the Galenic text, the author's anecdote introduces a discussion on a new topic, in Aetios' case, it functions as a concluding remark to his own discussion concerning the key attributes of the optimal wet nurse.[22]

Soranos' and Oribasios' similar discussions in the *Gynaecology* and *Medical Collections Incerti* (*Med. Coll. Inc.*) respectively,[23] on the other hand, do not include any anecdotes recounting either their own experiences or those of other medical authors. In a relatively long passage (*Gyn.* 2.19.2.1–2 (CMG 4, 66.12–13)), Soranos explains the logic behind each of his key prescriptions for choosing the optimal wet nurse, which are enumerated at the outset of his homonymous subchapter: her age, number of offspring, state of health, bodily *diaplasis*, breast and nipple size and shape, character, ethnicity, hygiene practices, and a number of other habits. Neatness and tidiness, again as prerequisites and primary obligations of the Soranian wet nurse, are stressed with just a brief justification on the potential impact of bad smell on the infant.[24] Bad odour is likewise condemned by Oribasios on the basis of the evil smell's potential damaging impact.[25]

All in all, as is the case with Soranos' simile vs Galen's anecdote concerning the bodily situation of the milk consumer, there are variations in the treatment of the *katharios* wet nurse in the examined medical authors. While Galen resorts to anecdote and Aetios follows this example by rewriting the Galenic text, Soranos and Oribasios choose to clarify their arguments by using a descriptive method. In contrast to Galen's abundant utilization of anecdotes, his contemporary Soranos resorts to figurative speech and to recollections of generic principles. In turn, Oribasios, Aetios, and later authors are seen to employ both strategies, although their anecdotes are less elaborate and less frequent than those in the Galenic corpus.

22 The same technique of condensation in rewriting a Galenic anecdote is followed by Aetios also in *Tetr.* 2.102.1–10 (CMG 8.1, 189.6–15). In the context of his discussion of the medical uses of cheese, Aetios provides in summary form Galen's anecdote concerning the use of cheese as a decoction to treat a man with arthritic problems (Gal. *On the Capacities of Simple Drugs* 10.9, 12.270.11–272.8K, ed. Kühn 1826, comprising 33 lines in Kühn's 1826 edition, next to the 10 lines of Olivieri's Aetian text).

23 Sections bearing the same subtitle in the two authors: Sor. *Gyn.* 2.19 (CMG 4, 66–68); Orib. *Med. Coll. Inc.* 31 (CMG 6.2.2, 121.10–124.26, ed. Raeder 1933).

24 "Lest the odor of the swaddling clothes cause the child's stomach to become weak and it lie awake on account of itching or suffer some ulceration subsequently" ("καθάριον δὲ δεῖ εἶναι τὴν τιτθήν, ἵνα μὴ διὰ τὴν τῶν σπαργάνων ὀσμὴν ὁ στόμαχος ἐκλύηται τῶν νηπίων ἀγρυπνῇ τε διὰ τοὺς ὀδαξησμοὺς ἤ τιν' ὕστερον ἕλκωσιν ὑπομένῃ," Sor. *Gyn.* 2.19.15.1–3 (CMG 4, 68.22–24); trans. Temkin 1956, 93–94). The bad smell ("δυσωδία") of unclean coverlets ("ἐπιβλήματα") is elsewhere commented on in Soranos: *Gyn.* 2.16.3–4 (CMG 4, 63). For the *katharios* nurse in Soranos and her affinities with Musonius' woman philosopher, see Chapter 2 in this volume.

25 "Let her wear clean clothes and be clean in the rest of her conduct, without having an ill-smelling skin" ("ἔστω δὲ καθάριος κατὰ τὴν ἐσθῆτα καὶ τὴν λοιπὴν δίαιταν, κατὰ τὸν αὐτῆς χρῶτα μὴ δυσώδης," Orib. *Med. Coll. Inc.* 32.4.1–3 (CMG 6.2.2, 124.33–35)).

Each author's rhetorical education and style may constitute important reasons for the divergences in the writing methods of Galen and Soranos. Galen, in particular, was not just a physician and medical author but also a philosopher.[26] The two authors' distinct conceptions of and approaches to medical theory and *praxis* are also reflected in their stylistic variation. In Galen's epistemological approach, reason and empirical adequacy are keys for the acquisition of medical knowledge, which, in turn, is applied according to the individuality of each disease and patient.[27] Both principles seem to shape Galen's tactics of argumentation. Anecdotes are indeed ideal for foregrounding both the value of a physician's practical experience and his diagnosis, which is based on the individuality of each disease and patient. Soranos' close adherence to the principles of the Methodic sect – which rejects experimental knowledge and aetiological research and adopts a generalized approach to the sick – on the other hand,[28] excludes recourse to the incorporation of anecdotes in medical writing.[29] Soranos' markedly figurative language and scientific explications primarily shape his own strategy of argumentation. As for Oribasios and Aetios and other later authors,[30] who are otherwise close followers of Galen's epistemology and stylistic choices, they do not refrain from incorporating anecdotes, Galenic or other, into their galaktology sections. Their anecdotes are invariably fewer and shorter. The synoptic and practical nature of the medical collection genre, within which both were operating, necessitates such an approach. Oribasios and Aetios are more interested in collecting and saving the medical knowledge of their times rather than engaging in their predecessors' experimentations with figurative language and genre.[31]

In both Galen and his followers, anecdotes function as economical ways of grounding medical opinion by interpreting and extracting generalities from case studies, without having to make many technical medical explications. Through anecdotes, a better understanding, an enhancement of the texts' mnemonic effect, and aesthetic pleasure are also achieved. Soranos' frequent use of figurative language, on the other hand, is appreciated through another lens: as a method compensating, in a sense, for the exclusion of anecdotes from his own work. Whereas the other medical authors enliven their scientific texts through the incorporation of anecdotes, Soranos actuates elaborate analogies from both the human and animal worlds via imagery and metaphor in order to add figurative meaning and maximize

26 See Xenophontos 2024, in press and 2023.
27 Hankinson (2008, 157–183) brings out reliance on reason and experience and emphasis on identifying a patient's individuality as key features of Galen's epistemology. Cf. Brain 1986, 14.
28 For Soranos as representative of the Methodic school of medicine and the key principles of Methodism, see Van der Eijk 1999, 397, 400–401; Lloyd 1983, 182–200; Temkin 1956, xxv–xxx.
29 Instead of needing to know the complex humoural balance of the individual patient, the Methodist doctor shaped his treatment based on commonalities.
30 Cf. e.g. Paul Aegin. *Epitome of Medicine* 7.25.1 (CMG 9.2, 401.6–10), ed. Heiberg 1921, rewriting a Galenic anecdote in condensed form.
31 For the brevity and practical applicability of the medical theory chosen for explication, functioning as defining prerequisites and characteristics of the early Byzantine medical compilations, see e.g. Bouras-Vallianatos 2018, 197; Van der Eijk 2010, 526.

the appeal of his own ideas and comments. The thematic focus of galaktological anecdotes, commonly revolving around the usage of milk as a dietetic or pharmaceutical product, may be another parameter defining the variation in the patterns of their usage between Soranos and the rest of our authors. Whereas therapeutic galaktology occupies a large part of Galen's, Oribasios', and Aetios' medical treatises, this is not the case with the Soranic text. Soranos acknowledges and comments upon the potential therapeutic impact of the nurse's milk on the infant, by repeatedly linking the milk's therapeutic powers to the regimen and diet of the wet nurse. Being exclusively interested in gynaecology and childrearing, Soranos does not discuss the use of milk in recipes and patient treatment.

Beyond offering enlightening insights into our authors' medical theory and praxis, as well as their writing and rewriting strategies, the detection and study of anecdotes, albeit within this limited span and focus on galaktology, is significant also in another sense. Anecdotes, as stocks of experiences and records of medical knowledge, allow a glimpse into the wider sociocultural context within which ancient and early Byzantine medical writing and rewriting acquired shape. We are referring to the common taboos and approaches of ancient and early Byzantine patients and to the dynamics of physician–patient interactions. Driven by their biases and taboos, patients, such as the man opting for donkey milk, might have rejected effective therapies, and in so doing, they prolonged their suffering. Patients' extended anguish might also have been the result of charlatans' interventions. A case in point is the old man whose body was dried up through unsuitable therapies before Galen came to his rescue. Furthermore, the existence of different medical schools (for example, Humorism and Methodism) led both physicians and patients to different challenges in the competitive and unstable medical "marketplace" of the examined times.[32] Our medical authors' resort to other people's customs and stories – what we label here "ethnography," which is discussed below – further widens our comprehension of both Greco-Roman and other cultural conceptions of and approaches to galaktology.

Ethnography

For this chapter's purposes, ethnography involves references to stories, customs, geography, and/or other descriptive material related to different peoples and places

---

32 The phrase "medical marketplace," which has been popularized by Nutton 1992, succinctly describes the open nature of the environment of medical theory and practice in Galen's age, where various professional, religious, magical, and practical practitioners coexisted. This is a condition magnifying the value of rhetorical dexterity as an essential asset for medical thinkers, who needed to establish their authority amidst this unstable pluralistic environment. For this characteristically open and competitive nature of medical discourse, as exemplified specifically via public experimentational practices and their writing in Galen, see Salas 2020, 55–102. For critique of the ignorance and frivolity of naïve upper-class patients as a recurrent feature in Galen's writings, see Nutton 2020, 98–101. See also below under "Saying."

in the galaktology sections of the examined works.[33] Of course, it is not our aim to interrogate the historical accuracy and validity of the ethnographical information provided in our corpus, but we seek to investigate the various forms and functions of ethnography in galaktology sections.[34] The examination of ethnography in ancient and Byzantine medical works is worthwhile for three essential reasons. First, it opens a window to the ways in which the authors under investigation engaged with the wider cultural milieu of their times and to how their works may have influenced contemporary conceptions of cultural differentiation. Second, ethnography, like anecdote and figurative language, provides a constructive lens for understanding the formation, formulation, and history of premodern galaktology. Finally, the following discussion reminds us that ethnography had wider uses in ancient and Byzantine cultures than we tend to believe; medical works constitute graphic examples of ethnography's non-historiographical applications.[35] In other words, what we would call "medical ethnography" is an essential element of galaktology, in particular, and of medicine, in general. However limited and short in span, the study of ethnography within the framework of galaktology attests to the multifarious and meaningful ways in which ethnography thrived as an auxiliary genre in ancient and Byzantine medical writing and rewriting.

Ethnographic material recurs in galaktology sections, particularly in discussions about breastfeeding, wet nurses, childrearing, and infant care practices. By juxtaposing Greek bathing practices with their German counterparts, for example, Galen aims at highlighting the superiority of Greek infant childcare while at the same time denigrating that of the barbarian Other. As Galen writes,

> Among the Germans, the little children are not nurtured well. But I am not now writing these things for Germans or other wild and barbaric people, any more than I am for bears, lions or wild boars, or any other wild animals, but for Greeks and for those born barbarians in race who emulate the practices of the Greeks. For who, of those dwelling among us, would tolerate an infant,

---

33 For the complexities involved in defining the oeuvre and key features of historiography, geography, ethnography, and other related disciplines in antiquity, see e.g. Nicolai 2015, 1090–1092 (see also pp. 1116–1124 for his focus on the evolution of geography as an independent discipline from the Hellenistic period onwards).

34 Historical objectivity is not foregrounded as a primary criterion in medical ethnographic excursions where no autopsy is claimed by the authors under investigation. What is more, either any indication of the authors' sources is completely absent or, most frequently, the authors present their ethnographic material as a popular and non-specified wider opinion; see e.g. Sor. *Gyn.* 2.44.1.3–4 (CMG 4, 85.9–10: "as some people say"; "καθὼς δέ τινες λέγουσι"); Gal. *San. Tu.* 1.10.18 (CMG 5.4.2, 24.28: "as they precisely say"; "καθάπερ φασὶ"); Orib. *Med. Coll.* 10.7.10.1–2 (CMG 6.1.2, 50.15, ed. Raeder 1929: "as I have heard"; "ὡς πυνθάνομαι").

35 Historiographical studies focussing primarily on Herodotus have dominated the study of ethnography in antiquity and beyond. Although the ways in which medical writing influenced or absorbed the influence of ethnographical and/or historical material have been discussed by scholars (e.g. Scalnon 2015, 70, 73; Kaldellis 2013, 190), there is no extensive study of medical authors' use of ethnography.

still warm from the birth, being immediately carried to the flowing waters of a river, and there, as they say the Germans do, in an attempt to test its nature and at the same time strengthen its body, being dipped into cold water, like red-hot iron? … Who then, in his right mind, who was not a total savage and a Scythian, would choose to subject his own infant to such a test in which failure means death and nothing of significance will be gained from surviving the test? Perhaps it might be a great good for an ass or some of the other irrational animals to have a thick and hard skin so as to be able to bear the cold without distress, but for man, a rational animal, what would be great about such a thing?

παρὰ μέν γε τοῖς Γερμανοῖς οὐ καλῶς τρέφεται τὰ παιδία. ἀλλ᾽ ἡμεῖς γε νῦν οὔτε Γερμανοῖς οὔτε ἄλλοις τισὶν ἀγρίοις ἢ βαρβάροις ἀνθρώποις ταῦτα γράφομεν, οὐ μᾶλλον ἢ ἄρκτοις ἢ λέουσιν ἢ κάπροις ἤ τισι τῶν ἄλλων θηρίων, ἀλλ᾽ Ἕλλησι καὶ ὅσοι τῷ γένει μὲν ἔφυσαν βάρβαροι, ζηλοῦσι δὲ τὰ τῶν Ἑλλήνων ἐπιτηδεύματα. τίς γὰρ ἂν ὑπομείνειε τῶν παρ᾽ ἡμῖν ἀνθρώπων εὐθὺς ἅμα τῷ γεννηθῆναι τὸ βρέφος ἔτι θερμὸν ἐπὶ τὰ τῶν ποταμῶν φέρειν ῥεύματα, κἀνταῦθα, καθάπερ φασὶ τοὺς Γερμανούς, ἅμα τε πεῖραν αὐτοῦ ποιεῖσθαι τῆς φύσεως ἅμα τε κρατύνειν τὰ σώματα, βάπτοντας εἰς τὸ ψυχρὸν ὕδωρ ὥσπερ τὸν διάπυρον σίδηρον; … τίς οὖν ἂν ἕλοιτο νοῦν ἔχων καὶ μὴ παντάπασιν ἄγριος ὢν καὶ Σκύθης εἰς τὴν τοιαύτην πεῖραν ἀγαγεῖν αὐτοῦ τὸ παιδίον, ἐν ᾗ θάνατός ἐστιν ἡ ἀποτυχία, καὶ ταῦτα μηδὲν μέγα τι μέλλων ἐκ τῆς πείρας κερδανεῖν; ὄνῳ μὲν γὰρ ἴσως ἤ τινι τῶν ἀλόγων ζῴων ἀγαθὸν ἂν εἴη μέγιστον, οὕτω πυκνὸν καὶ σκληρὸν ἔχειν δέρμα, ὡς ἀλύπως φέρειν τὸ κρύος· ἀνθρώπῳ δέ, λογικῷ ζῴῳ, τί ἂν εἴη μέγα τὸ τοιοῦτον; (Gal. *San. Tu.* 1.10.17–21 (CMG 5.4.2, 24.21–25.5); trans. with modifications Johnston 2018a, 75)

In a highly derisive and ironic tone, Galen assimilates the Germans to bears, lions, wild boars, or any kind of wild animals. As treated by the Germans, the newborn is likened to an ass or any similar irrational thick-skinned creature, while its very body is equated with a piece of red-hot iron. Through strong images, metaphors, similes, the repetitive use of words conveying the sense of an irrational wildness, and the accumulation of rhetorical apostrophes, Galen graphically condemns the alleged German practice of the newborn's cold bath as a cruel and absurd custom of likewise brutal, illogical, and savage people. His third apostrophe especially, metaphorically aligning the infant as treated by the barbarians to a donkey or any other irrational animal, carries a high degree of rhetorical energy. Galen's overall line of thought on the supremacy of Greek childrearing customs over the barbarians' perverse and ferocious practices is carried through with force and cynical sarcasm. Quoting Hippocrates' approach to transpiration in relation to the thinness or thickness of the body, Galen provides a medical explanation for his condemnation of the German practice: taking into consideration the softness of the newborn's body is essential during the first stages of infancy to secure the infant's best growth through breastfeeding and bathing with warm and sweet waters (*San. Tu.* 1.10.23–25 (CMG 5.4.2, 25.11–18)).

Soranos' and Oribasios' discussions of infant bathing, too, contain allusions to the bathing practices of Germans and other Northern peoples. Yet the character of these authors' ethnographic digressions is quite divergent, both in formulation and in rhetorical function. Referring to the practice of the first cold bath, Soranos attributes the custom not only to many barbarians, particularly Germans and Scythians, but also to some Greeks (*Gyn.* 2.12.1.1–2 (CMG 4, 59.10–11)). Soranos lists cold bathing with a number of other infant cleansing practices, such as washing with different types of wine and infant urine, which he considers unfitting (*Gyn.* 2.12.2.1 (CMG 4, 59.16)). Contrary to Galen's emphatic dwelling on the ethnic origins of the practice of cold bathing, Soranos' accent falls only on the medical explanation of its inappropriateness. As he explains, cold bathing should be avoided because it causes death, and for its harmful effects even on the infants who survive its deadly force.

The stress on the ethnic origins of infant bathing practices (Greek vs barbarian), although quite differently from that of Galen, returns in Oribasios' *Medical Collections* (*Med. Coll.*) where he comments on other peoples' practice of resorting to cold bathing during infancy in general ("τὰ γοῦν νήπια τοῖς μὲν βαρβάροις ἔθος ἐστίν, ὡς πυνθάνομαι, καὶ καθιέναι συνεχῶς εἰς τὸ ψυχρόν," *Med. Coll.* 10.7.10.1–2 (CMG 6.1.2, 50. 15–16)). The barbarian custom is juxtaposed with the reverse Greek tendency towards continuous warm bathing of the child:

> We, in contrast, continuously use warm bathing, being convinced by the nurses, who happily consider sufficient the children's sleep in their carriages after the exhaustion of bathing, arguing that boiling the children somewhat to softness via the frequent warm bathing ensures that they are not annoyed exceedingly during the night by turning sleepless.
>
> ἡμεῖς δέ γε καθεψῶμεν ταῖς συνεχέσι θερμολουσίαις, πειθόμενοι ταῖς τιτθαῖς, αἵτινες ἀσμενίζουσαι τῷ μετὰ τὴν ἐν τοῖς λουτροῖς ἀπαύδησιν [τῷ] κάρῳ τῶν παιδίων ἀποχρώντως τε ἔχειν νομίζουσιν ἑαυταῖς, εἰ μὴ πολλὰ διοχληθῇ † τῶν τε νύκτωρ δύσυπνα φάμεναι γίνεσθαι τὰ μὴ τακερωθέντα μικροῦ δεῖν ὑπὸ τοῦ πλήθους τῆς θερμολουσίας. (Orib. *Med. Coll.* 10.7.10.2–7 (CMG 6.1.2, 50.16–21))[36]

Thus, contrary to Galen's heated censure of barbarian childcare methods, the juxtaposition of Greek and foreign bathing habits is used by Oribasios to criticize the misjudgement and incompetence involved in Greek practices.

Moving from infant bathing to other childcare practices and to the need for a devoted wet nurse, Soranos uses ethnography to highlight and promote the suitability of Greek wet nurses. According to Soranos, the wet nurse should be Greek, for two important reasons. First, only Greek wet nurses can teach infants to speak

---

36 That the baby's peaceful and uninterrupted sleep constitutes an important manifestation of the wet nurse's good mothering is also suggested in philosophical works, such as "Myia's" *Letter to Phyllis*; see Chapter 2 in this volume.

the Greek language correctly (*Gyn.* 2.19.2, 2.19.15 (CMG 4, 66.12–16, 68.22–25)). Second, Greek women are the most experienced and devoted wet nurses. Roman women, by contrast, neither have the Greek wet nurses' great caring experience, nor are they sufficiently devoted to their mothering role as to pay good attention to all stages of the infant's development and to provide the necessary assistance (*Gyn.* 2.44.1–2.3 (CMG 4, 85.7–15)). Compared to Galen's binary dichotomy between the Greek self and the barbarian Other discussed above,[37] Soranos' comparisons between Greek and Roman women do not aim to prove the superiority of the first by demeaning the latter. His intention is rather to present himself as a devoted follower of Methodism, which was critical of the Romans' temper, than to argue for non-Greek women's inferiority as constructed through denigrating epithets and equation with animality.[38]

Concerning milk's dietetic and medical uses, which are mostly discussed by Galen, the use of ethnography acquires quite a different character. His reference to the milk-drinking Scythians, in his *Therapeutic Method to Glaucon* (*MMG*), for example, contains nothing of the pejorative rhetoric of the previously discussed passage about the bathing customs of the "savage animal-like peoples" of the North. In this case, ethnography is strongly associated with geography and climate. The Scythians' suitable milk diet, in combination with their region's cold climate, provides them with maximum immunity to elephantiasis (*MMG* 2.12, 11.142.7K, ed. Kühn 1826). The inhabitants of Alexandria, by contrast, a place with extremely high temperatures providing a diet rich in foods that generate thick melancholic humours (for example, gruel, lentil soup, salted fish), are quite susceptible to the disease (*MMG* 2.12, 11.142.3–9K). A similar reference to geography and climate conditions appears also in Galen's *Therapeutic Method*, where he discusses the therapeutic powers of the milk that is produced in Tabia due to the region's excellent geomorphology and climate conditions (Gal. *MM* 5.12, 10.363–366K).[39] The elevated position of this Roman province, along with the ambient dry air and the rich fertile pasture which is available to milk-producing animals (i.e. cows, asses, and goats), is described in minute detail, as they are considered the key reasons for Tabian milk's high quality. This is the very milk that Galen chooses for the treatment of the ulcer cases discussed above.

---

37 Galen's extremely pejorative tone for Northern peoples seems to be unique in medical writing. Searches in the *Thesaurus Linguae Graecae* (*TLG*) for "German" ("Γερμανός") and "Scythian" ("Σκύθης") in all their forms and derivatives in the whole extant corpuses of Soranos, Oribasios, and Aetios give much fewer results, which have a mild or neutral tone (Galen: 14 occurrences of "Γερμανός" and ten occurrences of "Σκύθης"; Soranos: one reference for each; Oribasios: one occurrence for "Γερμανός" and two occurrences for "Σκύθης"; Aetios: total absence of either ethnic term).

38 Disdain towards the temper of Roman people has been detected as a general characteristic of the Methodic sect to which Soranos belonged; see Temkin 1956, xxix.

39 For ancient conceptions (with potentially Hippocratic origins as well, if Hippocrates is indeed the author of the treatise *On Airs, Waters, and Places*) of climate's central role in the formation of a region's character and culture, see e.g. Romm 2010, 215–235.

All in all, the medical author most frequently using ethnography and providing the most elaborate and embellished presentations is Galen, who, as we have seen, also mostly favours the anecdote. Interestingly, for reasons that cannot be explained here, none of Galen's, Soranos', or Oribasios' ethnographic allusions figure in the works of Aetios. The first three authors resort to ethnographic digressions to support their galaktological epistemologies and to present various aspects under debate as either primarily socially and ethically fashioned or geographically and environmentally preconditioned phenomena. Despite their different uses of ethnographic material, our authors invariably appear to foreground a totally superior Greek nursing *ethos* in all respects, next to a milk quality and effectiveness in diet and therapy determined in relation to varying geographical and environmental factors. As is the case with the anecdote, our authors' shorter and longer ethnographic excursions, taking the form of brief references and detailed descriptions which are sometimes embellished with rhetorical devices, enrich the galaktology sections of their works, rendering them interesting and entertaining even for modern readers. At the same time, Galen's, Soranos', and Oribasios' ethnographies possibly provided audiences sharing a Greek culture with a feeling of satisfaction in their superiority as far as their nursing and childrearing practices and customs were concerned.

Saying

In antiquity and Byzantium, sayings were an educational, philosophical, theological, and literary pursuit, as attested by textbooks, school exercises,[40] sayings collections, and a considerable number of texts belonging to different genres.[41] Our authors' relatively frequent use of sayings shows that this small form was also an essential element of scientific – in this case medical – discourse. As expected, sayings are the shortest literary forms detected in the galaktology sections of our corpus. The shortest sayings consist of a couple of words, while the longest ones have a couple of sentences. Sayings are used in the form of extremely short units which the authors insert to their theoretical and explanatory sections, or they become parts of anecdotes and ethnographic digressions. The examined sayings might be attributed to a medical authority (for example, Hippocrates) or they might appear as words of general wisdom.[42] Through the use of sayings, as the following discussion

40 For the centrality of sayings in ancient and Byzantine education, see e.g. Morgan 1998.
41 See e.g. Branch-Trevathan 2020, 49–105; Larsen 2016; Lelli 2011; Lardinois 2000; Russo 1997; Gotoff 1981.
42 By focussing on short apophthegmatic quotes of previous medical material, our examination differs from previous studies on medical doxography that analyze all types of recording (verbatim or freely rephrased) of previous medical opinions. For studies focussing on medical doxography, see e.g. Manetti 2012 (Galen and Hippocrates); Van der Eijk 1999 (doxography in Methodism). Salas' (2020) analysis of Galen's anatomical works brings out nicely the way in which Galen's interpretations of previous authorities function as a competitive gesture for establishing his authority over his rivals (especially. 51–53, and 56–102), what Salas terms Galen's "doxographical polemic" (p. 12).

will show, medical authors attempt to establish the validity and timelessness of their theories and approaches, to prove the shortcomings of authors, doctors, and methods they disagree with, and to provide their texts with rhetorical power and aesthetic pleasure.

For reasons of space, we will examine a few instances of Galenic usage and (potential) Soranic allusion to Hippocratic maxims by mostly focusing on a single dictum: "opposites are cures for opposites" ("τὰ ἐναντία τῶν ἐναντίων ἐστὶν ἰήματα," Hippoc. et Hippoc. Corpus *On Winds* 1.25–26 (CMG 1.1, 92.7–8), ed. Heiberg 1927), which encapsulates a key principle of Hippocratic epistemology.[43] A search in the whole corpus of *TLG* for *enantios* ("opposite") and *iama* ("cure") in their various forms and in proximity (within the span of five words) substantiates the widespread endorsement of the saying as a valid and uncontested Hippocratic principle for diagnosing and curing disease via venesection and for comprehending medical art, treatments, and the workings of human and animal biology.[44] Statistics, returning only three instances of the saying before Galen and extracting 39 out of the 130 results from the Galenic corpus alone, suggest that Galen was the first and most significant author promoting this particular Hippocratic dictum. The present sample study, even though necessarily narrow in focus, provides an enlightening glimpse into some of our medical authors' recognition and varying exploitation of popular sayings.

In this chapter's first section, on the medical anecdote, we discussed a Galenic narrative regarding the behaviour of a prematurely delivered goat, which ends with the following words: "At this moment we all exclaimed loudly, since we recognized now what Hippocrates had described: 'The nature of the animals does not result from learning'" ("ἐν ᾧ καὶ ἀνεκεκράγαμεν ἅπαντες, ἐναργῶς ὁρῶντες ὅπερ Ἱπποκράτης ἔφη· φύσιες ζῴων ἀδίδακτοι." (Gal. *Loc. Aff.* 6.6, 8.443.15–17K; trans. Siegel 1976, 194)).

The sight of the baby goat opting for the bowl containing milk drives all bystanders to exclaim at once a Hippocratic dictum.[45] By incorporating the Hippocratic saying in this anecdote, Galen validates his experiment and pronounces in a marked, economical, and authoritative manner his own theory that nature provides all creatures with the ability to perform their proper functions. What is more, Galen's observations and interpretations are purported to be a meaningful mani-

---

43 For the doctrine of the treatment of diseases with their opposites as a key Hippocratic principle, see Lloyd 1966, 20–23; cf. Brain 1986, 7.

44 See e.g. Orib. *Med. Coll.* 9.21.3 (CMG 6.1.2, 20.26–29), on the humoral balance of bodily juices; Alex. Tralles, *Therapeutics* 10, 2.461.12–15, ed. Puschmann 1879, on the regulation of diet.

45 Hippoc. et Hippoc. Corpus, *On Nutriment (Alim.)* 39 (CMG 1.1, 82.28), ed. Heiberg 1927: "Φύσιες πάντων ἀδίδακτοι." The referent of the word *pantōn* as animal beings ("ζῷα," the word used by Galen) is indicated by the content of the preceding line: "inanimates get life, animates get life, the parts of animates get life" ("Ζωοῦται τὰ μὴ ζῷα, ζωοῦται τὰ ζῷα, ζωοῦται τὰ μέρεα τῶν ζῴων," *Alim.* 38 (CMG 1.1, 82.27); trans. Jones 1868, 358). *On Nutriment* (dated between the 5th c. BC and the 1st c. AD) is a short treatise discussing nutrition, the process of digestion, and the assimilation of food into the body. The book is composed of brief aphorisms, marked for their obscurity already in antiquity (Craig 2004).

festation of an otherwise obscure Hippocratic maxim.[46] In its new context, the pertinence of the Hippocratic principle is even further expanded to account for the interpretation of the structure and performance of each individual bodily organ. The sophistication and authority of source, text at hand, and medical author are mutually magnified. The Hippocratic proverbial phrase is most effective in its shortness, which renders it memorable and recitable by a group of people that operates as a choir. At the same time, the rhetorical devices seen in the rest of the anecdote (for example, repetitions, figures of speech, and imagery) effectively connect the maxim with the Galenic experiment.

As for Hippocrates' more popular dictum and aforementioned focus of our analysis ("opposites are cures for opposites"), Galen foregrounds in his *Bloodletting against Erasistratus* (*Ven. Sect. Er.*) the mechanics of milk production as the most illustrative example of nature's endorsement of the Hippocratic axiom in the way female physiology is designed and regulated by nature.[47] In this treatise, Galen aims at refuting Erasistratus' and his followers' rejection of bloodletting as the proper therapeutic treatment for evacuation of an excess of blood. Thus, Galen grounds a large part of his argumentation on demonstrating how the Hippocratic principle of cure via opposites constitutes a fundamental functioning of nature and a common doctrine of the physicians who rely on experience (including Hippocrates himself). To these ends, Galen uses examples from female, male, and animal bodily processes or behaviour.[48] Milk production, for example, is described in detail as one of nature's operations for eliminating the superfluity of blood in woman's body (*Ven. Sect. Er.* 5, 11.164.10–12K).[49] The Hippocratic saying itself is quoted thrice at different junctures of Galen's adjacent text: "Who does not know that **opposites are the cure for opposites**? This is not the doctrine of Hippocrates alone; it is the common belief of all men" ("τίς οὐκ οἶδεν ὅτι **τἀναντία τῶν ἐναντίων ἰάματα**;

---

46 For *On Nutriment*'s obscurity, which has also raised doubts about its Hippocratic authorship, see Craig 2004, 19.

47 This work is the first of three Galenic treatises dealing with the subject of venesection, presented together in translation in a monograph by Brain 1986: *Bloodletting against the Erasistrateans at Rome* (*Ven. Sect. Er. Rom.*); *Bloodletting* (*[Ven. Sect.]*). In the second of these works (*Ven. Sect. Er. Rom.* 1, 11.191–194K, ed. Kühn 1826), Galen explains how the strong resistance of doctors, followers of Erasistratus of Ceos (a physician practising in Alexandria in the 3rd c. BC), against the use of phlebotomy, led to this address, to refute their false argumentation. For Galen's critique of Erasistrateans, see Salas 2020, especially. 165–195, 227–264.

48 From the functions of male physiology, Galen refers, with less detail, to the elimination of excess black bile through haemorrhoids (*Ven. Sect. Er.* 5, 11.166.3–10K); regarding animal physiology and conduct, references are made to cranes and eagles (in the passages quoted below), to dogs, Egyptian birds, and other animals (at *Ven. Sect. Er.* 5, 11.167–168K).

49 Galen's emphasis on the close link between milk and blood through another Hippocratic saying is worth mentioning, albeit in passing: "Hippocrates says that breastmilk and menstruation are siblings" ("τὰ γάλακτα τῶν ἐπιμηνίων ἀδελφά φησὶν Ἱπποκράτης," Gal. *On the Function of the Parts of the Body* 14.8, 4.177.19–178.1K, ed. Kühn 1822). The saying, utilizing an animating metaphor, projects the image of menstrual blood and milk as "siblings." For the ancient and Byzantine medical conception of milk as double-processed blood, i.e. blood that turns into milk after parturition, see e.g. Pedrucci 2013, 260–291; Orland 2012; Yalom 1997, 206–207.

μὴ γὰρ Ἱπποκράτους ἡ γνώμη μόνου, κοινὴ πάντων ἀνθρώπων ἐστίν." (Gal. *Ven. Sect. Er.* 6, 11.167.6–8K, ed. Kühn 1826; trans. Brain 1986, 27; emphasis added)).

Who would be so stupid as not to call for the evacuation of blood? But it is clear that Erasistratus, because of his enmity towards Hippocrates, does not share the opinions that are common to all the rest of humanity; he turns out to be even more unintelligent than the cranes. Even these birds can be seen from afar, like eagles flying to the ends of the earth, escaping heat and cold in turn, and **curing opposites with their opposites in everything**.

τίς οὕτως ἀνόητος ὡς μὴ κένωσιν αἵματος εἰπεῖν; ἀλλ' Ἐρασίστρατος ὑπὸ τῆς πρὸς Ἱπποκράτη φιλονεικίας οὐδὲ τὰς κοινὰς ἁπάντων ἀνθρώπων ἐννοίας φαίνεται διασώζων, ἀλλ' ἔτι καὶ τῶν γεράνων ἀνοητότερος εὑρίσκεται. μακρῷ τοιγαροῦν καὶ ταύτας, ὡς ἀετοὺς μέχρι περάτων γῆς πετομένους ἐστὶν ἰδεῖν, ὑποφευγούσας ἐν μέρει κρύος τε καὶ θάλπος, **ἰωμένας τε διὰ παντὸς τοῖς ἐναντίοις τὰ ἐναντία**. (Gal. *Ven. Sect. Er.* 6, 11.168.8–15K; trans. Brain 1986, 28; emphasis added)

Merely to know that **opposites are the treatment for opposites**, and that evacuation is the opposite of *plethos*, does not impress me; even animals without reason have a share in such learning as that. But if you would undertake to open your ears, or, I should rather say, your mind, to receive the true doctrine, I might be prepared to overlook your hostility towards Hippocrates and tell you something worthy of that man's art.

τὸ δ' ὅτι χρὴ **τὰ ἐναντία τοῖς ἐναντίοις ἰᾶσθαι** καὶ ὡς τῷ πλήθει ἡ κένωσις ἐναντίον, τοσούτῳ δέω θαυμάζειν ὥστε καὶ τοῖς ἀλόγοις ζώοις μετεῖναί φημι τῆς ἐννοίας. εἰ δὲ βούλει μικρὸν ἀνοίξας τὰ ὦτα, μᾶλλον δὲ τὴν ψυχήν, ἀληθῆ λόγον καταδέξασθαι τῆς πρὸς Ἱπποκράτη δυσμενείας ἐπιλαθόμενος, εἴποιμ' ἄν σοί τι τῆς ἐκείνου τέχνης ἄξιον. (Gal. *Ven. Sect. Er.* 6, 11.169.7–13K; trans. Brain 1986, 28; emphasis added)

In between and through these quotations and via his resort to galaktology primarily – but also to other examples from human and animal physiology – Galen grounds the principle of balance via opposites as an operational law both of nature and of effective medical treatment. Once again, as in the goat anecdote above, Galen's rhetorical skills are clearly manifested. There is a strategic repetition of words, even of those included in the Hippocratic saying itself (for example, "ἐναντίος"). Galen also repeats certain rhetorical tropes, such as apostrophes and rhetorical questions (for example, "τίς οὐκ οἶδεν …;" "εἰ δὲ βούλει μικρὸν ἀνοίξας τὰ ὦτα"), functioning as irony markers. In his formulation of argumentation and paradigms, Galen employs the conceptual schema of antithesis (for example, "τῷ πλήθει ἡ κένωσις ἐναντίον"). He also uses ironic and animating similes that assimilate his medical opponent, Erasistratus, with animals or disabled people, like the blind who choose the long and difficult route without being able to see the direct and short one (*Ven. Sect. Er.* 4, 11.157.5–11K) and the deaf who do not hear the shouts of the town crier (*Ven. Sect. Er.* 5, 11.165.7–11K). As is the case with the goat anecdote, here too, the employment of Hippocrates' saying along with rhetorical tropes maximizes the impact and the overall force of Galen's argumentation and criticism of Erasistratus, which is established as legitimate and necessary.

Galen refers to the Hippocratic saying also in *Hygiene*, in the context of his discussion of infant physiology. Since the bodily situation of infants is moister than in later life stages, claims Galen, there is a need to maintain an accord with this very nature of infancy by adopting moist diets and giving baths in potable waters (*San. Tu.* 1.7.16 (CMG 5.4.2, 17.18–20)). However, there are physicians who, in their attempt to promote the opposite – a dry diet and regimen – employ the same Hippocratic maxim. In the following passage, Galen argues for these doctors' er-roneous understanding of Hippocrates:

> For there are those who think natures that are too moist always need to be dried, just as natures that are too cold always need to be heated, natures that are too dry to be moistened, and those that are too hot to be cooled, for each of the imbalances is increased by like things but corrected and reduced through the opposites – in short, "opposites are the cures of opposites." But they must not only know and remember Hippocrates' statement, that "opposites are the cures of opposites," but also that in which he says, "moist regimens are beneficial to all who are febrile, particularly children, and others who are accustomed to being so treated." Here he has obviously placed three things in juxtaposition – disease, stage of life and custom. From the disease, he takes the indication of opposites while from the stage of life and custom, he takes the indication of similars.
>
> εἰσὶ γὰρ οἳ νομίζουσιν ἀεὶ δεῖσθαι ξηραίνεσθαι τὰς ὑγροτέρας φύσεις, ὥσπερ γε καὶ θερμαίνεσθαι μὲν τὰς ψυχροτέρας, ὑγραίνεσθαι δὲ τὰς ξηροτέρας, ψύχεσθαι δὲ τὰς θερμοτέρας· ὑπὸ μὲν γὰρ τῶν ὁμοίων ἑκάστην τῶν ἀμετριῶν αὐξάνεσθαι, κολάζεσθαι δὲ καὶ καθαιρεῖσθαι πρὸς τῶν ἐναντίων, ἑνὶ δὲ λόγῳ "τὰ ἐναντία τῶν ἐναντίων" ὑπάρχειν "ἰάματα." ἐχρῆν δὲ αὐτοὺς μὴ τοῦτο μόνον Ἱπποκράτους ἀνεγνωκέναι τε καὶ μνημονεύειν [ὡς τὰ ἐναντία τῶν ἐναντίων ἐστὶν ἰάματα], ἀλλὰ κἀκεῖνα, δι' ὧν φησιν· "αἱ ὑγραὶ δίαιται πᾶσι τοῖσι πυρεταίνουσι ξυμφέρουσι, μάλιστα δὲ παιδίοισι καὶ τοῖσιν ἄλλοισι τοῖσιν οὕτως εἰθισμένοισι διαιτᾶσθαι." φαίνεται γὰρ ἐνταῦθα παράλληλα θεὶς ἐφεξῆς τὰ τρία, νόσημά τε καὶ ἡλικίαν καὶ ἔθος, ἀπὸ μὲν τοῦ νοσήματος ἔνδειξιν λαμβάνων τῶν ἐναντίων, ἀπὸ δὲ τῆς ἡλικίας τε καὶ τοῦ ἔθους τῶν ὁμοίων. (Gal. *San. Tu.* 1.7.10–12 (CMG 5.4.2, 16.33–17.9); trans. Johnston 2018a, 49–51)

According to Galen's argumentation, a moist regimen in infancy is the natural body state which must be preserved via similars, and not a disease which should be adverted via the application of opposites. Nature's wise forethought is again foregrounded as one of Galen's compelling arguments. In order to retain a moist regimen, nature provides for the foetus' and infant's analogous nutrition: blood while in utero, milk (along with the suckling mechanism, in order to distil it from the breast) after parturition (*San. Tu.* 1.7.17–21 (CMG 5.4.2, 17.24–18.6)). For the complaints of infants, moderate movement and a mild emulation of the carer's voice are likewise customary and fitting remedies (the word used is again *iamata*, *San. Tu.* 1.7.23 (CMG 5.4.2, 18.12)). The application of the third word of Hippocrates' saying, *iama*, to name the effect of similars, and the playful accumulated juxtapositions of the epithets *homoios–enantios* (in the quoted passage and elsewhere) are quite apt strategies for expounding in a lively way the differentiation of the function of similars and opposites in the context of Galen's new argumentative logic.[50]

Whereas in the previous cases, unanimity and singlemindedness concerning the meaning of the Hippocratic saying are variously stressed, content and meaning in this instance bring about a completely different rhetoric. Galen is minded to conditionalize the appropriate usage of the saying by those alluding to Hippocrates' authority to promote wrong medical approaches.[51] Otherwise, the saying runs the risk of misinterpretation and of losing its practical validity. Thus, another significant dimension of the use of sayings is graphically displayed here: splintering whole doctrines into a fleeting phrase, however sharp and memorable, can be misleading. The polysemy and various factors conditioning a saying's interpretation require meticulous attention to avoid its potential of misapprehension and misuse. Via his elaborated explanatory commentary on the Hippocratic saying, Galen succeeds both in grounding his doctrine regarding infant diet and regime on Hippocrates' wisdom and in staging his own intelligence as the ultimate interpreter of his most important precursor.[52]

Even though *TLG* returns no results of a verbatim citation of the Hippocratic saying in *Gynaecology*, Soranos sometimes develops an argumentation with markedly proverbial-sounding phrases which play around the same notion of antithesis

---

50 Cf. e.g. Gal. *San. Tu.* 1.7.12 (CMG 5.4.2, 17.7–9): "From the disease, he takes the indication of opposites while from the stage of life and custom, he takes the indication of similars" ("ἀπὸ μὲν τοῦ νοσήματος ἔνδειξιν λαμβάνων τῶν ἐναντίων, ἀπὸ δὲ τῆς ἡλικίας τε καὶ τοῦ ἔθους τῶν ὁμοίων;" trans. Johnston 2018a, 49); *San. Tu.* 1.7.13–14 (CMG 5.4.2, 17.10–15): "whereas in children (for in them it is not in fact a disease but a stage of life and accords with nature), what is most similar is most helpful. It is also the same with customs, as these produce certain acquired natures in bodies for which the exhibition of opposites is very harmful" ("τοῖς δὲ παιδίοις (οὐ γὰρ νόσημα τούτοις γε, ἀλλὰ κατὰ φύσιν ἢ ἡλικίαν) τὸ ὁμοιότατον ὠφελιμώτατον. οὕτω δὲ καὶ τοῖς ἔθεσιν, ὡς ἂν καὶ αὐτοῖς ἐπικτήτους τινὰς ἐν τοῖς σώμασι φύσεις ἐργαζομένοις, ἡ τῶν ἐναντίων προσφορὰ βλαβερωτάτη" (trans. Johnston 2018a, 49)).

51 Concern for the proper comprehension of this particular Hippocratic maxim recurs elsewhere in Galen's work; cf. e.g. within the same work *San. Tu.* 5.52–57 (CMG 5.4.2, 159.21–160.8), 5.12.23–26 (CMG 5.4.2, 166.30–167.12); *MM* 11.11, 10.761K.

52 Note how in Gal. *Ven. Sect. Er.* 6, 11.169.7–13K, quoted above, diligent study of the doctrine from which the principle is extracted is again a point that Galen stresses to start explicating the particulars of the practical application of Hippocrates' method of bloodletting. Cf. also Galen's complaint about the common neglect on the part of many medical thinkers of a comprehensive study of the previous material, under "Anecdote." For the exceptional way Galen uses Hippocrates to define and authorize his own position, see the revealing comments in Gill et al. 2012, 7–12. For Galen's reception of the Hippocratic corpus more generally, see Lloyd 2012; Manetti 2012; von Staden 2012.

and balance as key definer of what is simultaneously natural and medically sound.[53] A case in point is the following passage that concerns the physiology of the uterus and the mechanics of menstruation:

> Now one should not treat those without disease for whom it is physiological not to menstruate because of their age. For they are not troubled in any way and besides, to change nature is either impossible or not easy and sometimes even dangerous. For **if the pathological state is the opposite of the physiological**, the physiological if changed into **its opposite** necessarily becomes pathological.
>
> τὰς μὲν οὖν δίχα πάθους μὴ καθαιρομένας δι' ἡλικίαν [οὐ] φυσικῶς οὐ δεῖ θεραπεύειν. οὐδὲν γὰρ ἐνοχλοῦνται, καὶ ἄλλως μεταθεῖναι φύσιν ἢ ἀδύνατον ἢ οὐ ῥάδιον, ἔσθ᾽ ὅπου δὲ καὶ ἐπισφαλές. εἰ γὰρ **ἐναντίωται τῷ κατὰ φύσιν τὸ παρὰ φύσιν**, ἀνάγκη τὸ κατὰ φύσιν μεταλαμβανόμενον **εἰς τὸ ἐναντίον** γενέσθαι παρὰ φύσιν. (Sor. *Gyn.* 3.9.1–2.1 (CMG 4, 98.22–26); trans. Temkin 1956, 134; emphasis added)

Syntax and repetition of words and phrases in parataxis (i.e. the repeated ἢ ... ἢ structures), with the use of the epithet *enantios* and the concept of nature/natural order, provide for concision and swift flow in Soranos' discourse, endowing his argument with a decidedly apophthegmatic relish.[54] Such epigrammatic-sounding expressions figure also elsewhere in Soranos and other medical writers.[55] Expressing a generalized reality and marked by terseness, cohesion, and velocity, these phrases become notable, having the status of freestanding isolated sayings. Since there is no indication about the source(s) of such apophthegmatic phrases, we cannot convincingly argue either that a medical authority is implied or that contemporary audiences treated them as sayings. Only a systematic study of examples such as the Soranian passage above could establish with more certainty influences and implied sources. Suffice it to state here that our authors employ succinct and pithy language to inject proverb-like wisdom and a sense of a long and largely accepted experience lurking behind their advice and doctrines.

---

53 Regarding the galaktological sections of the other authors discussed in this chapter, a *TLG* search gives only one result for Oribasios, one result for Alexander of Tralles, and no results for Aetios and Paul of Aegina.

54 The opposition to Erasistratus' views and those of his followers also form part of Soranos' discussion in Book 3 (e.g. *Gyn.* 3.2.1, 3.4 (CMG 4, 94.16–95.5, 96.3–20)).

55 To mention just a few examples from galaktology sections, cf. e.g. Sor. *Gyn.* 1.42.2.3–4 (CMG 4, 29.22–23): "As a matter of fact if a thing is useful, it is not in every case healthful as well" ("οὐ πάντως γε μὴν εἴ τι ὠφέλιμόν ἐστιν, τοῦτο καὶ ὑγιεινόν;" trans. Temkin 1956, 41); Sor. *Gyn.* 1.60.2.3–4 (CMG 4, 45.10–11): "moreover, because it is the specific task of medicine to guard and preserve what has been engendered by nature ..." ("καὶ ὅτι τῆς ἰατρικῆς ἐστιν ἴδιον τὸ τηρεῖν καὶ σῴζειν τὰ γεννώμενα ὑπὸ τῆς φύσεως ...;" trans. Temkin 1956, 63); Orib. *Med. Coll. Inc.* 39.3.5–6 (CMG 6.2.2, 138.32–33): "the remission and happiness of the soul contributes greatly to the well-being of the body" ("ἡ δ᾽ ἄνεσις καὶ χαρὰ τῆς ψυχῆς εἰς εὐτροφίαν σώματος μεγάλα συμβάλλεται.").

All in all, common types of sayings and the mode of their use reveal how the examined authors' engagement with previous (medical) tradition is a process invested with rhetorical skill. Through sayings, reiteration of earlier material turns into a profoundly rhetorical strategy for enlivening medical writings, amplifying their aesthetic pleasure and deepening the understanding and persuasiveness of the authors' arguments. Our authors' employment of Hippocratic sayings, in particular, places them in a chain of medical writing that goes back to the most authoritative ancient medical author. One could certainly argue that, although the shortest and simplest of all discussed literary forms, saying is equally central in medical writing and rewriting.

Conclusions

As the previous discussion has amply demonstrated, the medical author of simple literary forms *par excellence* is Galen. His abundant use of anecdotes documenting his experiences with patients foregrounds his authority as a medical practitioner and a thinker, and exemplifies his literary style. Likewise, Galen's use of sayings make manifest his powerful rhetoric and diligent awareness of earlier (particularly Hippocratic) medical knowledge, which he artfully incorporates into his texts to highlight the weaknesses of rival doctors and thus to prove the correctness of his own doctrines and methods. The markedly pejorative tone of Galen's critique against others characterizes not only his anecdotes and sayings but also the ethnographical digressions that further enrich his works' literariness.

Embellished with a denigrating irony against the barbarian Other, Galen's descriptions of variant nursing customs sustainedly serve to enforce the supremacy of the Greek nursing paradigm in the same way as our author attempts to stress his own supremacy as author and physician through his use of anecdotes and sayings. In their ethnographies, both Soranos and the later authors, by contrast, converge in a more nuanced formulation of ethnic polarities concerning nursing customs and in a milder anti-barbarian rhetoric. While a sense of the pre-eminence of the Greek nursing *ethos* invariably permeates all the discussed authors' galaktologies, the vehemence of Galen's propaganda on the primitiveness of divergent barbaric custom is unparalleled by the other examined authors.

In general, anecdote, ethnography, and saying are less frequently employed by Soranos, Oribasios, and Aetios. Soranos' galaktology is chiefly served by figurative language – mostly similes – detailed descriptions, and medical exegesis rather than by anecdotes, ethnography, or sayings. Oribasios and Aetios, on the other hand, resort both to descriptive comments and to anecdotal evidence, often reusing Galenic anecdotes, but in shorter and simpler versions. As in the Galenic paradigm but to a lesser extent, Oribasios and Aetios use sayings, primarily of earlier medical authorities, such as Hippocrates and Galen himself.

In sum, the mere presence of simple genres, such as anecdote, ethnography, and saying, in ancient and early Byzantine medical writing and rewriting constitutes an eloquent testimony of the cultures in which the examined texts were produced. These texts are the products of deliberate and rich rhetorical cultures that perceived them not as merely practical expositions of scientific evidence but as artful performative persuasion in the classical sense of the term.[56] What is more, the study of anecdotes, ethnography, and sayings unravels both the markedly literary character of medical (re)writing and the intermeshing of medical thinking with the larger scientific, social, ethnic, and wider cultural contexts of the authors' times. Thus, the examination of simple literary forms in medical works allows us to acknowledge and to clarify the complexities of ancient and early Byzantine scientific writing. Our analysis has brought to the fore a number of important issues that require further investigation: the pluralism and competitiveness of ancient and Byzantine medical epistemologies; the complex dynamics of the interaction between doctor and patient; sociocultural taboos and factors complicating the application of milk doctrines in therapy; and wider social and ethnic ideologies about lactating women and infants that link the biology of breastfeeding with gender and ethnicity politics in interesting ways. As we begin to decode the literary embellishment of ancient and early Byzantine medical (re)writing, more threads and layers than these, not necessarily related to purely medical treatements, begin to disentangle.

References

Texts: Editions and Translations

Brain, P. trans. 1986. *Galen on Bloodletting: A Study of the Origins, Development and Validity of His Opinions, with a Translation of the Three Works*. Cambridge: Cambridge University Press.

Heiberg, J.L. ed. 1921. *Paulus Aegineta, Libri I–IV, edidit J.L. Heiberg*. Corpus Medicorum Graecorum 9.1. Leipzig and Berlin: Teubner.

———. ed. 1927. *Hippocratis Indices librorum, Iusiurandum, Lex, De arte, De medico, De decente habitu, Praeceptiones, De prisca medicina, De aere locis aquis, De alimento, De liquidorum usu, De flatibus, edidit J.L. Heiberg*. Corpus Medicorum Graecorum 1.1. Leipzig and Berlin: Teubner.

Ilberg, J. ed. 1927. *Sorani Gynaeciorum libri IV, De signis fracturarum, De fasciis, Vita Hippocratis secundum Soranum, edidit J. Ilberg*. Corpus Medicorum Graecorum 4. Leipzig and Berlin: Teubner.

Johnston, I. ed. and trans. 2018a. *Galen: Hygiene*, vol. 1: *Books 1–4*. Loeb Classical Library 535. Cambridge, MA: Harvard University Press.

———. ed. and trans. 2018b. *Galen: Hygiene*, vol. 2: *Books 5–6*. Loeb Classical Library 536. Cambridge, MA: Harvard University Press.

Jones, W.H.S. trans. 1868. *Hippocrates Collected Works*. Vol. 1. Cambridge, MA: Harvard University Press.

Koch, K., G. Helmreich, C. Kalbfleisch, and O. Hartlich. eds. 1923. *Galeni De sanitate tuenda libri IV, edidit K. Koch. De alimentorum facultatibus libri III, edidit G. Helmreich. De bonis malisque sucis liber, edidit idem. De victu attenuante liber, edidit C. Kalbfleisch.*

---

56 The ways in which rhetoric pervades all ancient genres as a mode of performance and a style of writing are variously elucidated in Gill et al. 2012, 19–114. See also Salas 2020 (with a focus on Galen's anatomical writings as rhetorical performative texts); Taub 2017 (a study on the variety of formats for communicating ancient scientific, mathematical, and technical writing).

De ptisana liber, edidit O. Hartlich. Corpus Medicorum Graecorum 5.4.2. Leipzig and Berlin: Teubner.

Kühn, C.G. ed. 1822. *Claudii Galeni Opera omnia*. Vol. 4. Leipzig: Knobloch.

———. ed. 1824. *Claudii Galeni Opera omnia*. Vol. 8. Leipzig: Knobloch.

———. ed. 1825. *Claudii Galeni Opera omnia*. Vol. 10. Leipzig: Knobloch.

———. ed. 1826. *Claudii Galeni Opera omnia*. Vols 11–12. Leipzig: Knobloch.

Olivieri, A. ed. 1935. *Aetii Amideni Libri medicinales I–IV, edidit A. Olivieri*. Corpus Medicorum Graecorum 8.1. Leipzig and Berlin: Teubner.

Puschmann, T. ed. 1879. *Alexander von Tralles: Original-Text und Übersetzung nebst einer einleitenden Abhandlung: Ein Beitrag zur Geschichte der Medicin*. Vol. 2. Vienna: Wilhelm Braumüller.

Raeder, J. ed. 1929. *Oribasii Collectionum medicarum reliquiae, libri IX–XVI, edidit J. Raeder*. Corpus Medicorum Graecorum 6.1.2. Leipzig and Berlin: Teubner.

———. ed. 1933. *Oribasii Collectionum medicarum reliquiae, libri XLIX–L, libri incerti, eclogae medicamentorum, edidit J. Raeder*. Corpus Medicorum Graecorum 6.2.2. Leipzig and Berlin: Teubner.

Siegel, R.E. trans. 1976. *Galen on the Affected Parts*. Basel and London: Karger.

Temkin. O. trans. 1956. *Soranus' Gynecology*. Baltimore: Johns Hopkins University Press.

Secondary Works

Bouras-Vallianatos, P. 2018. "Reading Galen in Byzantium: The Fate of *Therapeutics to Glaucon*," in P. Bouras-Vallianatos, and S. Xenophontos (eds) *Greek Medical Literature and Its Readers: From Hippocrates to Islam and Byzantium*. New York: Routledge, 180–229.

Branch-Trevathan, G. 2020. *The Sermon on the Mount and Spiritual Exercises. Novum Testamentum* Supplements 178. Leuven: Brill.

Constantinou, S. 2020. "*Metaphrasis:* Mapping Premodern Rewriting," in S. Constantinou, and C. Høgel (eds) *Metaphrasis: A Byzantine Concept of Rewriting and Its Hagiographical Products*. The Medieval Mediterranean 125. Leiden and Boston: Brill, 3–60.

Constantinou, S., and A. Skouroumouni-Stavrinou. 2022. "Premodern 'Galaktology': Reading Milk in Ancient and Early Byzantine Medical Treatises," *Journal of Late Antique, Islamic and Byzantine Studies* 1 (1–2): 1–40.

———. 2024. "The Other Mother: Ancient and Early Byzantine Approaches to Wet Nursing and Mothering," *Journal of Hellenic Studies*, in press.

Craig, M. 2004. "Printed Medical Commentaries and Authenticity: The Case of 'De alimento,'" *Journal of the Washington Academy of Sciences* 90 (4): 17–28.

Eijk, P. van der. 1999. "Antiquarianism and Criticism: Forms and Functions of Medical Doxography in Methodism (Soranus, Caelius Aurelianus)," in P. van der Eijk (ed.) *Ancient Histories of Medicine: Essays in Medical Doxography and Historiography in Classical Antiquity*. Leiden: Brill, 397–452.

———. 2010. "Principles and Practices of Compilation and Abbreviation in the Medical 'Encyclopaedias' of Late Antiquity," in M. Horster (ed.) *Condensing Text – Condensed Texts*. Stuttgart: Steiner, 519–554.

Gill, C., T. Whitmarsh, and J. Wilkins. eds. 2012. *Galen and the World of Knowledge*. Cambridge: Cambridge University Press.

Gotoff, H.C. 1981. "Cicero's Style for Relating Memorable Sayings," *Illinois Classical Studies* 6: 294–316.

Gourevitch, D. 2013. *Limos kai Loimos: A Study of the Galenic Plague.* Paris: De Boccard.

Hankinson, R.J. ed. 2008. *The Cambridge Companion to Galen.* Cambridge: Cambridge University Press.

Jolles, A. 2017. *Simple Forms.* Translated by P.J. Schwartz. London and New York: Verso.

Kaldellis, A. 2013. *Ethnography after Antiquity: Foreign Lands and Peoples in Byzantine Literature.* Philadelphia: Pennsylvania State University Press.

Kazantzidis, G., and N. Tsoumpra. 2018. "Morbid Laughter: Exploring the Comic Dimensions of Disease in Classical Antiquity," *Illinois Classical Studies* 43 (2): 273–297.

Kim, L. 2017. "The Trouble with Calasiris: Duplicity and Autobiographical Narrative in Heliodorus and Galen," *Mnemosyne* 72 (2): 229–249.

Kokoszko, M., and J. Dybała. 2016. "Medical Science of Milk Included in Celsus' Treatise *De medicina*," *Studia Ceranea* 6: 323–353.

Kokoszko, M., K. Jagusiak, Z. Rzeźnicka, and J. Dybała. 2018. "Pedanius Dioscorides' Remarks on Milk Properties, Quality and Processing Technology," *Journal of Archaeological Science Reports* 19: 982–986.

Lardinois, A.P.M.H. 2000. "Characterization through *gnomai* in Homer's *Iliad*," *Mnemosyne* 53 (6): 641–661.

Larsen, L.I. 2016. "Early Monasticism and the Rhetorical Tradition: Sayings and Stories as School Texts," in P. Gemeinhardt, L. Van Hoof, and P. Van Nuffelen (eds) *Education and Religion in Late Antique Christianity: Reflections, Social Contexts and Genres.* London and New York: Routledge, 13–33.

Lelli, E. 2011. "Proverbs and Popular Sayings in Callimachus," in B. Acosta-Hughes, L. Lehnus, and S.A. Stephens (eds) *Brill's Companion to Callimachus.* Leiden and Boston: Brill, 384–403.

Lloyd, G.E.R. 1966. *Polarity and Analogy: Two Types of Argumentation in Early Greek Thought.* Cambridge: Cambridge University Press.

———. 1983. *Science, Folklore and Ideology.* Cambridge: Cambridge University Press.

———. 2008. "Galen and His Contemporaries," in Hankinson 2008, 34–48.

———. 2012. "Galen's Un-Hippocratic Case-Histories," in Gill, Whitmarsh, and Wilkins 2012, 115–131.

Manetti, D. 2012. "Galen and Hippocratic Medicine: Language and Practice," in Gill, Whitmarsh, and Wilkins 2012, 157–174.

Morgan, T. 1998. *Literate Education in the Hellenistic and Roman Worlds.* Cambridge: Cambridge University Press.

Nicolai, R. 2015. "Historiography, Ethnography, Geography," in F. Montanari, S. Matthaios, and A. Rengakos (eds) *Brill's Companion to Ancient Greek Scholarship.* 2 vols. Leiden: Brill, 1090–1125.

Nutton V. 1992. "Healers in the Medical Market Place: Towards a Social History of Graeco-Roman Medicine," in A. Wear (ed.) *Medicine in Society: Historical Essays.* Cambridge: Cambridge University Press, 15–58.

———. 2020. *Galen: A Thinking Doctor in Imperial Rome.* London: Routledge.

Orland, B. 2012. "White Blood and Red Milk: Analogical Reasoning in Medical Practice and Experimental Physiology (1560–1730)," in M. Horstmanshoff, H. King, and C. Zittel (eds) *Blood, Sweat and Tears: The Changing Concepts of Physiology from Antiquity into Early Modern Europe.* London: Brill, 443–478.

Pedrucci, G. 2013. "Sangue mestruale e latte materno: Riflessioni e nuove proposte. Intorno all'allattamento nella Grecia antica," *Gesnerus* 70 (2): 260–291.

Petit, C. 2018. *Galien de Pergame ou la rhétorique de la providence.* Leiden: Brill.

Romm, J. 2010. "Continents, Climates, and Cultures: Greek Theories of Global Structure," in K.A. Raaflaub, and R.J.A. Talbert (eds) *Geography and Ethnography: Perceptions of the World in Pre-Modern Societies*. Malden, MA: Wiley Blackwell, 215–235.

Russo, J. 1997. "Prose Genres for the Performance of Traditional Wisdom in Ancient Greece: Proverb, Maxim, Apothegm," in L. Edmunds, and R.W. Wallace (eds) with a preface by M. Bettini, *Poet, Public, and Performance in Ancient Greece*. Baltimore, MD: Johns Hopkins University Press, 49–64.

Rzeźnicka, Z. 2016. "Milk and Dairy Products in Ancient Dietetics and Cuisine According to Galen's *De alimentorum facultatibus* and Selected Early Byzantine Medical Treatises," in I. Anagnostakis, and A. Pellettieri (eds) *Latte e latticini: Aspetti della produzione e del consumo nelle società Mediterranee dell'Antichità e del Medioevo*. Verneta: Grafica Zaccara, 49–72.

Rzeźnicka, Z., and M. Kokoszko. 2020. *Milk and Dairy Products in the Medicine and Culinary Art of Antiquity and Early Byzantium (1st–7th Centuries AD)*. Series of the Department of Byzantine History of the University of Łódź 38. Łódź and Kraków: Łódź University Press and Jagiellonian University Press.

Salas, L.A. 2020. *Cutting Words: Polemical Dimensions of Galen's Anatomical Experiments*. Studies in Ancient Medicine 55. Leiden and Boston: Brill.

Scalnon, T.F. 2015. *Greek Historiography*. Malden, MA: Wiley Blackwell.

Staden, H. von. 2012. "Staging the Past, Staging Oneself: Galen on Hellenistic Exegetical Traditions," in Gill, Whitmarsh, and Wilkins 2012, 132–156.

Taub, L. 2017. *Science Writing in Greco-Roman Antiquity: Key Themes in Ancient History*. Cambridge: Cambridge University Press.

Thumiger, C. 2018. "The Professional Audiences of the Hippocratic Epidemics: Patient Cases in Hippocratic Scientific Communication," in P. Bouras-Vallianatos, and S. Xenophontos (eds) *Greek Medical Literature and Its Readers: From Hippocrates to Islam and Byzantium*. London: Routledge, 48–58.

Xenophontos, S. 2023. "Galen as a Storyteller of Didactic Tales," in S. Constantinou, and A. Andreou (eds) *Storyworlds in Short Narratives: Approaches to Late Antique and Early Byzantine Tales*. Leiden and Boston: Brill in press.

———. 2024. *Medicine and Practical Ethics in Galen*. Cambridge: Cambridge University Press, in press.

Yalom, M. 1997. *A History of the Breast*. New York: Ballantine Books.

Part III

Art and Literature

7 Images of Breastfeeding in Early Byzantine Art

Form – Context – Function*

Maria Parani

Introduction

Images of women nursing in the art of the fourth down to the seventh century in the lands of an increasingly Christianized Roman Empire are rare. A number of these have been identified as representations of the Virgin Mary suckling the baby Jesus in an iconographic type that has become known as the *Galaktotrophousa* or *Virgo Lactans*.[1] The origins, geographic distribution, and meaning of this type in relation to Christological dogma on the one hand and the rise of the cult of the Virgin on the other have monopolized the interest of scholars down to the present day. Images of other female figures nursing have received comparatively little attention, with the exception of the effigy of Empress Fausta nursing one or two of her sons on coinage of the reign of Constantine I.[2] Recently Grace Stafford has included images of ordinary women breastfeeding in her discussion of the representation and polyvalent signification of nudity in late antique art.[3] Though Lucia Langener has compiled a helpful list of late Roman and early Byzantine representations of nursing figures other than the Virgin,[4] and, while Mati Meyer has explored such images as reflecting the realities of women's actual and emotive experiences at the time,[5] there is no specialized study on the theme of the ordinary nursing woman in early Byzantine art exploring in a systematic way its pictorial treatment, the contexts in which it

* This study benefitted greatly from the expert advice of Mat Immerzeel, Mati Meyer, and Pagona Papadopoulou, whom I here gratefully acknowledge. All shortcomings and mistakes remain my own. The chapter was written while the author was a member of the project "Network for Medieval Arts and Rituals" (NetMAR), which has received funding from the European Union's Horizon 2020 research and innovation programme under grant agreement nr 951875. The opinions expressed in this chapter reflect only the author's view and in no way reflect the European Commission's opinions. The European Commission is not responsible for any use that may be made of the information it contains.
1 Selectively: Immerzeel 2016; Mathews and Muller 2005; Bolman 2005 and 2004; Langener 1996; Cutler 1987.
2 Centlivres Challet and Bähler Baudois 2003; Vanderspoel and Mann 2002.
3 Stafford 2022, especially 341, 343.
4 Langener 1996, 147–152, 162–163, 217–220.
5 Meyer 2009, 81–88.

DOI: 10.4324/9781003265658-10

occurs, the semiotic discourse in which it participates, and, not least, the reason why such a common, natural, and necessary act of caregiving was so rarely represented. The purpose of the present study is to take a step towards filling this gap.

In contrast to the situation just outlined, in recent decades, specialists in Etruscan, classical Greek, and Roman art have been scrutinizing the representation of the naked female breast and the act of breastfeeding in their respective periods, with some thought-provoking results.[6] *Mutatis mutandis*, by inspiring alternative ways of looking at the early Byzantine pictorial material, their insights can help disengage the discussion of the later images that are of concern for us here from a mere search for their assumed pagan origins and earlier artistic models. To begin with, what these studies make clear is that the image of the ordinary nursing woman, as opposed to the divine nursing figure, was relatively rare in the arts of classical Greece and Rome.[7] As opposed to the nursing goddesses, whose images proliferated down to the late Roman period, not only in Egypt, but also in Italy, Gaul, and Germany, representations of ordinary women nursing were uncommon. Apropos of the art of classical Athens, Larissa Bonfante attributed the scarcity of images of ordinary nursing mothers to the fact that the Athenian elite considered breastfeeding as a primitive, "uncivilized" act, associated primarily with animals, barbarians, but also with women of low social status and slaves, from the ranks of which came the wet nurses who breastfed the children of the upper classes. According to her, when the image of a mortal woman nursing was introduced into classical art, it appeared in contexts that implied vulnerability and fear of impending violence and death. Not least, she suggested, given the religious and magical potency of the image of the nursing goddess, who through her milk was thought to bestow divinity upon the suckling as well as life and protection, breastfeeding was "too important a gesture to be used with impunity" as a simple genre theme.[8]

As for the Roman period down to the fourth century AD, Claude-Emmanuelle Centlivres Challet suggested that the scarcity of representations of ordinary, mortal women nursing may be explained to a certain extent by the disinterest of the elite consumers of Roman art in this act that was mostly entrusted to wet nurses of inferior social status. Indeed, when it came to scenes inspired by daily life, it was mostly male activities that were preferred rather than exclusively female ones. Elaborating further on this gendered approach informed by current anthropological and psychological research, Centlivres Challet went on to propose that in patriarchal Roman society, where women were relegated to a subaltern role, elite men attempted to control the empowering act of breastfeeding, from which they were naturally excluded. This they attempted to do, she claimed, not only by introducing restrictions and regulations through medical treatises written by male doctors, but

6 See e.g. Centlivres Challet 2017; Carroll 2014; Beerden and Naerebout 2011; Rothe 2011; Koloski-Ostrow and Lyons 1997; Bonfante 1989, 567–569.
7 Having said this, images of nursing mothers are encountered in the funerary arts of the Roman provinces; see Carroll 2014.
8 Bonfante 1997, especially 187 for the quotation.

also by manipulating the artistic representation of the theme, which, in most cases when it does occur, serves a symbolic or allegoric function aiming to promote the dominant male discourse – also internalized by the women of the elite – on the ideal roles of women, motherhood, and family.[9]

When it comes to the period that concerns us here, that is, from the fourth century down to the seventh century AD, even allowing for losses of material brought about by the passage of time, it becomes obvious that the image of the ordinary nursing woman was never popular. I was able to locate around ten securely identified instances of the theme. In this reticence, early Byzantine art seems to be following the pattern of Greco-Roman art – whether for the same or other reasons remains to be seen. Still, despite their small number, representations of ordinary women nursing appear in a variety of media, from mosaic pavements to a textile roundel, and, in diverse settings, both private and public. Indeed, for a subject apparently so rarely depicted, the nursing theme seems to have been put to a variety of uses, as the range of contexts in which it occurs intimates. For the purposes of the present study, I have selected for discussion five examples,[10] taken from the funerary, the secular, and the religious sphere, which will serve as the basis for exploring the function and significance of this theme in early Byzantine art, before attempting to gauge the reasons behind its rare occurrence. In each case, the analysis will take into account both the specific iconographic context into which the image was introduced and its pictorial treatment therein. Contextualizing the image will help us gauge its meaning and function and, ultimately, trace those practices, ideas, and perceptions associated with breastfeeding that may have informed its representation in early Byzantine art.

The Funerary Sphere

We will begin our discussion with an image from the funerary sphere, which straddles the divide between the secular and the religious. As we turn to examine it, however, it would help to keep in mind that funerary representational art moves in between the real and the ideal, both seen and presented through an emotional lens tinged by loss, the grief of separation, and hope for the afterlife. Prior to the fourth century AD, funerary monuments in which the deceased mother was presented nursing her child were uncommon, especially in Rome; likewise, images of nursing

---

9 Centlivres Challet 2017.
10 Given that the focus is on ordinary women, I chose to exclude from the discussion mythological and biblical nursing figures, as well as those whose identification is uncertain. For a group of terracotta figurines of nursing female figures from Beth Shean, Israel (4th–6th c. AD), which have been recently identified as Nysa nursing Dionysos, see Hagan 2013. For Eve nursing Abel(?) in the sixth-century *Ashburnham Pentateuch* (Paris, Bibliothèque nationale de France, *nouvelle acquisition latine* 2334, fol. 6r), see Narkiss 2007, 65 (image), 339 (commentary). The images in this chapter may be juxtaposed with those discussed in Chapter 3 in this volume, which represent inversions of the theme of breastfeeding: serpents biting the breasts of female sinners in an inversion of the life-giving action of nursing infants.

were only exceptionally introduced into biographical cycles on children's funerary monuments.[11] When we turn to the fourth century AD and later, the situation continues more or less the same.[12]

The only securely identified funerary portrait of a nursing mother that has come down to us from the period under consideration is an engraved and painted limestone stele from Medina al-Fayum in Egypt, dated to the fourth or fifth century (Figure 7.1).[13] The portrayal is reminiscent of a Christian icon in its solemnity. If it were not for the painted inscription – no longer visible to the naked eye – on either side of the female figure, which reveals her as a 21-year-old mother, one would have been inclined to identify her with the Virgin *Galaktotrophousa*, given her reserved pose, the way she is put on display in front of a green curtain framed by the two columns, and the presence of the two crosses on either side of her head. The young mother is portrayed frontally, seated on a folding stool with a cushion. She wears a long, ochre tunic and a dark blue mantle that also covers her head. She offers her left breast to the naked child supported by her left hand, while a curved engraved line denotes her right breast. The posture of the child seems awkward, lying supine in the mother's embrace, rather than turning towards her, with its left hand hanging listlessly over the mother's supporting arm. The child seems to be looking up at the face of the mother, who inclines her head slightly towards the left, though it is unclear whether she is actually looking at her offspring or not. The mother's unfocused gaze and her restrained pose and the child's limp posture seem to evoke, however subtly, the separation brought about by the mother's death. Irrespective of whether the young woman ever breastfed her child or would have done so if she had lived, the nursing image is employed here to proclaim motherhood as the main achievement of her short life, while at the same time visualizing the sorrow caused by her death, which left her child without her supportive, nourishing presence. Somewhat later, similar feelings at the loss of a young mother, whose death deprived her children of her milk, were expressed in words rather than images in a sixth-century Christian funerary inscription from Athens.[14]

The Secular Sphere

When we turn to the secular figure, I was able to locate only two instances in which a nursing figure appears as a genre theme in early Byzantine iconographic cycles inspired by life in the countryside. Against this background – and taking

---

11 Carroll 2014; Huskinson 1996, 10–11, 15–16. For the Egyptian tombstone of 21-year-old Sarapous nursing her son Hierax (2nd c. AD), now in the National Museum in Warsaw, see Parlasca 2007, 324, Figure 2.

12 No nursing scenes were reported on Christian children's sarcophagi of the fourth century by Jastrzebowska 1989.

13 Parlasca 2007; Effenberger and Severin 1992, nr 66 (153–154); Effenberger 1977, especially 164–167, for the Greek inscription: "*name?* 21 years old. No one is immortal. Be of good courage [*or*, farewell], good one" ("ευμν/ημα (?)/ἔτῳ[ν]/κα οὐ/δίς/ἀθάνα/τος | εὐψύ/χι/ἀγα/θέ"). Translations, unless otherwise indicated, are mine.

14 Papanikola-Mpakirtzē 2002, nr 658 (484–485) (entry by C.B. Kritzas).

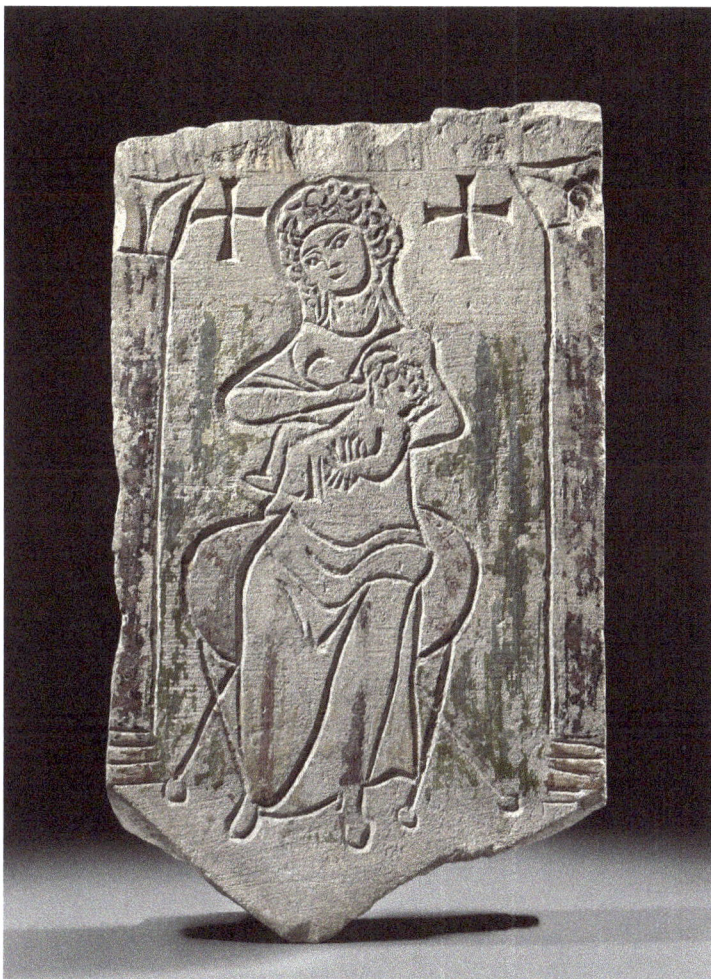

Figure 7.1 Berlin, Museum für Byzantinische Kunst, inv. 4726. Limestone tombstone of a nursing mother, engraved and painted. Medina al-Fayum, fourth or fifth century AD. Photo: bpk/Skulpturensammlung und Museum für Byzantinische Kunst, SMB/Antje Voigt.

into account the Roman hesitation to portray actual, as opposed to divine, women nursing, which was even more pronounced outside a funerary context – to discover an empress represented as a nursing mother was rather startling. The reference is to Empress Fausta (ca. AD 290–326), wife of Constantine I (AD 306–337), with whom she had three sons and two daughters.[15] Fausta appears nursing one of her sons on the reverse of a double solidus medallion issued by the mint of Trier in AD

15 Gwynn 2018.

324/325, following her being raised to the rank of Augusta (Figure 7.2).[16] On the obverse, the bust of Fausta appears in profile, following long-established conventions for the representation of empresses on imperial coinage. The reverse type, however, is unique, with no direct antecedents in earlier Roman imperial coinage.[17] True, in bronze issues of the Antonine period (AD 164–169), Lucilla, the wife of Lucius Verus (AD 161–169), is accompanied on the reverse by the seated personification of Fecunditas (Fertility) nursing one child and surrounded by two others.[18] Earlier Roman empresses, however, are not represented nursing. Furthermore, the treatment of the theme on the Fausta medallion is strikingly different in its gravity, turning the whole composition into one of glorification of the nursing mother empress, accentuated by the wreaths – traditional symbols of honour and victory – presented to her by the two *genii* at the feet of her throne. It should be noted here

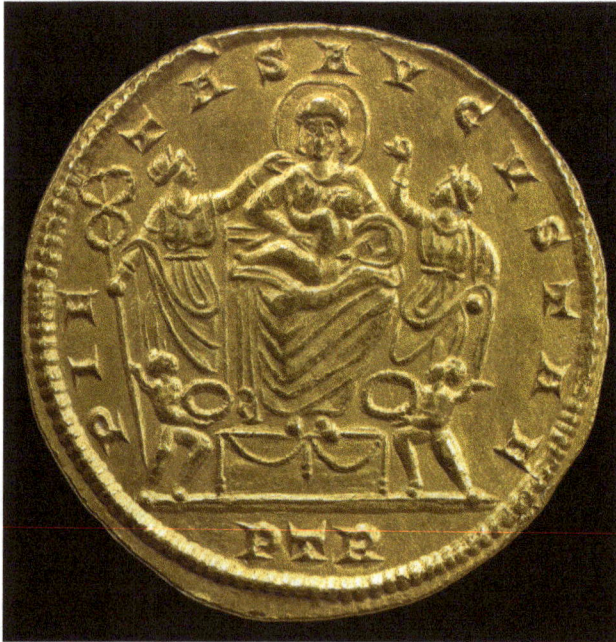

Figure 7.2 London, British Museum, inv. 1896,0608.100. Double-solidus medallion of Fausta (ca. AD 290–326), reverse: Fausta enthroned, nursing a child, flanked by Felicitas (left) and Pietas (right), with a pair of *genii* at the feet of the throne. Trier, AD 324/325. Photo: © The Trustees of the British Museum.

16 Bruun 1966, 203, nr 443. Note that in the online catalogue of the British Museum, the medallion is misleadingly listed as a single solidus, British Museum. "Coin; medallion." https://www.britishmuseum.org/collection/object/C_1896-0608-100. Accessed 26 March 2022.
17 This uniqueness has already been pointed out by Centlivres Challet and Bähler Baudois 2003, especially 275.
18 British Museum. "Coin." https://www.britishmuseum.org/collection/object/C_R-14503. Accessed 26 March 2022.

that this image should not be perceived as an actual portrait, since it is unlikely that the empress would have nursed her children herself. Besides, Constantine II and Constantius II were eight and seven years old respectively at the time, while the youngest, Constans, who may have been born as early as AD 320, was also probably too old to be represented as a suckling.[19]

The empress, frontal and nimbate, is seated on a throne placed on a raised platform and staring straight ahead. She is fully covered by her draped garment. She has a child in her lap, who is suckling from her left breast while grasping at her garment. The empress is flanked by the personifications of Felicitas (Happiness) to the left, holding a *caduceus*, a symbol of peace and prosperity, and of Pietas (Dutifulness) to the right, while the whole is surrounded by the inscription "PIETAS AUGUSTAE." Here, the nursing theme is employed to proclaim the empress' devotion to and fulfilment of her duty to the empire by the production and raising of heirs to the throne, thus ensuring the state's stability and, by extension, the happiness and prosperity of its subjects. Issued at the end of a period of internal strife and wars, which resulted in Constantine's becoming the uncontested sole ruler of the empire, the medallion served as a promise of a new, glorious age of security and peace, which was ensured by the establishment of a new dynasty thanks to the empress' *pietas* and fecundity.

Still, that the image of the empress nursing was chosen to convey these ideas, rather than the more traditional personifications of Fecunditas or Pietas surrounded by children seen on certain Antonine issues, remains puzzling.[20] Allusion to nursing is also discernible on coin issues of the same date associated with Fausta and her role in ushering in an era of stability and prosperity for the empire due to her motherhood (Figure 7.3).[21] On the reverse of these issues, the empress is represented standing, turned towards the left, holding two children at her breasts, while surrounded by the legend "SALUS REI PUBLICAE" ("safety/welfare of the state") or "SPES REI PUBLICAE" ("hope of the state"). John Vanderspoel and Michelle Mann have suggested that these other issues attempt to assimilate Fausta with a *dea nutrix* (nursing goddess), and indeed the iconographic similarity with terracotta figurines of a goddess nursing two infants, quite widespread in the Western Roman provinces at the time, is suggestive (Figure 7.4).[22]

I would agree that the imagery on Fausta's coins and medallion was informed by elements of the cult of nursing goddesses or, possibly, of the Egyptian goddess Isis nursing her son Horus, but I think we still need to explain why the creators of these types turned specifically to nursing imagery and not the more traditional ways of promoting the empress' role in securing the welfare of the empire through her motherhood. The nursing images of Fausta appear at a turning point, which marked a shift in the mode of government of the empire. After abolishing the tetrarchy,

---

19 Vanderspoel and Mann 2002, 352.
20 Centlivres Challet and Bähler Baudois 2003, 270.
21 Discussed by Vanderspoel and Mann 2002.
22 Vanderspoel and Mann 2002.

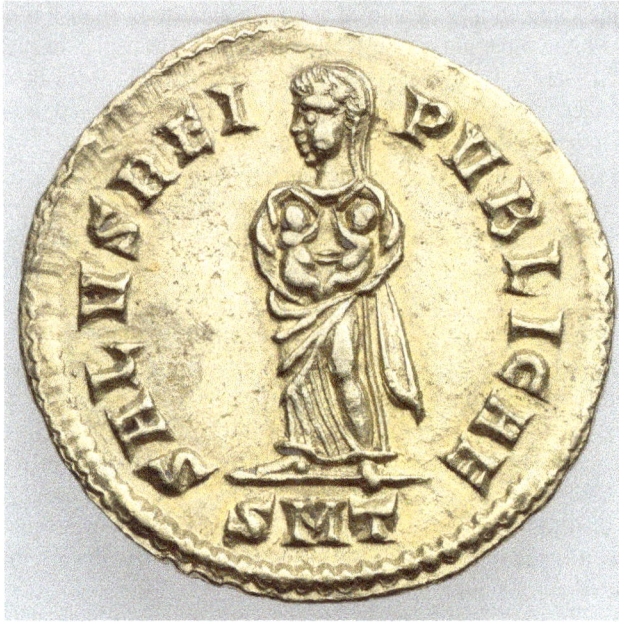

Figure 7.3 Boston, Museum of Fine Arts, Theodora Wilbour Fund in memory of Zoë Wilbour, inv. 2009.2288. Solidus, reverse: Fausta, standing, nursing two children. AD 324/325. Photo: © 2023 Museum of Fine Arts, Boston.

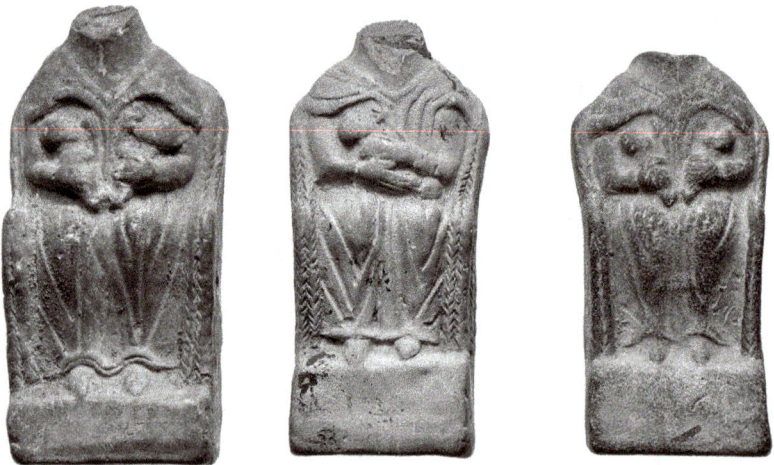

Figure 7.4 Museum of London, inv. 2088, A243, A244. Clay figurines of *deae nutrices* with one or two infants suckling at their breasts, heads missing. Second century AD(?). Photo: © Museum of London.

Constantine I promoted administering the state by means of dynastic succession. Fausta, daughter and wife of emperors, like Isis and the *deae nutrices* to whom she was visually compared, transferred to her sons the authority to rule through her milk. It is perhaps concern for such pagan associations, rather than Fausta's dramatic fall from grace and death in AD 326, that led to the abandonment of the powerful and empowering type of the nursing empress from the coinage of a progressively Christianized empire, where the right to rule was believed to be bestowed by God's favour rather than by the milk of a human empress. As suggested by Matthew Immerzeel (pers. comm.), the emergence by the later fourth century of the type of the Virgin *Galaktotrophousa*, first securely attested on a marble krater from Constantinople,[23] and a concomitant desire to avoid any "competition" or conflation between the human empress and the *Theotokos* (the one who gave birth to God), may also have informed the decision not to employ the type of the enthroned nursing empress on imperial coinage after Fausta.

Moving away from this exceptional use of the nursing theme in Constantinian dynastic discourse as expressed through coinage, we turn to the two other extant occurrences of the subject in the secular sphere that I was able to discover. Both are introduced into cycles of romanticized rural life. Though encountered in different media, from different regions, and separated by more than 100 years from each other, they display contextual and, I would suggest, functional similarities, which raise the tantalizing possibility that the theme may have enjoyed a wider distribution than the evidence currently available allows us to believe. The earlier of the two is the image of a nursing woman on a tapestry roundel from an unknown Egyptian context, dated to the fifth century AD (Figure 7.5). The roundel forms part of a set of four, which must have once adorned a tunic (Figure 7.6).[24] Due to the lack of archaeological context, the age and gender of the tunic's owner, as well as the original arrangement of the roundels on the garment, remain unascertained. Nonetheless, the appearance of images associated with childhood and childcare in three of the four roundels – a rare occurrence – could imply that the intended owner of the garment was a child.

The roundels are adorned with scenes set in an idealized pastoral setting. We see shepherds tending their flocks and watering their animals, a man and, elsewhere, a boy playing the flute, a group of half-naked youths enjoying an outdoor meal, a toddler playing with a dog looking at a shepherdess carrying a child on her back, and a reclining mother with a naked child on her lap. A potential danger – in the form of a snake wound around a tree trunk – that threatens this peaceful, idyllic existence is attacked by a man with a hoe. It is into this bucolic cycle that the image of the nursing woman is introduced. Whether she is a mother or a wet nurse

---

23 Severin 1970.

24 Stafford 2022, 341; Brett 1950. Brooklyn Museum. "Roundel." https://www.brooklynmuseum.org/opencollection/objects/56953. Accessed 26 March 2022.

Figure 7.5 New York, Brooklyn Museum, Charles Edwin Wilbour Fund, 44.143b. Tapestry roundel with bucolic scenes, including a nursing woman. Linen, wool, 12.2 × 10.9 cm (4 13/16 × Diam. 4 5/16 in.). Coptic, fifth century AD. Photo: Brooklyn Museum.

we cannot tell, since her headdress is not distinctive enough to offer a clue.[25] She is shown seated cross-legged on the ground, her body fully covered by her long tunic, with the exception of her left breast, which appears rather incongruously coming out of the side of her garment. She cradles a naked child in her arms, though her attention is elsewhere, her head turned towards the left; what has her distracted we do not know. Apparently left to its own devices, the child seems to be pushing the dress back to get to the lactating breast, a charmingly vivid image. When compared to the woman with the baby on her knees (Figure 7.6, roundel to the lower left),

25 See below, n. 34.

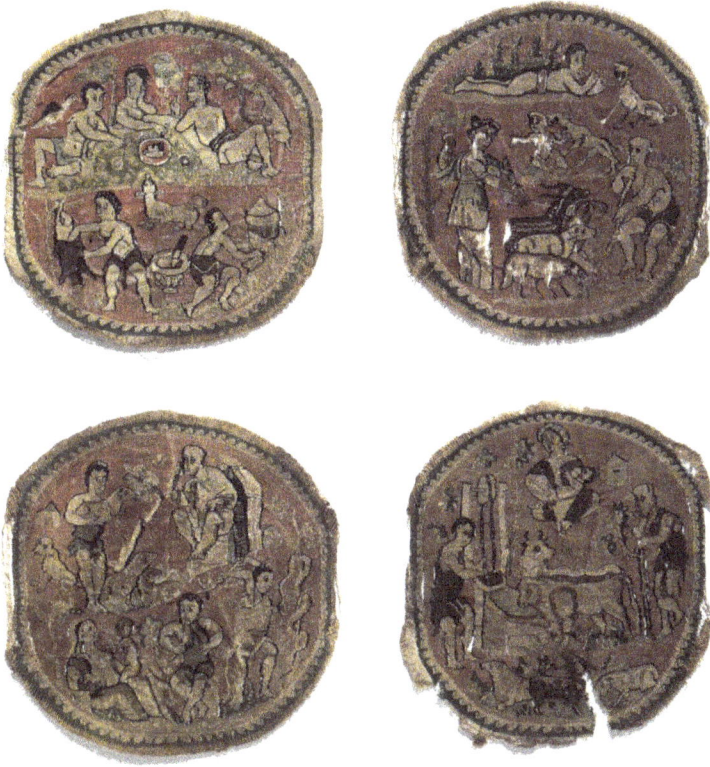

Figure 7.6 New York, Brooklyn Museum, Charles Edwin Wilbour Fund, 44.143a, 44.143b,
44.143c, 44.143d. Four tapestry roundels with bucolic scenes. Linen, wool,
11.9 × 12.1 cm (4 5/8–4 13/16 × Diam. 4 5/16–4 3/4 in.). Coptic, fifth century
AD. Photo: Brooklyn Museum.

our nursing group appears endowed with an animating tension that is absent from
the other group.

In certain late Roman funerary contexts, we find a nursing figure associated with
pastoral themes, there meant to provide comfort with the promise of a tranquil and
protected existence for the soul in the afterlife.[26] More likely than not, the Brooklyn
roundels were recovered from a funerary context. However, there is no way for us to
know whether the tunic they once adorned was made specifically for funerary use or
whether it followed its wearer to the grave. Be this as it may, studies of the decoration of early Byzantine dress have demonstrated that themes, such as the pastoral

26 E.g. Rothe 2011, Figures 1, 3: limestone tombstone of the wet nurse (*nutrix*) Severina from Cologne
(AD 220–250), with the image of a shepherd on the front side and Severina nursing her charge on
the right side; Weitzmann 1979, nr 237 (255) (entry by J. Weitzmann-Fiedler): fragment of a child's
marble sarcophagus from Rome (3rd or early 4th c. AD) with a nursing scene in a bucolic setting.

idyll on the roundels, evoking abundance, prosperity, and a pleasurable existence were meant not simply as a celebration of "the good life," but also as a means of invoking it for the wearer and of protecting them from the dangers that could threaten the prospect of a prosperous, long existence.[27] The leitmotif of protection seems to me to be quite strong on the Brooklyn roundels, with the shepherds guarding their flocks and, notably, the man attacking the snake (Figure 7.6, roundel to the lower left). Within this context, I would suggest that the figure of the alert nursing woman, prominently placed at the top of the roundel, encompasses the concepts of nourishment and protection, essential for the growth and survival of children. It is these life-affirming and protective aspects – simultaneously acknowledging human vulnerability – that made the image of the nursing woman appropriate for use both at the home and in the tomb.

In my view, protection is also central in the third occurrence of the theme in a secular context, though its setting is dramatically different. I am referring to the floor mosaics brought to light in Constantinople by the Walker Trust of the University of St Andrews (excavations: 1935–1938 and 1952–1954).[28] This is one of the most famous and most controversial works bequeathed to us by early Byzantine art. Considering the many uncertainties surrounding the creation and function of the mosaics, to say nothing of their date, variably ascribed from the fourth down to the ninth century AD, I opt for the more neutral designation "Walker Trust mosaics," since the moniker "Great Palace Mosaics" by which they are more commonly known tempts one to seek an imperial reading that may not be appropriate in this specific case.[29] As for the dating, I am inclined to agree with those assigning the ensemble to the late sixth or first half of the seventh century on the basis of limited and, admittedly, inconclusive, archaeological evidence.[30]

Spread over the covered porticoes of a large open peristyle court, the mosaics comprise a series of independent vignettes set against a neutral white background, arranged in four parallel, superimposed zones, with no formal separation between them. Their repertoire is diverse, comprising animals and animal combat, bucolic imagery, scenes of daily life, hunting scenes, and staged animal hunts in the hippodrome, as well as a small number of mythological figures. There have been numerous attempts to find an overarching unifying theme behind this selection, with varying degrees of success. James Trilling recognized three basic categories of subject matter, "rural or idyllic life, animal violence, and protection,"[31] while Katherine Dunbabin saw in them "a vision of the secular world" "characterised principally by the bounties of peaceful nature on the one hand, and on the other by its violence and ferocity: man must fight to preserve order and tranquillity."[32]

27 Ball 2016, 56, 59; Maguire 1999.
28 Trilling 1989.
29 For the view that the Walker Trust buildings were not part of the Great Palace of the Byzantine emperors, see Featherstone 2015, 592–593.
30 Bardill 2006, 12–20.
31 Trilling 1989, especially 58 for the quotation.
32 Dunbabin 1999, 232–235, especially 235 for the quotations.

It is in this fantastic array that the image of a nursing woman was inserted, the only currently known attestation of this theme in a secular early Byzantine floor mosaic (Figure 7.7). The image is located roughly at the centre of the peristyle's northeast portico. The woman is seated on a wooden stool, turning towards the right. Her head is covered by a grey head-kerchief, while her blue-grey-draped garment (not a tunic) leaves her shoulders, breasts, and right leg bare; she is barefoot. Her partial nudity is unique among Roman and early Byzantine images of nursing women; even mythological figures, such as the nymphs nursing Dionysos, have both their legs covered.[33] It is not possible to know whether, in his rendering of this half-covered female body, the mosaicist was referencing a now-lost antique model,[34] whether he wished to evoke a primitive, "natural" way of life, or whether he meant to imply violence.[35] In her lap, the woman holds a small child, dressed in a short dark ochre tunic. With its right leg crossed beneath its left leg, the child suckles from the woman's breast

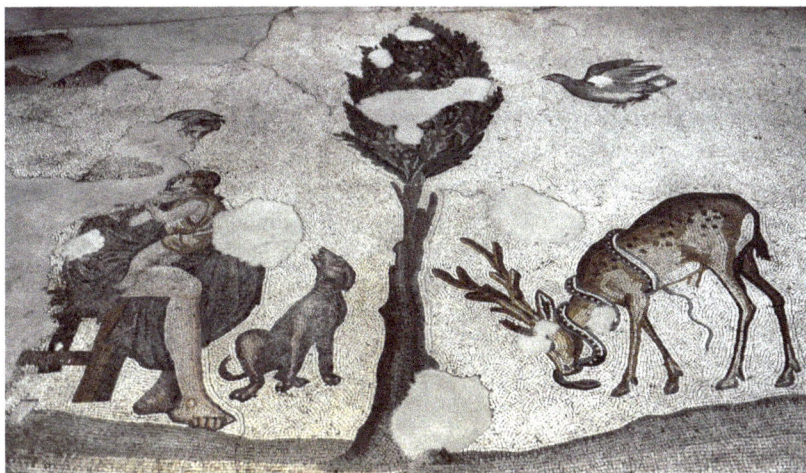

Figure 7.7 Constantinople, Walker Trust Excavations, peristyle court. North-east portico, mosaic pavement, detail: nursing woman with dog (left) and stag attacking a snake (right) on either side of a tree. Late sixth–first half of seventh century AD(?). Photo: PRISMA ARCHIVO/Alamy Stock Photo.

33 E.g. Dunbabin 1978, Figure 178: floor mosaic from the so-called *Maison de Bacchus*, Cuicul (Djémila), Algeria, depicting a nymph of Mount Nysa nursing the infant Dionysos (2nd c. AD).

34 As suggested by the figure's head-kerchief, which is reminiscent of the headdress of wet nurses in Roman funerary sculpture, see Zanker and Ewald 2012, ill. 65; Weitzmann 1979, nr 237 (255).

35 See also Stafford 2022, 341. For nudity evoking connotations of powerlessness, vulnerability, but also violation in classical art, see Cohen 1997; Bonfante 1989. For early Byzantine images of women breastfeeding among defeated barbarians, providing poignancy to the theme, and perhaps encapsulating the concept of the subjugation of an entire people to imperial might, see Stafford 2022, 343. For the two representations in question, see Delbrueck 1929, 87–93 (nr 2: consular ivory diptych, today in Halberstadt, 5th c. AD), 196–200 (nr 49: imperial ivory triptych, today in Milan, 6th c. AD); also discussed by Volbach 1976, 42–43 (nr 35) and 48–49 (nr 49) respectively.

while grasping her right arm. The woman cups the child's face with her right hand in a gesture of tenderness, yet her eyes seem to be upon the seated dog to her right, who is staring back at her. The woman's whole stance, when seen together with her garment that leaves her body half-exposed, imparts to the figure an air of exquisite vulnerability, which is nonetheless sublimated into care and concern for the child.

As already noted, the individual vignettes of the peristyle mosaics seem to be independent from each other. However, our nursing image may have been exceptional in this respect, as it shares the same band of soil with the episode represented immediately to the right. Though they are separated by a tree in between, the common strip of earth that they both share, the symmetrical arrangement on either side of the tree, and the direction of the woman's gaze invite us to look at the two scenes as pendant images. To the right of the tree, and below a bird flying towards it, we see a stag, turning left, attacking a snake; one cannot help but remember the iconography of the Brooklyn roundels discussed above. The belief that deer attack and kill snakes is well-attested in Roman sources, while by the fourth century AD the motif had already been invested with Christian symbolism, as an allegory of Christ defeating Satan.[36] However, it is not necessary to insist on a specific Christian reading for the stag with the snake in the Walker Trust mosaics. Following Trilling,[37] the stag attacking the snake could be understood as a powerful image of protection against the dangers, both physical and spiritual, that lurk even in the most idyllic environments and that threaten frail human existence, the fragility of which is delicately displayed in the image of the half-naked woman lovingly nursing the child to ensure its survival and growth. As in the case of the Brooklyn roundels, so in the case of the Walker Trust mosaics, the image of the nursing woman is not so much about fertility and nourishment, as about protecting and nurturing life in order for it to reach its full potential.

The Religious Sphere

There is only one other known representation of a nursing woman in an early mosaic pavement, which takes us into the religious sphere. There too, it was incorporated into a wider cycle of pastoral and rural themes, drawing from the same standard antique and early Byzantine repertoire of such imagery as the Brooklyn roundels and the Walker Trust mosaics. Once again, however, subtle differences in the treatment and contextualization of the theme suggest potential differences in function. As in the two secular examples we have examined above, the image of the nursing woman is accorded a central position within the wider composition. In fact, it would have been the first figure that one saw as one entered the central nave of the rural church of Saint Stephen at Ḥorvat Be'er-Shem'a in Israel, dated to the last third of the sixth century (Figure 7.8).[38] The mosaic pavement in question belongs

---

36 Shemesh 2019, 14–17; Trilling 1989, 59.
37 Trilling 1989, 59.
38 Gazit and Lender 1993. The nursing image is briefly commented upon by Stafford 2022, 341 and Hachlili 2009, 171. I am deeply grateful to Dr. Lihi Habas, who very generously shared with me photographs for study and a detailed description of the Ḥorvat Be'er-Shem'a mosaic pavement.

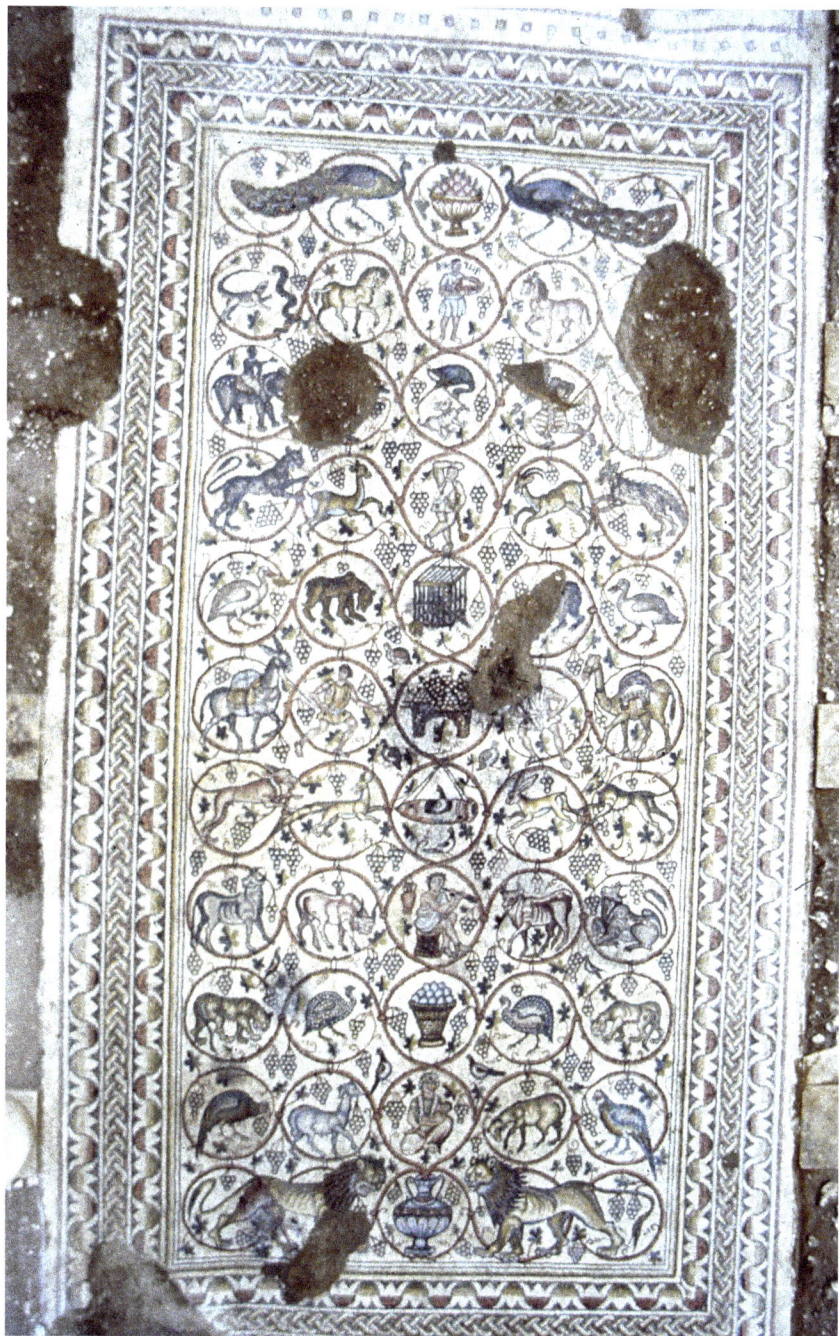

Figure 7.8 Ḥorvat Be'er-Shem'a, Saint Stephen's Church, nave, general view of mosaic pavement. Last third of sixth century AD. Photo: Yael Yolovitch, courtesy of the Israel Antiquities Authority.

to the type known as an inhabited scroll, where the figural decoration is organized into medallions created by the stalks of a vine, which in this example spring from a krater flanked by two striding lions. Above the krater, the vines create ten rows of five medallions each, populated with birds and animals (predatory, domesticated, and exotic), men engaged in pastoral and other activities, and allegorical images, like the bird in a cage. Our nursing figure is the only woman represented in the pavement, and she appears in the central medallion of the first row, immediately above the krater from which the vine sprouts.

The woman is seated cross-legged on the ground (Figure 7.9). She wears a long, ample sleeveless tunic and, above it, what seems to be a sleeveless green vest with unusual chequered *clavi* (vertical decorative bands) and a thin neckband for decoration. While she is barefoot, her coiffure is rather elaborate, surprisingly reminiscent of hairstyles associated with upper class women of the fifth and sixth centuries AD.[39] Golden earrings hang from her ears, while a bracelet and a pair of armbands adorn her naked right arm. As in the case of the nursing woman on the Brooklyn roundel, her naked left breast appears through the left side of her garment. With her arms and left leg, she supports the nursing child lying in her lap. The child wears a short, ochre sleeveless tunic; a golden bracelet and a golden anklet adorn its left wrist and ankle respectively. The child seems to be grasping at a red band, the function, however, of which is unclear. Neither woman nor child looks at each other, both having their gaze turned towards the right. Whether they are looking at the sheep in the medallion immediately to the right, or the lion directly below, is unclear. The medallion immediately to the left side encloses the image of a sheep, while those at either end of the same row enclose images of pheasants. In the medallion directly above the figure of the nursing woman, there is a basket filled with fruit.

Within the context of early Byzantine Christian basilicas, such intricate figured mosaic carpets, with vignettes inspired by the natural world and a variety of human activities, both peaceful, like the tending of flocks and the harvest, and violent, like the hunt, have been interpreted by scholars as a composite rendering of Creation in all its bounteous variety aimed at glorifying the Creator, as well as an image of the earthly world being saved by Christ.[40] Numerous such pavements have come down to us especially from the Eastern Roman provinces. To my knowledge, no other contains an image of a nursing woman. In the absence of comparanda from the same sphere, interpretation becomes a challenge. Should the figure be interpreted "literally," as a genre theme, however uncommon, associated with daily life in the countryside, where peasant women nursed their children or served as wet nurses, even while fulfilling their other duties, like tending their sheep? Or should one seek an allegorical interpretation for the pair? Admittedly, the elaborate dress of the nursing woman and the golden adornment of the child could intimate that these are not ordinary figures, yet the woman's bare feet and her being seated on the ground seem to contradict the impression of elevated status. Truth be told, we

39 E.g. Harlow 2004, Figures 7, 10.
40 Maguire 2012, 11–22.

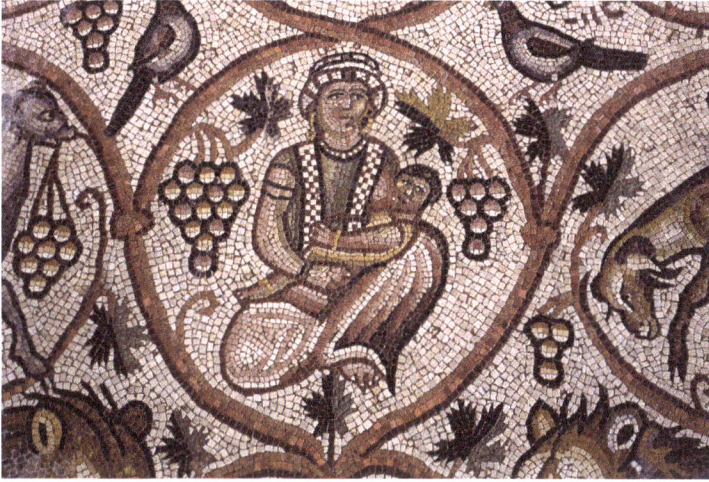

Figure 7.9 Ḥorvat Be'er-Shem'a, Saint Stephen's Church, nave, mosaic pavement, detail: medallion with nursing woman. Last third of sixth century AD. Photo: Yael Yolovitch, courtesy of the Israel Antiquities Authority.

do not know enough about local female attire of the peasant classes at the time to be able to ascertain whether the ensemble here was meant to be authentic or not. On the other hand, the adornment of the child with jewellery seems to be a realistic touch, as confirmed by both archaeological and written evidence.[41]

The rather ornate attire of the figures, in combination with the placement of the image, seems to imply that the latter was important, but where does that importance lie? In the special meaning that it may have held for the donor(s) of the mosaic,[42] or in its wider implications? Perhaps the image of the nursing woman was deemed appropriate to be placed at the root of the inhabited scroll as alluding to birth and life's new beginnings. Framed by sheep, birds, and the basket full of fruit, it could likewise be an evocation of the fertility and bounty of God's Creation. An image of care and protection, it could indeed offer reassurance of God's parental concern for humanity. Not least, this image of nursing, being an image of nourishment, encircled as it is by vines and grapes, may have been imbued with Eucharistic associations: just as the woman's milk gives life to the child, so the Eucharist sustains and opens the path to salvation and everlasting life to the faithful entering to worship in the church. However, if the image indeed had such a wide-ranging and powerful semiotic potential, why was it not more widely used in religious contexts? At the moment, I can offer no satisfactory answer, only some thoughts for future consideration at the end of the "Conclusions" below.

41 Pitarakis 2009, 187–195.
42 The ten Greek inscriptions located in the church, including one immediately to the west of the mosaic pavement of the nave, remain unpublished. According to Gazit and Lender 1993, 274, they contain "numerous names of men and women."

Conclusions

Having reached the end of our survey of images of ordinary women nursing, the great discrepancy between art and actual practice becomes apparent. While, in reality, breastfeeding was an act as common as it was necessary, it was very rarely represented in art, and this was obviously not for lack of suitable iconographic contexts. It is their rarity that makes the few extant examples of nursing images so compelling. As we have seen, these images were not meant to be simple domestic scenes. Rather, they were meant to serve a symbolic or an allegorical function, be it to identify a woman as a mother in funerary portraiture, to promote dynastic claims on imperial coinage, or to articulate ideas about fertility, nurture, vulnerability, dependency, and protection, sometimes hopeful, sometimes precarious, and always poignant. The centrality accorded to images of nursing women in the mosaics at Constantinople and Ḥorvat Be'er-Shem'a, as well as on the Brooklyn roundel, intimates that both creators and intended audience were sensitive to the image's semiotic potential and power.

In their pictorial treatment of the topic, early Byzantine artists occasionally seem to fall back on earlier Roman artistic prototypes, as suggested by the occurrence of the distinctive head-kerchief of Roman nurses in the Walker Trust mosaic at Constantinople. Depicting contemporary, practical aspects of the act realistically does not appear to have been a requisite for them. It is not clear, for instance, how the breasts were divested of their clothing for nursing. In the case of the women on the Brooklyn roundel and the Ḥorvat Be'er-Shema mosaic, whose garments evoke current fashions more closely, the implication is that the breast was accessed through a side opening or even through the broad sleeves of the female tunic once they were pulled back. However, in these examples, as in all other cases of fully dressed nursing figures, the lactating breast, represented incongruously against an otherwise fully covered torso, appears detached, deprived of an organic connection to the female body, with its potential sexual connotations neutralized.[43] This mode of representation draws attention to the breast as the nurturing organ, a function further highlighted by the woman's offering it to the child. In a society that viewed especially public human nakedness as shameful,[44] isolating the breast from the rest of the female body in a way that focused attention on the nurturing act rather than its physicalness may have also been a means to maintain the nursing woman's dignity, as well as ensuring that the viewer was not distracted from the point being made by the embarrassment of looking upon a partially naked female form.

In four out of the five representations we have examined, it is her left breast that the woman offers to the child.[45] In this, early Byzantine art follows a long-established preference that can be traced all the way back to the art of classical Greece.[46] Christian views, such as those reflected in the *Life of Symeon Stylite the*

---

[43] Cf. Ventura 2015, 217.

[44] Meyer 2009, 279, with additional references. See also the nuanced discussion by Stafford 2022.

[45] Because of damage, this particular detail is unclear in the mosaic from Constantinople.

[46] Bonfante 1997, 196, n. 73; Cohen 1997, 79.

Younger (*LSSY*; 6th/7th c.AD), according to which the infant Symeon refused to receive milk from his mother's left breast, but would only suckle from the right, "because the child is of the right (things),"[47] apparently had no obvious impact on the traditional preference of depicting an infant nursing from the left breast of ordinary women in art. As a whole, postures and gestures conveyed the function of the woman not only as the nurturer, caregiver, but also as the protector of the child in her arms. In some examples, certain gestures and the direction of the gaze evoked the sentimental bond between the woman and the child that developed as a result of the act of breastfeeding, as also acknowledged in related medical writings.[48] Often, however, the woman did not gaze at her charge. In some examples, she gazes at the viewer, endowing the composition with an iconic rather than a narrative function. In others, she gazes to the side, implying some form of disturbance or potential danger that enhances the impression of the fragility of human life epitomized by the child in her arms. The child's dependency on the woman for its survival is vividly displayed by the way that it is often shown grasping at her. Sometimes naked, sometimes dressed in a simple short, sleeveless tunic, its gender remains undefined. A nursling was perhaps deemed too young to participate in the gender discourse of its society and to be ascribed distinct gender characteristics, at least in art. Nonetheless, this "unformed" quality was a dynamic one, as it contained the promise of growth and development under the woman's nurturing care.

If one considers the potential of such nursing images to promote the ideal of woman as mother, nurturer, and carer for children, which was the primary role ascribed to women in the construction of the female gender at the time, the question of why they were not more frequently depicted becomes even more puzzling. My own impression is that there were different factors at play, artistic and social, as well as religious. To begin with, early Byzantine artists may have been restrained in their use of this image because it did not occur often in the earlier models to which they turned for inspiration; it was certainly not as popular as other themes inspired by daily life in the antique artistic vocabulary to which they had recourse. On the other hand, their sometimes novel treatment of this theme indicates that early Byzantine artists were not confined by tradition and that suitable settings for its introduction could be found if there was demand.

As for potential patrons, they may have been disinterested in this theme, given the social realities associated with the actual practice, specifically that upper class women would not often nurse their own offspring, relegating the activity to women of low social status, including slaves. The moral ambivalence surrounding the figure of the wet nurse, a woman, as astutely pointed out by Stavroula Constantinou and Aspasia Skouroumouni-Stavrinou, in a sense selling her body for money, may

---

47 "τῶν γὰρ δεξιῶν ἐστι τὸ παιδάριον" (*LSSY* 3.9–10, ed. Van den Ven). This passage has been discussed by Chevallier Caseau 2009, 147.

48 For ancient and early Byzantine medical writings pertaining to lactation, see Chapters 4–6 in this volume.

have fed into this reticence.[49] Likewise, patrons and viewers, who included both men and women, may have found the theme somewhat embarrassing and awkward, considering current attitudes to ordinary human nakedness, and thus may have wished to avoid it, especially in public contexts away from the more personal and emotional setting of the tomb. Given that we lack information on the identity of the persons who commissioned the images we are discussing, there is no way to estimate whether there might have been a gender bias involved; one should, however, avoid making any assumptions about female preference for the theme, as opposed to male indifference or conscious avoidance, simply because of its content.

Finally, considering that patrons and viewers lived in a progressively Christianized world, one cannot help but wonder whether there may have been a Christian wariness towards the theme of the nursing woman, given its frequent association with the pagan cults of mother goddesses, *deae nutrices*, and Dionysos. We have nothing from the period that we have been examining that could compare to the second-century AD rabbinic ban against "a nursing female image," admittedly from a time when such cults were still going strong on imperial soil.[50] In the centuries that followed, memory may have survived the cults themselves and the theme may have been avoided, especially in religious contexts, at least until it could accumulate a new set of associations that would allow for its use without suspicion. But this is a different story, and mine stops here.

References

Texts: Editions and Translations
Ven, P. van den. ed. 1962. *La vie ancienne de S. Syméon Stylite le jeune (521–592)*. Subsidia Hagiographica 32. Brussels: Société des Bollandistes.

Secondary Works

Ball, J.L. 2016. "Charms: Protective and Auspicious Motifs," in T.K. Thomas (ed.) *Designing Identity: The Power of Textiles in Late Antiquity*. Princeton, NJ: Princeton University Press, 55–64.
Bardill, J. 2006. "Visualizing the Great Palace of the Byzantine Emperors at Constantinople: Archaeology, Text, and Topography," in F.A. Bauer (ed.) *Visualisierungen von Herrschaft: Frühmittelalterliche Residenzen – Gestalt und Zeremoniell*. Byzas 5. Istanbul: Ege Yayınları, 5–45.
Beerden, K., and F.G. Naerebout. 2011. "Roman Breastfeeding? Some Thoughts on a Funerary Altar in Florence," *Classical Quarterly* 61 (2): 761–766.
Bolman, E.S. 2004. "The Coptic Galaktotrophousa Revisited," in M. Immerzeel, and J. Van der Vliet (eds) *Coptic Studies on the Threshold of a New Millennium: Proceedings of the*

---

49 See Chapter 2 in this volume and Constantinou and Skouroumouni-Stavrinou 2024, in press.
50 Friedheim 2003.

Seventh International Congress of Coptic Studies. Leiden, August 27–September 2, 2000.
2 vols. Orientalia Lovaniensia Analecta 133. Louvain: Peeters, 1173–1184.

———. 2005. "The Enigmatic Coptic Galaktotrophousa and the Cult of the Virgin Mary in
Egypt," in M. Vassilaki (ed.) *Images of the Mother of God: Perceptions of the Theotokos
in Byzantium.* London: Ashgate Publishing, 13–22.

Bonfante, L. 1989. "Nudity as a Costume in Classical Art," *American Journal of Archaeology* 93 (4): 543–570.

———. 1997. "Nursing Mothers in Classical Art," in Koloski-Ostrow and Lyons 1997,
174–196.

Brett, G. 1950. "The Brooklyn Textiles and the Great Palace Mosaic," in *Coptic Studies in
Honor of Walter Ewing Crum = The Bulletin of the Byzantine Institute* 2: 433–441.

Bruun, P.M. 1966. *The Roman Imperial Coinage*, vol. 7: *Constantine and Licinius, A.D.
313–337.* London: Spink and Son Ltd.

Carroll, M. 2014. "Mother and Infant in Roman Funerary Commemoration," in M. Carroll,
and E.-J. Graham (eds) *Infant Health and Death in Roman Italy and Beyond. Journal
of Roman Archaeology* Supplementary volume 96. Portsmouth, RI: Journal of Roman
Archaeology, 159–178.

Centlivres Challet, C.-E. 2017. "Roman Breastfeeding: Control and Affect," *Arethusa* 50
(3): 369–384.

Centlivres Challet, C.-E., and M. Bähler Baudois. 2003. "Les femmes sur les monnaies
impériales romaines: Quelles influences à l'origine de la monnaie de la Fausta trônante?"
in R. Frei-Stolba, A. Bielman, and O. Bianchi (eds) *Les femmes antiques entre sphère
privée et sphère publique: Actes du Diplôme d'études avancées, Universités de Lausanne
et Neuchâtel, 2000–2002.* Bern: Peter Lang, 269–279.

Chevallier Caseau, B. 2009. "Childhood in Byzantine Saints' Lives," in Papaconstantinou
and Talbot 2009, 127–166.

Cohen, B. 1997. "Divesting the Female Breast of Clothes in Classical Sculpture," in
Koloski-Ostrow and Lyons 1997, 66–92.

Constantinou, S., and A. Skouroumouni-Stavrinou. 2024. "The Other Mother: Ancient and
Early Byzantine Approaches to Wet Nursing and Mothering," *Journal of Hellenic Studies*
145, in press.

Cutler, A. 1987. "The Cult of Galaktotrophousa in Byzantium and Italy," *Jahrbuch der Österreichischen Byzantinistik* 37: 335–350.

Delbrueck, R. 1929. *Die Consulardiptychen und verwandte Denkmäler.* Berlin: De Gruyter.

Dunbabin, K. 1978. *The Mosaics of Roman North Africa: Studies in Iconography and Pa-
tronage.* Oxford: Clarendon Press.

———. 1999. *Mosaics of the Greek and Roman World.* Cambridge and New York: Cambridge University Press.

Effenberger, A. 1977. "Die Grabstele aus Medinet el-Fajum: Zum Bild der stillenden Gottes-
mutter in der koptischen Kunst," *Forschungen und Berichte* 18, *Archäologische Beiträge*:
158–168.

Effenberger, A., and H.-G. Severin. 1992. *Das Museum für Spätantike und Byzantinische
Kunst.* Mainz: Staatliche Museen zu Berlin – Zabern.

Featherstone, M. 2015. "Space and Ceremony in the Great Palace of Constantinople under the Macedonian Emperors," in *Le corti nell'Alto Medioevo: LXII Settimana di studi
della Fondazione Centro italiano di studi sull'alto Medioevo, Spoleto, 24–29 aprile 2014.*
Spoleto: Fondazione Centro italiano di studi sull'Alto Medioevo, 587–607.

Friedheim, E. 2003. "Who Are the Deities Concealed behind the Rabbinic Expression 'A
Nursing Female Image'?" *Harvard Theological Review* 96 (2): 239–250.

Gazit, D., and Y. Lender. 1993. "The Church of St. Stephen at Ḥorvat Be'er-Shem'a," in Y. Tsafrir (ed.) *Ancient Churches Revealed*. Jerusalem: Israel Exploration Society, 273–276.

Gwynn, D.M. 2018. "Fausta," in O. Nicholson (ed.) *The Oxford Dictionary of Late Antiquity*. 2 vols. Oxford: Oxford University Press, 587.

Hachlili, R. 2009. *Ancient Mosaic Pavements: Themes, Issues, and Trends. Selected Studies*. Leiden and Boston: Brill.

Hagan, S. 2013. "Death and Eternal Life at Beth Shean," *Expedition* 55 (1): 33–36.

Harlow, M. 2004. "Female Dress, Third–Sixth Century: The Messages in the Media?" *Antiquité Tardive* 12: 203–215.

Huskinson, J. 1996. *Roman Children's Sarcophagi: Their Decoration and Its Social Significance*. Oxford: Clarendon Press.

Immerzeel, M. 2016. "Coptic–Ethiopian Artistic Interactions: The Issues of the Nursing Virgin and St George Slaying the Dragon," *Journal of the Canadian Society for Coptic Studies* 8: 95–118.

Jastrzebowska, E. 1989. "Les sarcophages chrétiens d'enfants à Rome au IVe siècle," *Mélanges de l'Ecole française de Rome. Antiquité* 101 (2): 783–804.

Koloski-Ostrow, A.O., and C.L. Lyons. eds. 1997. *Naked Truths: Women, Sexuality, and Gender in Classical Art and Archaeology*. London and New York: Routledge.

Langener, L. 1996. *Isis lactans, Maria lactans: Untersuchungen zur koptischen Ikonographie*. Altenberge: Oros Verlag.

Maguire, H. 1999. "The Good Life," in G.W. Bowersock, P. Brown, and O. Grabar (eds) *Late Antiquity: A Guide to the Postclassical World*. Cambridge, MA: Belknap Press of Harvard University Press, 238–257.

———. 2012. *Nectar and Illusion: Nature in Byzantine Art and Literature*. Oxford: Oxford University Press.

Mathews, T., and N. Muller. 2005. "Isis and Mary in Early Icons," in M. Vassilaki (ed.) *Images of the Mother of God: Perceptions of the Theotokos in Byzantium*. London: Ashgate Publishing, 3–11.

Meyer, M. 2009. *An Obscure Portrait: Imaging Women's Reality in Byzantine Art*. London: Pindar Press.

Narkiss, B. 2007. *El Pentateuco Ashburnham. La ilustración de códices en la antigüedad tardía: Introducción al facsímil*. Valencia: Patrimonio Ediciones.

Papaconstantinou, A., and A.-M. Talbot. eds. 2009. *Becoming Byzantine: Children and Childhood in Byzantium*. Washington, DC: Dumbarton Oaks Research Library and Collection.

Papanikola-Mpakirtzē, D. ed. 2002. *Καθημερινή Ζωή στο Βυζάντιο*. Athens: Υπουργείο Πολιτισμού.

Parlasca, K. 2007. "Pseudokoptische Grabreliefs aus Ägypten," *Chronique d'Egypte* 82 (163–164): 323–329.

Pitarakis, B. 2009. "The Material Culture of Childhood in Byzantium," in Papaconstantinou and Talbot 2009, 167–251.

Rothe, U. 2011. "Der Grabstein der Severina Nutrix aus Köln: Eine neue Deutung," *Germania: Anzeiger der Römisch-Germanischen Kommission des Deutschen Archäologischen Instituts* 89 (1–2): 191–214.

Severin, H.-G. 1970. "Oströmische Plastik unter Valens und Theodosius I," *Jahrbuch der Berliner Museen* 12: 211–252.

Shemesh, A.O. 2019. "The Deer, the Snake and the Water: Jewish Medieval Interpretations of Psalm 24.1," *European Journal of Science and Theology* 15 (4): 9–22.

Stafford, G. 2022. "Privilege, Pleasure, Performance: Reading Female Nudity in Late Antique Art," in M.E. Stewart, D.A. Parnell, and C. Whately (eds) *The Routledge Handbook on Identity in Byzantium*. London: Routledge, 333–362.

Trilling, J. 1989. "The Soul of the Empire: Style and Meaning in the Mosaic Pavement of the Byzantine Imperial Palace in Constantinople," *Dumbarton Oaks Papers* 43: 27–72.

Vanderspoel, J., and M.L. Mann. 2002. "The Empress Fausta as Romano-Celtic Dea Nutrix," *Numismatic Chronicle* 162: 350–355.

Ventura, G. 2015. "Breastfeeding, Ideology and Clothing in Nineteenth-Century France," in S.-R. Marzel, and G.D. Stiebel (eds) *Dress and Ideology: Fashioning Identity from Antiquity to the Present*. London and New York: Bloomsbury, 211–229.

Volbach, W. 1976. *Elfenbeinarbeiten der Spätantike und des frühen Mittelalters*. Mainz: Philipp von Zabern.

Weitzmann, K. ed. 1979. *Age of Spirituality: Late Antique and Early Christian Art, Third to Seventh Century*. New York: Metropolitan Museum of Art.

Zanker, P., and B.C. Ewald. 2012. *Living with Myths: The Imagery of Roman Sarcophagi*. Translated by J. Slater. Oxford: Oxford University Press.

8 Empowering Breasts

Women, Widows, and Prophetesses-with-Child at Dura-Europos

Barbara Crostini

Introduction: Bare Breasts at Dura-Europos

Two sets of bare breasts are prominently displayed in the lower panels of the paintings of the West Wall in the synagogue at Dura-Europos (ca. AD 240). To the right of the Torah niche, a frontal bather, identified as Pharaoh's daughter, stands in the River Nile at the centre of an elaborate composition relating the narrative of Moses' rescue (cf. *Exodus* (*Ex*) 2). To the left of the Torah niche, a mother in distress has torn the upper garment of her black robes and exposed her bosom as a sign of mourning for her dead son (cf. 1 *Kings* = 3 *Kingdoms* (1 *Kg* (3 *Kg*)) 17.17–24).[1] These scenes were not tucked away to be seen by few: this register of paintings is the closest to the viewer's level, and the West Wall is the most important side of the interior space. Along this register, which takes into its visual field the Torah arch, a total of 14 female figures are represented. Even accounting for some duplicate characters, this overwhelming number of female figures calls for consideration in the interpretation of the message of the West Wall.[2]

Despite their prominence, the presence of these women has gone largely unremarked in scholarship, with one notable exception.[3] The captions by which the scenes are known typically erase the women's role in the action by describing these panels with reference to male biblical heroes, such as "Pharaoh and the Infancy of Moses" and "Elijah Revives the Widow's Child."[4] Such labels confirm patriarchal expectations from a Jewish milieu, spectacularly failing to appreciate the impact of the women portrayed at the centre of this space.

Some attention, however, has been paid to the breasts of Pharaoh's daughter. According to classicist Warren Moon, "For members of the congregation the frontal nudity of Pharaoh's daughter must have had a risqué connotation."[5] Moon

---

1 Translations of the Bible, unless otherwise indicated, are taken from the *New King James Version* (*NKJV*). Copyright © 1982 by Thomas Nelson, Inc. https//www.biblestudytools.com/nkjv/. Accessed 16 June 2022.
2 Xeravits 2017b does not advance the discussion in this sense.
3 Steinberg 2006.
4 Kraeling 1956, 143, 169.
5 Moon 1992, 596.

DOI: 10.4324/9781003265658-11

emphasizes the contrast between Hellenistic nakedness and Jewish prudishness, attributing unequivocal condemnation for such flesh-exposing images "even to a hellenized (*sic*) Jew."[6] Moon's judgement disregards ambivalence towards the breast in ancient cultures, where eroticism is accompanied by celebrations of fertility.[7] It also sweepingly sets aside a whole biblical tradition in which the erotic connotations of women's breasts are inscribed. Explicit celebrations of women's bodily attractiveness in the Bible should caution against accepting at face value Moon's concern about the inappropriateness of nakedness within sacred liturgical space. The tradition of the *Song of Songs* (*S of S*) springs to mind as the clearest example of the incorporation of erotic sensual experience in the spiritual realm. As Annette Schellenberg has shown,[8] the encounter of the woman with her bridegroom is a profoundly physical sensory experience, in which breasts are described as two gazelles (*S of S* 4.5, 7.3), evoking their delicate curvature, or as two towers, alluding to the erectility of aroused sexual organs (*S of S* 8.10). Moreover, the voice of this woman frames and drives the narrative of erotic encounter. Her initiative is in striking contrast to the male-oriented sexuality of the Bible, where sex is contemplated only from the point of view of men and concerns women only to the extent that they are men's property.[9] In contrast, the *S of S* attributes a prominent role to women. Its performance would not have been alien to an environment similar to that surviving at Dura.[10]

Just as the sensuality of the *S of S* is not aberrant to the biblical canon, so is the depiction of breasts in the women of the Dura synagogue paintings integral to its painterly programme. In this chapter, I argue that, far from needing to avert our eyes from such a display of nudity, we need to sharpen our sight to capture this mark of women's presence and power. Focusing on Pharaoh's daughter and the widow of Sarepta, I argue that exposure of their breasts in the Dura synagogue, far from being a matter of shame, is purposefully designed to draw attention to these women's active and prophetic role in Israel. While the identification of Pharaoh's daughter with the fertility goddess Anahita proposed by Erwin Goodenough has been rightly rejected,[11] nevertheless his comparison captures the numinous aura of this woman at the centre of the painted panel, endowed with as much power as ancient breastfeeding divinities.[12] As for the widow, her relation to Elijah is far from subordinate. Robert du Mesnil du Buisson remarked that her stance is comparable to later images of the Virgin Mary with child.[13] The coupling of these women to their children unleashes their capacities as special witnesses to the di-

---

6 Moon 1992, 595.
7 Iavazzo et al. 2009.
8 Schellenberg 2018 and 2016.
9 Carr 2000, 237–241.
10 Schellenberg 2016, 114.
11 Xeravits 2017a, 268–269.
12 Moon 1992, 588.
13 Mesnil du Buisson 1939, 114. For the imagery of the Virgin Mary with child, and in particular the *Galaktotrophousa* motif, see Chapter 7 in this volume.

vine in the world: partaking in God's act of creation, they enact salvation, foresee future outcomes, and contribute in a determinant way to leading the community in the right direction. Thus, sexual attributes are here exposed in order to highlight these women's roles as life givers and nourishers. In particular, these women are unlike the majority of biblical female prophet figures, who are without child; on the contrary, they are bound to their children as an important marker of their prophetic identity. Thus, their role as mothers is not confined to the domestic sphere because of childbirth; rather, their offspring enhance the women's contribution to the community. Children do not steal the limelight from their mothers, leaving these women as mere instruments of their coming into existence.

In order to understand how these images do not conform to the trend of mitigating female initiative through the confines of motherhood, I highlight two factors: (1) how the status of these women is uncoupled from male presence, even concerning the origin of their offspring, and (2) how mothers are responsible for their children's education. After exploring their relationship to the category of female prophets-with-child, I further highlight how these women, who are neither sterile nor inviolate, are portrayed as single mothers. Contrary to conventions of well-ordered family structures still largely upheld today,[14] their husbandless solitude is not stigmatized, nor is their fertility – of which the breasts are an evident boast – branded as immoral. Without a partner or guardian, these women's agency comes across as more encompassing and comprehensive than in a regular family hierarchy. Freed from men's possession, just as real Durene women attested from contemporary documents on papyrus were, these biblical heroines reflect the unexpected face of women's power in a late ancient setting.

Turning to the real women around town, women's roles in the community and in society at large display independent traits, including equality of legal rights with men. Situating the daughter of Pharaoh and Elijah's widow in contemporary context, I show that the synagogue's paintings displayed no radically different attitude to women than what was acceptable in that society. The attitude of Jewish prophetesses thus contributed to reinforce and justify women's legal freedom as practised under the Severi. I conclude that it was precisely as single mothers that the status of the women depicted in these paintings was enhanced and their contribution as seers appreciated. Despite the certain presence of a male priestly caste at Dura, a mantic "proto-priestly" function of women-with-child is also envisaged. Against this background, these single women-with-child (and without husband), fully comprised of their creative powers in body and mind, can be considered as forerunners of the Virgin Mary, devoid of the connotations of asexual or anti-sexual *encratism* associated with her figure.[15]

Like the use of images in a Jewish setting, the idea that women were no less worthy of spiritual authority after producing a child, whether in or outside wedlock, whether the male partner was temporarily absent or permanently gone, and

14 But see O'Reilly 2019.
15 Clayton Croy and Connor 2011.

whatever the reasons for the latter – death or neglect and abandonment – breaks free of expectations. These unconventional, real-life scenarios in which women could become lone actors are covered by the meaning of the word "widow" in ancient Greek (*chēra*) and Latin (*vidua*), terms that describe a state of singleness, whatever the causes.[16] Being a "widow," or a single mother, was no reason for shame, but rather deserved special consideration and status beyond that of becoming the object of charitable benefactions. Exposing the beautiful female body in open proclamation of that special condition, the paintings of the Dura synagogue attest to a place (the Roman Eastern *limes*) and a time (the first half of the 3rd c. AD) where female agency was pivotal to the Jewish faith. Their outspokenness may contribute to explaining the backlash found in Scriptures aimed at restraining controversy on this front. This process is observed not only in the Hebrew Bible but also in New Testament writings, resulting in the coexistence of both liberal and conservative traditions concerning women.[17] For this reason, Steinberg's claim that women's status was enhanced in the paintings in order to entice modern-thinking Jewish women to remain in the synagogue, rather than defect to the Christian competition because it was offering them a better deal, expresses an interesting, but ultimately unpersuasive, theory.[18]

Prophetess-with-Child: Isaiah's Exception to the Rule

In a well-argued and careful article, Esther Hamori observes a pattern of female diviners in the Bible who are not also depicted as mothers. The distinction stands out as a contrast to the overwhelming emphasis on fertility and motherhood as a sign of God's favour in Israel.[19] There are only four women explicitly designated as prophetesses: Miriam, Huldah, Deborah, and Noadiah. Miriam's family relationships are designated only with respect to male relatives, her brothers Moses and Aaron, as we shall see further below.[20] Deborah and Huldah are married, but there is no mention of children in the text (*Judges* 4.4 and 2 *Kings* = 4 *Kingdoms* (2 *Kg* (4 *Kg*)) 22.14 respectively).[21] Reference to Noadiah is too brief to draw conclusions (*Nehemiah* 6.16).[22] Other women who prophesy, such as the two wise women of Tekoa (2 *Samuel* 14), use metaphors of motherhood in their prophecies but are not said to be mothers themselves.[23] Hamori stresses that her conclusions may not relate to the reality of these women, but are confined to their presentation in the text,

---

16 Maier 2021, 59: "The Greek term 'χήρα' could refer to any woman who chose to live without a man, whether one whose husband had died or a single woman"; see also Lehtipuu 2017.
17 Zamfir 2020 for the New Testament; Schellenberg 2018 for the Hebrew Bible.
18 Steinberg 2006, 482, 487.
19 Hamori 2013.
20 Hamori 2013, 170.
21 Hamori 2013, 171–172.
22 Hamori 2013, 172.
23 Hamori 2013, 173–174.

which seemingly creates "an observable pattern of female diviners not also being depicted as mothers."[24]

The exception to the rule of childless women is the case of one anonymous prophetess (as the Bible designates her) mentioned in *Isaiah* (*Is*) 8.3,[25] with whom the prophet conceived a son. Exegetes are embarrassed about Isaiah's role, since his occasional sexual collaboration does not justify calling this woman the prophet's wife. This subordinate role was once suggested for all biblical prophetesses, whereas more recent studies have given women full credit for this role. Williamson calls her Huldah's predecessor, placing her in the succession of prophets from Moses.[26] Others have suggested that the role of this woman as prophet be downgraded because "she does not even speak."[27] To this objection, Hamori counters that "[w]hat she does in the story, she does only through her reproductive capacity: she bears a sign-child. This woman literally delivers an oracle."[28] Hamori also stresses the woman's active involvement in this provision of the baby oracle: "The text overtly describes the birth of the sign-child as prophetic symbolic action, and ... *most of this action is hers*."[29]

A general trend from classical antiquity common to Middle Eastern civilizations and, it would seem, also to the biblical tradition, separated women's divination from traditional family roles. For example, Apollo's Pythia was a permanent virgin or, at most, a postmenopausal "widow."[30] The nameless prophetess of *Isaiah* represents a very different trend by equating birth and motherhood with the very powers of prophecy: her prophetic words are enfleshed in her childbearing. This alternative strand does not require sexual abstinence but rather values the experience of childbirth as a kind of initiation into life's most vital mechanisms. The bringing forth of new life provides the essential depth of emotional experience that enables clarity of vision into the fundamentals of existence. The Dura scenes that we will now examine uphold this kind of understanding endorsed by *Isaiah*. They do not shy away from attributing independent powers as prophets and seers to women-with-child (and without husbands).

Acting Motherly: Miriam, Jochebed, and Pharaoh's Daughter

The scene of the rescue of Moses from the Nile, described by Kraeling as "Pharaoh and the infancy of Moses" (panel WC4: Figure 8.1), occupies a rectangular surface 4 m long and 1.29 m high, making it the largest panel on this row and one of the largest in the whole synagogue.[31] It displays nine women, of which one, centrally

24 Hamori 2013, 170.
25 Nissinen 2013, 30, n. 16.
26 Williamson 2010, 75.
27 Ackerman 1998, cited by Hamori 2013, 172.
28 Hamori 2013, 172.
29 Hamori 2013, 172. Emphasis added.
30 Hamori 2013, 180.
31 Kraeling 1956, 169–178.

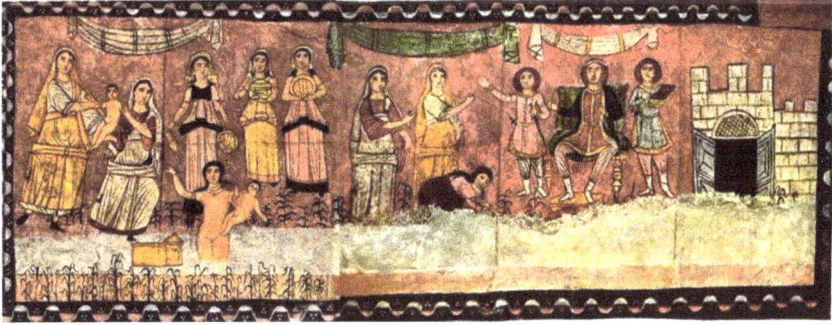

Figure 8.1 Miriam, Jochebed, and the daughter of Pharaoh rescue Moses from the Nile (left); the three maid attendants (centre); the introduction of Moses at Pharaoh's court (right). Fresco on the West Wall of the synagogue at Dura-Europos, Syria, ca. AD 240. After Goodenough, E.R. 1964. *Jewish Symbols in the Greco-Roman Period.* Toronto: Pantheon Books. Vol. 11, p. 9. Original photo: Fred Anderegg. Via https://www.reed.edu/humanities/hum110/dura_images04/dura.htm.

positioned in the middle-front plane of the panel, is standing naked in the river with baby Moses on her hip. The identity of each of these women is not completely certain. After reviewing the current understanding of the panel, I propose a different interpretation that highlights agency by the women depicted.

The movement of the action was envisaged, according to Kraeling, from right to left, bringing the viewer's attention towards the Torah niche at the centre of this wall and paralleling the flow of the river through the length of the panel from one edge to the other. Kraeling, peculiarly, also adds a horizontal division of the space into foreground and background planes indicated by the nearer and farther banks of the river, even though extensive damage to the lower right portion of the panel makes the exact shape of the nearer bank hypothetical.

Kraeling describes the group represented on the far bank of the river as "a king seated upon a throne attended by two courtiers, [and] a group of standing women."[32] The king's throne lacks the details, such as lions, proper to Solomon's throne.[33] Moreover, although the city gate framing the scene to the right stands for Egypt as in the *Exodus* panels above, the king, i.e. Pharaoh, is dressed in the Persian manner. Kraeling confidently identifies the two women as midwives, relating the scene to the order, imparted by Pharaoh, to kill male Hebrew babies while they are being delivered.[34] *Exodus* 1.15–16 even names these women as Shiphrah and Puah. Weitzmann and Kessler follow this identification, noting that the midwives' objection of conscience to Pharaoh's orders is key to the salvation of the Hebrew children.[35]

32 Kraeling 1956, 170.
33 Moon 1992, 606.
34 Kraeling 1956, 173.
35 Weitzmann and Kessler 1990, 27–28.

This explanation of the midwives as supporters of the Jewish nation explains why God protects them from Pharaoh's wrath, but sits in tension with the rescue of Moses and with their tale of deceit. The midwives tell Pharaoh that they have not managed to kill all the male Hebrew babies because Hebrew mothers are so capable and healthy that they give birth before the midwives can arrive. While the midwives' names designate them as Semitic women of slave descent in Egypt,[36] their interaction with Pharaoh and their unexpected moral integrity towards the commandment not to kill would make better sense if their loyalty to Egypt were underpinned by their Egyptian identity. In fact, their dilemma and ethical course raise precisely those issues of belonging in a multi-ethnic society that are further developed in the Moses story. However, Moses' survival does not depend directly on their action. Rather, his escape confirms a version of their story – which is meant to be false in the midwives' retelling – namely, that Jewish women use subterfuge to save male babies. Thus, from a narrative viewpoint, the midwives' scene is not essential to the dynamics of Moses' rescue.

Identifying the scene to the right with the text of *Exodus* 1.15–16 leaves out of the explanation the woman bending down to the ground between the midwives. Since the biblical account mentions only two midwives, this third presence must be eliminated from that ensemble. Thus Kraeling considers that she belongs to the foreground, removing her from the threesome. Imagining her near to the riverbank (which is now destroyed), Kraeling identifies her as Jochebed, the mother of Moses, floating her baby in the basket – as the Bible describes it in *Exodus* 2.3.[37]

This action confirms that the river would be flowing from right to left: placed on the water, Moses' casket would have floated downstream. But since the woman standing naked in the water is turned towards her right as she lifts up Moses, in this reconstruction the casket would have floated all the way past her before she reached out to it. This dynamic is implausible. There is no doubt that this woman should be identified with Pharaoh's daughter, who picks up and holds the naked baby Moses on her hip. Behind her are three maidservants holding ceremonial objects for the purpose of ablutions: a pitcher, two fluted metal bowls, and a casket, possibly of ivory.[38] In the scene, Pharaoh's daughter's nakedness is therefore exclusively displayed for the eyes of the women who surround her. Coming from the front, the viewer intrudes into an intimate moment of bathing, likely with ritual connotations, albeit in a public place, the river. The intrusion is justified because this moment coincides with Moses' rescue from the Nile. As described, the story of Moses would then unfold towards the left.

Again to the left of the central group of maidens, another two women are standing on the far shore.[39] These women are Miriam, who was in charge of watching the baby as it lay in the reeds, and Moses' mother Jochebed, who is named only at

36 Albright 1954, 229, nr 21 for Shiphrah. Puah is a Canaanite name.
37 Weitzmann and Kessler 1990, 28–29; Kraeling 1956, 173–174.
38 Weitzmann and Kessler 1990, 30; Kraeling 1956, 175 with drawing of these objects, Figures 47–50.
39 Weitzmann and Kessler 1990, 31–32; Kraeling 1956, 177.

Exodus 6.20, where she is described as the aunt of her husband Amram; both are from the house of Levi, as specified by *Exodus* 2.1.[40] In their expressive gestures, Moses' dramatic story is condensed. Miriam talks Pharaoh's daughter into handing her baby Moses, asking permission for him to be nursed by one of the Hebrew women. Her ruse reunites Moses with his mother Jochebed and saves him from death.

Despite scholarly consensus in favour of this interpretation, this reading from right to left does violence to the visual presentation of this panel. The movement of the bodies strongly suggests the opposite progression. Moreover, the need to create a split between a foreground and background in order to explain the court scene to the right is unconvincing. It divides what appears to be a unitary scene with a group of three women. The woman bowing in *proskynesis* is currently interpreted as consigning baby Moses to the current flowing downstream, but, as we have seen, this dynamic does not make sense of the pose of Moses' rescuer. She is rather best understood as an integral part of the imperial audience, bowing to the king. She only needs to be subtracted from the scene to force it into matching the *Exodus* passage (*Ex* 1.15–22), where only the two midwives are supposed to be present. Moreover, the dress of the two standing women presumed to be midwives precisely matches that of Miriam and Jochebed as depicted on the far left of the panel, strongly suggesting their identity. Intriguingly, a Talmudic interpretation names the midwives Miriam and Jochebed, ignoring the biblical names, but perhaps responding to this precise visualization of the scene.[41] The presence of Miriam and Jochebed casts doubt over the identification of the court scene with Pharaoh's orders to the midwives.

A progression from the court scene to the Nile episode, right to left, diminishes the prominence of the key scene, Moses' rescue, and with it the role of the women involved in it. Diluting the identity of the nine women across a range of different characters that includes the midwives also takes the focus away from the principal actors: Miriam, Jochebed, and Pharaoh's daughter. On the other hand, it is not possible to accept the identification of the women in the court scene with Jochebed and Miriam and at the same time consider them as the midwives of the biblical narrative.[42] This kind of interpretative violence to the images in order for them to comply with the biblical narrative sequence and details has been severely criticized by Annabel Wharton.[43] Supplementary midrashic sources have been identified for many scenes,[44] as in the case of the initiative by Pharaoh's daughter to go to the rescue of the baby herself rather than send her handmaid, as specified in *Exodus* 2.5.[45]

---

40 On Levite endogamy, see Tervanotko 2015.
41 *Talmud Sotah* 11b. https://halakhah.com/sotah/index.html. Accessed 28 May 2022.
42 Weitzmann and Kessler 1990, 27.
43 Wharton 1994.
44 Laderman 1997.
45 *Targum Onkelos* to *Ex.* 2.5: "And the daughter of Pharaoh came down to wash at the river, and her damsels walked on the river's bank; and she saw the ark in the flood, and reached out her arm and took it." Hebrew text at https://www.sefaria.org/texts/Tanakh/Targum/Onkelos. Accessed 27 June

It may not be enough, however, to bring in midrash as a source for the images in the Dura synagogue. Considering the court scene, there may be another occasion on which the relatives of Moses, and not the midwives, are having an audience with Pharaoh. I would like to suggest that the source underlying this panel is to be found in the rewriting of the book of *Exodus* in Ezekiel the Tragedian's *Exagoge* (Ezek.).[46] Connecting the scene with the dramatic *mise-en-scène* of the biblical narrative changes the entire approach to these paintings, further foregrounding women as main protagonists.

Dramatic Women in Ezekiel the Tragedian's *Exagoge*

Ezekiel the Tragedian's work, the *Exagoge*, is understood as a dramatic rewriting of the book of *Exodus*. Little is known about the author, and his dating is uncertain. The extant text, moreover, survives in a fragmentary state.[47] However, the episode of Moses' rescue is preserved. Ezekiel's theatrical version shares with the Targumin the prominent role given to the Egyptian princess (Ezek. vv. 19–31, ed. Lanfranchi 2006). It is she who picks up the baby, realizing that he is a Hebrew by birth. This moment, depicted at the centre of the fresco, dramatizes the recognition by showing the baby's genitals frontally. It would seem probable, then, that one should interpret the princess' understanding about the baby's origin as coming from her realization that he was circumcised.[48] Miriam is placed near the riverbank and mediates the transfer of the baby into the arms of his real mother, after a verbal exchange with the princess which concludes with the princess' gesture of hasty despatch (her right arm stretched out). Both the placing of Miriam close to the riverbank (Ezek. v. 18) and the mother's embracing of her baby (Ezek. v. 27) are details added by Ezekiel.[49] The image of the baby is repeated to mark a development in the narrative, a visual device also found in the widow of Sarepta's panel.

Strictly speaking, the horizontal curtain above the scene brackets the sequence of the discovery by the bathing princess, followed by the delivery of Moses back to his biological mother via Miriam, together with only one of the princess' servants. This servant holds both pitcher and bowl, one in each hand. It is possible that these washing instruments signal the naming of Moses by the princess at the time of his rescue, a detail anticipated by Ezekiel in the river scene, which underscores the etymology of the name.[50] To the right of the princess, two maidservants fall between curtain hangings: the one to the left holds a casket, while that to the right is dressed identically to the servant under the canopy and holds the same golden

---

2022; cited by Weitzmann and Kessler 1990, 29 (after Kraeling); Kraeling 1956, 176–177 and nn. 680–681.

46 Van der Horst (1987, 21, n. 21) is perhaps the first to note a similarity between Dura and Ezekiel, though he does not develop it.

47 Lanfranchi 2006 and 2003.

48 *Contra* Lanfranchi 2006, 137.

49 As noted by Lanfranchi 2006, 136–137.

50 Lanfranchi 2006, 138.

bowl to her chest. Although the biblical text speaks of three maids, this may not be reflected in the image. In Ezekiel's version, Pharaoh's daughter is accompanied by her "favourite slaves" (*havrais*, Ezek. v. 19; trans. Lanfranchi 2006, 113) without their number being specified. The dative plural may even be used as a dual.

The detail of the floating ark on the fresco, in the shape of a temple sarcophagus, has attracted a good deal of attention. It is a miniature of Noah's Ark. In addition, its shape resembles early Christian reliquaries or first-century Jewish ossuaries, the functions of which overlapped.[51] I suggest that the word used by Ezekiel, *kosmos*, which has much puzzled critics,[52] is clarified in the fresco's representation of Moses' basket as an ark, itself the image of the cosmos. Jochebed's chosen vessel is not the practical watertight basket described by the Bible. Her interpretation of what she needs to provide for the baby's safety encompasses a symbolic dimension: it is an ark, a tabernacle, which alone can be the sign of a positive outcome for her son. This awareness has passed through Miriam's prescience of Moses' future.

Miriam's pivotal role in the rescue reflects her prescience of the fate of Moses, imparted to her in a dream.[53] Although a sister, Miriam takes on a motherly role in protecting her brother and at the same time in preparing their parents for the unusual fate of their special child.[54] As in Ezekiel, Moses' father Amram has no role to play.[55] This is a women's world, where women's emotions motivate action and ultimately determine the survival and well-being of this child despite all odds.[56] While the nakedness of Pharaoh's daughter (who was bathing) visually contrasts with the long flowing garments of the Hebrew women on the shore, her heathen breasts react to the baby's presence in the same compassionate way as the baby's own mother. Thus, if exposure of the flesh marks the princess as non-Jew,[57] this is hardly the only function of the depiction. Rather, her naked breasts powerfully underline how salvation comes through women's bodies.

Ezekiel the Tragedian's work was modelled on Euripides, whose heroines take centre stage.[58] Seen through the eyes of the dramatist, the women who populate this scene are not accessory presences, but the very fulcrum of the story. Although not entirely different from the biblical account of *Exodus*, nevertheless the nuances of Ezekiel's poetry highlight women's roles as mothers and prophetesses, thus clarifying the biblical designation of Miriam as a divine seer. Ezekiel, and not *Exodus*, explicitly names Miriam in this episode.[59] Although Miriam is not herself

---

51 Kazan 2015, especially 83, n. 36; O'Connor 2013.
52 Lanfranchi 2006, 136–137.
53 Tervanotko 2013.
54 Tervanotko 2013, 162. Cf. the case of Perpetua and her own protective role for her brother Dinokrates (see Chapter 1 in this volume).
55 Lanfranchi 2006, 135 and n. 54.
56 The similarly different dynamics of maternal and paternal agency in the healing of children in miracle stories are explored in Chapter 10 of this volume.
57 Moon 1992, 598: "the use of nudity in the synagogue panels must surely have been intentionally iconographic."
58 Bryant Davies 2008, 406–407 (with thanks to Ted Kaizer for this precious reference); Powell 1990.
59 Lanfranchi 2006, 136.

described in the Bible as a mother, she is here the pivot of a mother-baby story that plays between the concepts of birth mother and adoptive parent.[60] By performing an exceptional role as "sister," she impacts the fate of her people in a major way, being herself chosen as leader of the Hebrew women at the time of the flight from Pharaoh.

Women's Educational Role

A reconsideration of the court scene to the right, bracketed by two overhanging curtains, in the light of Ezekiel's drama provides an alternative to the interpretation based on the description of midwives in *Exodus*. Following on from the rescue scene, Ezekiel develops the narrative of the introduction of Moses at the court of Pharaoh (Ezek. vv. 32–38). Among the various versions designating how old Moses was when he was given back to his adoptive mother, under whose protection alone he would be allowed to flourish, Ezekiel chooses a midpoint: Moses was a "νήπιος," which, as Lanfranchi explains, "peut designer un enfant jusqu'à la puberté."[61] I propose identifying the young man standing to the right of Pharaoh as Moses, gesturing goodbye to his sister and mother, who have just presented him at court. Between the Jewish women, it is Pharaoh's daughter who – her head uncovered as in the bathing scene, her hair flowing – implores her father to forgive her weakness. Presumably, she is acknowledging the baby as her own rather than confessing the fact that she let a Hebrew male child live. The presence of Miriam and Jochebed, purely as mediators and thus temporary caretakers of the infant, is thus explained. Yet their presence is also a reminder not only of the miraculous rescue that happened exclusively through their providential scheme but also of the education that Moses had so far received at home. Again, it is Ezekiel who attributes the function of teaching Moses the customs of the Hebrews exclusively to Moses' mother.[62] It is through her that Moses learnt about his own rescue from the Nile, about the history of the patriarchs and about the "gifts" of God.[63] Young Moses is standing to the right of Pharaoh, at once bidding farewell to his carers and proclaiming the blessings he received from them. To the left of Pharaoh stands a scribe, wax tablet and stylus in hand: he will impart a different knowledge to the adopted child of Pharaoh's daughter, but will not remove his initial imprint.

With this final scene, Moses takes his place at the court of Pharaoh, a development much more significant than the midwives' actions preceding his rescue story. There, he will continue to be educated and assume his Egyptian identity alongside that of his Jewish origins. This kind of discourse is essential to the message of the synagogue's walls: Moses' *paideia* "sums up Ezekiel's dual commitment to the

---

60 Reinhartz 1998, 109–110. I owe this reference to Rebecca Grose.
61 Lanfranchi 2006, 139.
62 Lanfranchi 2006, 139.
63 Horbury 1986.

Jewish people and to Greek culture,"[64] a feature that is perfectly suited to the multicultural atmosphere at Dura. Lanfranchi points out that Ezekiel is the first source to mention Moses' royal education, a detail that would be used again by Philo and in the *Acts of the Apostles* (*Acts*) (7.22).[65] The role of women in imparting religious education is picked up in the *Pastoral Epistles*, where Lois and Eunice, Timothy's grandmother and mother, are inserted in the narrative (perhaps as a pseudepigraphical element) to bring out women's contribution to a line of cultural transmission besides the biological one.[66]

The Widow of Sarepta as Prophetic Single Mother

Like Pharaoh's daughter,[67] but unlike Miriam and Jochebed, the widow of Sarepta (or Zarephath) is one of the unnamed women of the Bible.[68] Her Scriptural invisibility contrasts with her prominent presence on the panel to the left of the Torah niche at Dura, on the same register as Moses' Nilotic scene (see Figure 8.2). Even though the prophet Elijah is placed at the centre of this panel, it is the widow who moves forward the narrative. She performs the main actions that bookend the male prophet at centre stage: on the left, she mourns her dead son and forcefully presents him to Elijah for healing; on the right, she receives her healed son in triumph and gives praise to God. The colours of her garments underscore this dramatic change. At first, she is dressed in black with the neckline of her tunic pushed down so as to expose her breasts. After the prophet has resurrected the baby, the brightness of her yellow clothes marks her change of mood from mourning to joy. Not unlike the way Pharaoh's daughter held Moses rescued from the river, the widow of Sarepta proudly poses with her healed child sitting upright on her hip. An image of her baby is thus repeated three times, at each stage of the scene, just as baby Moses is repeatedly represented in the Nile scene.

Commentators have variously appreciated the narrative dynamic of this panel. Kraeling praised the panel's display of "artistic stenography" devised in order to "save space,"[69] while Weitzmann and Kessler lamented the inability of this panel to mirror details of the biblical narrative effectively, as these were sacrificed to aesthetic principles in order to achieve a balanced composition.[70] All readings premise the written biblical text as foundational in the making of the image. However bound we are to that point of reference for understanding these paintings, we need not limit ourselves to matching the images to the biblical text. As we have seen in the case of the Nile scene, a dramatic performance may underlie the depiction. Its essential components structure this composition as a *tableau vivant* in three still

64 Lanfranchi 2006, 140, quoting Barclay 1996, 138.
65 Lanfranchi 2006, 140.
66 Zamfir 2020, 186–187 and n. 14.
67 Reinhartz 1998, 126, 180–181.
68 Reinhartz 1998, 22, 113, 93.
69 Kraeling 1956, 389.
70 Weitzmann and Kessler 1990, 108.

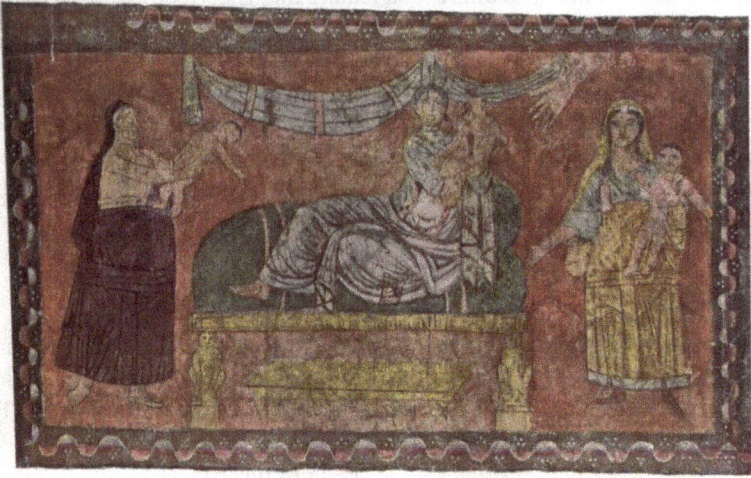

Figure 8.2 The widow of Sarepta begs Elijah to revive her lifeless child (left); Elijah prays to God in his room to effect the healing of the child (centre); the widow rejoices at her son's return to life (right). Fresco on the West Wall of the synagogue at Dura-Europos, ca. AD 240. Wikimedia Commons.

poses. These moments are specifically chosen to evoke in the mind of the viewer the speeches uttered by these characters, rather than to demonstrate the practical dynamics of the actions unfolding.[71]

The words spoken by the widow are revealing of her prophetic role. Her task is to draw attention to the perilous predicament of mortals and to model trust in the "man of God" ("ἄνθρωπος θεοῦ" – as quoted below in 1 *Kg* (3 *Kg*) 17.18, 17.24) who had come to visit her house. After the resuscitation of her son, she affirms Elijah's status as a true prophet (1 *Kg* (3 *Kg*) 17.24: "ῥῆμα κυρίου ἐν στόματι σου ἀληθινόν"), at the same time showing proof of his miracle to the audience. A graffito scratched on the painting's surface summarizes effectively how her message was received by visitors to the synagogue, even foreign ones: "Praise to the gods, praise! Since life, life eternally has been given." Steven Fine calls this writing an "assertively performative" theological inscription.[72]

The widow of Sarepta is a figure of contradiction, as her appearance in the Gospel of Luke brings out (*Luke* 4.24–26). She is a non-Jew to whom Elijah, one of the greatest Jewish prophets, turned for safety. The indignation her mention causes to Jesus' audience at Nazareth, as narrated in the pericope of Luke, may not be simply due to geographical or ethnic preoccupations. Her relationship with Elijah, who decides to live together with the widow and her child following God's order, remains somewhat ambiguous. Above all, her previous life is ominously foreshadowed in

71 Crostini forthcoming.
72 Fine 2011, 311–312.

her rebuke to the prophet during the dramatic moments of her son's death, when she retorts, "What have I to do with you, O man of God? Have you come to me to bring my sin to remembrance, and to kill my son?" (1 *Kg* (3 *Kg*) 17.18: "Τί ἐμοὶ καὶ σοί, ἄνθρωπε τοῦ θεοῦ; εἰσῆλθες πρός με τοῦ ἀναμνῆσαι τὰς ἀδικίας μου καὶ θανατῶσαι τὸν υἱόν μου;"). The Sareptian is here keeping her distance from the man she has welcomed under duress, a miracle worker whose moral high ground risks shaming her humble state and crushing her life. This child's life was the only consolation for her "sin." The phrase is unlikely to connote the sexual act itself. Rather, it may indicate that the boy had been born of a passing, unsanctioned union that had quickly left her a "widow," that is, a single mother. The fact that the widow is poor and has just one child (in this version of the story) would seem to confirm this possibility.

Rewriting the Widow of Sarepta's Story

Redactional changes to the widow of Sarepta's story as applied to Elisha in 2 *Kings* (4 *Kingdoms*) Chapter 4 confirm the discomfort with the original version. In the reprise, now featuring Elijah's disciple Elisha as protagonist, all potential ambiguities are dispelled. The two original episodes, the welcome of Elijah by the Sareptian resulting in the miracle of the multiplication of food, and the miracle of her son's healing, become two consecutive but distinct narratives, each concerning a different unnamed woman: a widow (2 *Kg* (4 *Kg*) 4.1–7) and the Shunammite woman (2 *Kg* (4 *Kg*) 4.8–37).

The changes ensure that neither could be (mis)construed as single or be suspected of having sexual relations with the prophet. The woman who welcomes Elisha to her house specifies that she is a widow because of her husband's recent death (2 *Kg* (4 *Kg*) 4.1), thus giving ample credentials of a regular marital union. She receives Elisha's multiplication miracle as charity for her poverty, as a woman deprived of the income a husband brings to the household. She represents all widows in this respect, as worthy objects of the community's charity, initiating the paradigm of the "poor widow" developed in the New Testament (*Mark* 12.41–44; *Luke* 21.1–4).

On the other hand, the Shunammite woman, a wealthy but infertile matron, has a husband who is an (almost) integral part of the story. The Shunammite decides, with her husband's consent, to make a place for Elisha in her house (2 *Kg* (4 *Kg*) 4.9–10). Elisha rewards her hospitality by promising that she will beget a son within the year (2 *Kg* (4 *Kg*) 4.16). The miraculous nature of this conception is guaranteed by the vigilant presence of the prophet's servant, Gehazi: unlike Elijah and the Sareptian, the Shunammite may visit the prophet's upper room, but she is never alone with him. Hers is certainly not the offspring of sin, but God's miracle, even though "her husband is old" (2 *Kg* (4 *Kg*) 4.14: "ὁ ἀνὴρ αὐτῆς πρεσβύτης"). At the key moment of the boy's illness, the husband is out in the fields and confidently passes the care of the boy to his wife. It is she who bears the entire burden of anxiety and shows deep faith in the prophet Elisha. The initiative to fetch the holy man is entirely the woman's. Nonetheless, the boy's father gives permission for the journey and provides the donkey, all the while being kept blissfully oblivious of the drama of his son's death. Even more remarkably, he does not re-enter the scene at its happy conclusion. When his task as guarantor of the woman's virtue is completed, he is no longer part of the action.

The care taken in 2 *Kings* to divide the original episodes at Sarepta between two different women, and to highlight the presence, or the cause of absence, of their respective husbands, reveals an anxiety about normalizing the situation. Manless women are a threatening presence, their morality is perceived as tenuous. Yet Jesus, in *Luke* 4, chooses to mention the more controversial of these stories. Only the "widow" of Sarepta acts completely on her own. Yet, her namelessness may be intentional in pointing to her situation as paradigmatic of a larger group. Being known by the toponym of her city, she acts as a representative for an entire geographical area, the coastal region of Syria Phoenicia. Confirmation of women's integration into the ecclesial structure in areas along the Mediterranean coast has been secured by recent finds at Azotos Paralios.[73] This excavation may reflect the testimony of the *Acts of the Apostles* 8.40, recording the activity of the apostle Philip, who "had four virgin daughters (*parthenoi*) who prophesied" (*Acts* 21.9: "τούτῳ δὲ ἦσαν θυγατέρες τέσσαρες παρθένοι προφητεύουσαι").

But while *Luke* 4 clearly refers to Jesus' preference for Sareptian-type women, other parts of his Gospel tone down women's independence, as for example in the episode rewriting the resurrection of the widow of Sarepta's son (*Luke* 7.11–17). Jesus enters Nain as Elijah had once entered Sarepta, but the scene is choral here, and the meeting is only fortuitous: Jesus stumbles across a funeral procession, accompanied by a large crowd, where the dead person is the only son of a mother, herself a widow. The mother's distress moves Jesus to pity, but she does not have a role to play in her son's restoration to life. It is Jesus who takes the initiative for the miracle and gives the child back to his mother. As a result of this resurrection, the crowd recognizes and proclaims Jesus a prophet.[74]

In Luke's reading, agency has totally passed to the male. Jesus' designation as prophet parallels the deeds of Elijah, while the widow of Nain is but a pale shadow of her predecessor from Sarepta. Even though the Sareptian's tale needed to be "purified," in Elisha's case, too, the female remained the protagonist of her offspring's salvation. While the prophets may act as healers, it is the mothers' foresight that is operative in obtaining the restoration of the miracle of life. The widow of Sarepta's explicit motherly role is paradigmatic in upholding and amplifying the model of Isaiah's nameless prophetess (*Is* 1.8). In contrast to other biblical prophetesses, whose children are not mentioned, her resurrected child, whatever his origin, is at once the sign and the proof of her prophetic activity as purveyor of salvation.

Real-Life Durene Women: Legal Status and Childbirth

In contrast to the subordinate place of women in society that was the norm in certain quarters, places, and times, women's agency and parity are consistent with the Macedonian Hellenistic ideal.[75] This ideal was continued or, more probably,

---

73 Bäbler and Fantalkin 2023, 107, 112-117; David 2021.
74 Brooke 2009, 43.
75 Carney 2000.

was consciously revived by the women of the Severan dynasty, who hailed from Syria.[76] These female rulers claimed power through their children, having sidelined their husbands or acted after their husbands' death, and were atypically involved in the military at provincial locations.[77] From the area of the Temple of Artemis at Dura comes an inscription commemorating Julia Domna (ca. AD 160–217) as mother of the assembly and of the holy troops: "The council of the Aurelian Antonine Europeans to Julia Domna Augusta mother of the assembly and of the sacred troops" ("Ἰουλίαν Δόμναν | Αὐγοῦσταν τὴν μητέρα | συγκλήτου καὶ τῶν | ἱερῶν στρατευμάτων | Αὐρηλ. Ἀντωνιανῶν Εὐρωπαίων ἡ βουλή").[78] While the extension of Roman citizenship to the inhabitants of Dura through the Antonine Constitution (11 July AD 212) and the elevation of the town to the status of Roman colony are discussed in scholarship with reference to the male emperors of the Severan dynasty, the role of Julia, of Syrian birth, should also be taken into account. A gypsum statue of Julia may have belonged together with the inscription.[79]

Another gypsum statue, of a veiled woman, was discovered in the stepped room of the Temple of Artemis. Cumont likens her to Roman personifications of Pudicitia, while considering her the portrait of a benefactress.[80] Her attire recalls the long robes of the Hebrew women as depicted in the synagogue.[81] By contrast, Pharaoh's daughter's nudity (see Figure 8.1) has been compared with the shapely female body of a plaster relief of Aphrodite, a type that was found in several places onsite, including the stepped room of Artemis' temple.[82] Aphrodite's relief is understood as marking the entrance to the town's brothel.[83] However, such stereotypical associations cannot be true of all the other 20 or so similar images found in both domestic and cultic contexts at Dura.[84] Downey suggests that "the Venus of the plaques was the tutelary divinity of a guild of entertainers and prostitutes," thus accounting for its proliferation in multiple settings.[85] Baird notes how the type of the naked woman, without a label, may have served multiple identifications.[86] This observation is certainly borne out by the similarity with the synagogue's fresco. These multivalent images possessed a universal communicative capacity that was the essence of their usefulness. It makes sense to envisage a large presence of women's licentious sexual establishments in a town populated in large proportion by military troops.[87]

---

76 Melone 2015; Rowan 2011.
77 Boatwright 2021, 248–249.
78 My translation; see Leriche 1999, nn. 21 and 28; Rowell 1930.
79 Baird 2018, 196, n. 169.
80 Cumont 1926, 205–206 and pl. 73, 79.
81 Baird 2018, 196, n. 168.
82 Baird 2018, Figure 6.9; Moon 1992, 596; Cumont 1926, 206–207 and pl. 80–81.
83 Baird 2018, caption to Figure 6.9; see Miles 2006.
84 Baird 2018, 146.
85 Moon 1992, 596; Downey 1977, 162–164.
86 Baird 2018, 146.
87 On the substantial and pervasive presence of troops in the city in Roman times, see James 2019. On prostitution, see Strong 2016.

At the same time, precisely this situation necessitated special protection for these women, who were as likely, if not more likely, to undergo pregnancies than married matrons. The choice of representing the goddess Venus, albeit in seated pose, on the reverse of the gold aureus of Septimius Severus, with Julia Domna's bust on the obverse, sheds a different light on the role of this deity, inscribed as "VENUS GENETRIX."[88] Thus, the childbearing properties of female bodies, whose breasts constitute the essential nourishment of the newborn, are here celebrated and advertised. This ambivalence needs to be kept in mind when evaluating the role of women at Dura. The X-shaped straps across Aphrodite's chest on the gypsum relief, which has attracted speculation about its symbolism from archaeologists, may well have been an ancient nursing bra rather than a tempting item of lingerie.[89]

Written papyrus records about women in the region of Dura demonstrate that they acted with an unusual measure of legal freedom, often receiving in their own hands assets to perform their duties as carers to their children. Although provincial citizens, they could invoke the *ius trium liberorum* – the right of three children – by which a woman gained the right to run her own business without the tutelage of a male relative.[90] Besides these documents, other tangible traces of Durene women are found in inscriptions of special stepped *odeon*-shaped rooms, the *salles à gradins*, dated to the first and second centuries AD. The function of these rooms within cultic precincts dedicated to the goddesses Artemis, Atargatis, and Azzanathkona is not absolutely clear.[91] The triad of "A" names could indicate three aspects of the Greek goddess Artemis, with the third name alluding specifically to a local deity.[92] Since Artemis was patroness of childbirth, a connection between these temple rooms and birthing practices can be postulated. In these inscriptions on the steps, the dedicatees, often fathers to their daughters or husbands to their wives, are concerned with good wishes for unborn heirs and celebrate genealogical lines.[93] The interpretation offered by Rostovtzeff and endorsed by Klaver, that these seats are similar to inscribed pews in modern churches, fails to explain these particular features.[94] It is more likely that the seats' dedications commemorated safe deliveries within notable families.

Moreover, even the shape of the rooms suggests that they could have had a practical use as birthing places. The *Augustan History* (*Hist. Aug.*) declares that Alexander Severus was born in a sacred precinct:

> He was given the name Alexander because he was born in a temple dedicated
> to Alexander the Great in the city of Arca [Akkar, Lebanon], whither his

---

88 Mattingly 1950, 28, nr 55. https://www.metmuseum.org/art/collection/search/246886. Accessed 25 May 2022; Rowan 2011, 250, Figure 1 for the proportion of different designs; Boatwright 2021, 144, n. 106 (stressing the fecundity value of coins with nudes), 166, Table 4.2.

89 Downey 1977, 164; the straps were sometimes chains.

90 Boatwright 2021, 24; Sommer 2016, 64–65.

91 Baird 2018, 104–105 and Figure 5.10.

92 Klaver 2019, 45–46.

93 Klaver 2019, 37–38.

94 Klaver 2019, 40, citing Rostovtzeff 1932, 179.

father and mother had chanced to go on the feast-day of Alexander for the purpose of attending the sacred festival.

Alexandri nomen accepit quod in templo dicato apud Arcenam urbem Alexandro Magno natus esset, cum casu illuc die festo Alexandri cum uxore pater isset sollemnitatis implendae causa, cui rei argumentum est quod eadem die natalem habet hic Mamaeae. (*Hist. Aug.* 18.3.1–2, ed. and trans. Magie 1924, 187)

While the unplanned birth of Alexander is meant to be full of ominous resonances, its concrete setting in a temple should not be overlooked. The mysterious Durene stepped rooms, in the shape of an amphitheatre (recalling 16th c. AD dissecting theatres), could have provided suitable spaces within sacred precincts, thus "in a temple." One can imagine a situation analogous to Alexander's birth taking place at Dura, where feasts were celebrated regularly, as attested in a military calendar known as the *Feriale Duranum*, which includes a celebration of Alexander's birthday in its list of feasts.[95]

Three lists of names without any honorific titles scratched on the wall of the Artemis *odeon* may well be a spontaneous record of such births.[96] Female personnel would have fulfilled both a cultic and a practical purpose in assisting with this delicate moment in a woman's life, giving birth,[97] when she most needed the goddess' protection. While scholarship has so far ignored women's contributions because of the simultaneous presence of male names and male cultic personnel,[98] with few exceptions,[99] observations about the prominence of women as mothers in the synagogue frescoes should embolden research on the active role of women in this town and allow their presence and activities to be reflected in the interpretation of the architectural evidence.

Conclusions

The independent women-with-child who articulate the negotiation of life and survival on the West Wall of the Dura synagogue find an appropriate setting in the general context and environment of Dura as a Roman colony. The infancy of Moses is a story of salvation negotiated around the instincts of preservation and care that mothers have, whether biological or acquired. This aspect is emphasized in Ezekiel's tragic rewriting and in the dramatic painting of the long panel at Dura. In the case of the "widow" of Sarepta, her interaction with the prophet Elijah portrays her as the woman in charge of the house. She is the one who leads the exchange, pilots the action, and proclaims its consequences, showing throughout her emotional involvement as mother in the fate of her child. Openness and interaction, the

95 Welles et al. 1959, 195–201.
96 Leriche 1999, 730.
97 Tsoucalas et al. 2014; French 1987.
98 Yon 2016; Leriche 1999.
99 Klaver 2019.

breaking of norms and entrenched customs, are women's doings. Unsurmountable cultural barriers break down in the name of life and children. Ezekiel's title, the *Exagoge*,[100] equally marks this outward movement that is fitting for the multicultural environment of the city of Dura.

Through these examples, childbirth, once a private, dangerous, and even jealously guarded endogamous event, became a door to the other, a way to initiate interaction, and a proof of communal solidarity and of intercultural initiative. As generations passed, integration was a natural process. Adopting the other's babies was a motherly first step, with long-ranging consequences.

The performative space of the synagogue mirrors the streets of Dura, exuding the same air of Hellenistic openness. The likely presence of associations of female entertainers and prostitutes in town enhanced the pastoral need for a concern about women's well-being and foregrounded childbirth as a redeeming, liberating opportunity. Moreover, this situation generated the need for charitable birthing institutions, the operations of which underpinned the values of maternity and life expressed in strong religious and cultic terms. Their premises were therefore probably connected to temple precincts. The importance of metaphors of erotic love in the *S of S* and the recurring role of prostitutes in Jewish stories make sense against this background.[101] The fame of Babylon as whore is probably also hanging in the balance of Dura's identity in this respect. Yet there is another aspect to the single-mother prophetesses at Dura when acknowledged as background to the developing Christian figure of Mary as a single, husbandless prophetess.[102] The comparison may help clarify aspects of her cult, such as the obsessive affirmation of her virginity and the limited success of her breastfeeding image.

References

Texts: Editions and Translations
Horst, P.W. van der. ed. 1987. *Joods-hellenistische Poëzie: De fragmenten der gedichten van Ezechiël Tragicus, Philo Epicus, Theodotus en de varvalste dichtercitaten*. Kok: Kampen.
Lanfranchi, P. ed. and trans. 2006. *L'Exagoge d'Ezéchiel le Tragique*. Leiden: Brill.
Magie, D. ed. and trans. 1924. *Historia Augusta*, vol. 2: *Caracalla. Geta. Opellius Macrinus. Diadumenianus. Elagabalus. Severus Alexander. The Two Maximini. The Three Gordians. Maximus and Balbinus*. Loeb Classical Library 140. Cambridge, MA: Harvard University Press.

Secondary Works

Ackerman, S. 1998. "Isaiah," in C.A. Newson, and S.H. Ringe (eds) *Women's Bible Commentary*. Louisville: Westminster John Knox Press, 161–168.
Albright, W.F. 1954. "Northwest-Semitic Names in a List of Egyptian Slaves from the Eighteenth Century B.C.," *Journal of the American Oriental Society* 74 (4): 222–233.

---

100 Lanfranchi (2006, 7) shows that Aristoboulos and Philo also called *Exodus* "Exagoge."
101 Hezser 2017.
102 Clayton Croy and Connor 2011.

Baird, J. 2018. *Dura-Europos*. London: Bloomsbury.

Barclay, J.M.G. 1996. *Jews in the Mediterranean Diaspora: From Alexander to Trajan (323 BCE–117 CE)*. Edinburgh: Clark.

Boatwright, M.T. 2021. *The Imperial Women of Rome: Power, Gender, Context*. Oxford: Oxford University Press.

Brooke, G.J. 2009. "Prophets and Prophecy in the Qumran Scrolls and the New Testament," in R.A. Clements, and D.R. Schwartz (eds) *Text, Thought, and Practice in Qumran and Early Christianity*. Leiden: Brill, 31–48.

Bryant Davies, R. 2008. "Reading Ezekiel's *Exagoge*: Tragedy, Sacrificial Ritual, and the Midrashic Tradition," *Greek, Roman, and Byzantine Studies* 48: 393–415.

Bäbler, B., and A. Fantalkin. 2023. "Azotos Paralios (Ashdod-Yam, Israel) during the Periods of Roman and Byzantine Domination: Literary Sources vs. Archaeological Evidence," in C. Horn, and B. Bäbler (eds) *Word and Space. Interacting in Palestine in Late Antiquity: Towards a History of Pluridimensionality.* Chesterfield, MI: Abelian Academic, 89–120.

Carney, E. 2000. "The Initiation of Cult for Royal Macedonian Women," *Classical Philology* 95 (1): 21–43.

Carr, D. 2000. "Gender and the Shaping of Desire in the Song of Songs and Its Interpretation," *Journal of Biblical Literature* 119 (2): 233–248.

Clayton Croy, N., and A.E. Connor. 2011. "Mantic Mary? The Virgin Mother as Prophet in Luke 1:26–56 and the Early Church," *Journal for the Study of the New Testament* 34 (3): 254–276.

Crostini, B. forthcoming. "Performing the Bible at Dura: A Panel of Elijah and the Widow of Sarepta as *tableau vivant*," in N. Tsironi (ed.) *Performance in Late Antiquity and Byzantium*. Princeton: Center for Hellenic Studies.

Cumont, F. 1926. *Fouilles de Doura-Europos (1922–1923)*. Paris: Geuthner.

David, A. 2021. "Byzantine Basilica with Graves of Female Ministers and Baffling Mass Burials Found in Israel," *Haaretz*, November 15. https://www.haaretz.com/archaeology/2021-11-15/ty-article-magazine/byzantine-basilica-with-female-ministers-and-baffling-burials-found-in-israel/0000017f-e722-dc7e-adff-f7af11070000

Downey, S. 1977. *The Stone and Plaster Sculpture: Excavations at Dura-Europos*. Los Angeles: University of California-Los Angeles Press.

Fine, S. 2011. "Jewish Identity at the *Limus*: The Earliest Reception of the Dura Europos Synagogue Paintings," in E.S. Gruen (ed.) *Cultural Identity in the Ancient Mediterranean*. Los Angeles: Getty Research Institute, 303–320.

French, V. 1987. "Midwives and Maternity Care in the Greco-Roman World," in M. Skinner (ed.) *Rescuing Creusa: New Methodological Approaches to Women in Antiquity*. Lubbock: Texas Tech University Press, 69–84.

Hamori, E.J. 2013. "Childless Female Diviners in the Bible and Beyond," in J. Stökl, and C.L. Carvalho (eds) *Prophets Male and Female: Gender and Prophecy in the Hebrew Bible, the Eastern Mediterranean, and the Ancient Near East*. Atlanta: Society of Biblical Literature, 169–192.

Hezser, C. 2017. "Prostitution in Early Judaism," in C. Hezser (ed.) *Oxford Encyclopedias of the Bible*. Oxford Biblical Studies Online. https://www.oxfordreference.com/display/10.1093/acref/9780197669402.001.0001/acref-9780197669402-e-26.

Horbury, W. 1986. "Ezekiel Tragicus 106: δωρήματα," *Vetus Testamentum* 36: 37–51.

Iavazzo, C.R., C. Trompoukis, I.I. Siempos, and M.E. Falagas. 2009. "The Breast: From Ancient Greek Myths to Hippocrates and Galen," *Reproductive BioMedicine Online* 19 (2): 51–54.

James, S. 2019. *The Roman Military Base at Dura-Europos, Syria: An Archaeological Visualisation*. Oxford: Oxford University Press.

Kazan, G. 2015. "Arks of Constantinople, the New Jerusalem: The Origins of the Byzantine Sarcophagus Reliquary," *Byzantion* 85: 77–125.

Klaver, S. 2019. *Women in Roman Syria: The Cases of Dura-Europos, Palmyra, and Seleucia on the Euphrates*. Amsterdam: University of Amsterdam.

Kraeling, C.H. 1956. *The Excavations at Dura-Europos Conducted by Yale University and the French Academy of Inscriptions and Letters: Final Report VIII, Part I: The Synagogue*. New Haven, CT: Yale University Press.

Laderman, S. 1997. "A New Look at the Second Register of the West Wall of Dura Europos," *Cahiers archéologiques* 45: 5–18.

Lanfranchi, P. 2003. "L'*Exagogè* d'Ezéchiel: Du texte biblique au texte théâtral," *Perspectives: Revue de l'Université Hébraïque de Jérusalem* 10: 15–32.

Lehtipuu, O. 2017. "To Remarry or Not to Remarry? 1 Timothy 5:14 in Early Christian Ascetic Discourse," *Studia Theologica* 71 (1): 29–50.

Leriche, P. 1999. "Salle à gradins du temple d'Artémis à Doura-Europos," *Topoi* 9 (2): 719–739.

Maier, H.O. 2021. "The Entrepreneurial Widows of 1 Timothy," in J.E. Taylor, and I.L.E. Ramelli (eds) *Patterns of Women's Leadership in Early Christianity*. Oxford: Oxford University Press, 59–73.

Mattingly, H. 1950. *Coins of the Roman Empire in the British Museum*, vol. 5: *Pertinax to Elagabalus*. London: Trustees of the British Museum.

Melone, C. 2015. "Pushing the Limit: An Analysis of the Women of the Severan Dynasty." *Honors Projects* 5. http://digitalcommons.iwu.edu/grs_honproj/5. Accessed 15 May 2022.

Mesnil du Buisson, R. du. 1939. *Les peintures de la synagogue de Doura-Europos, 245–256 après J.-C.* Rome: Pontificio Istituto Biblico.

Miles, M.R. 2006. *Carnal Knowing: Female Nakedness and Religious Meaning in the Christian West*. Eugene, OR: Wipf & Stock.

Moon, W.G. 1992. "Nudity and Narrative: Observations on the Frescoes from the Dura Synagogue," *Journal of the American Academy of Religion* 60 (1): 587–658.

Nissinen, M. 2013. "Gender and Prophetic Agency in the Ancient Near East and in Greece," in J. Stökl and C.L. Carvalho (eds) *Prophets Male and Female: Gender and Prophecy in the Hebrew Bible, the Eastern Mediterranean, and the Ancient Near East*. Atlanta: Society of Biblical Literature, 27–58.

O'Connor, A. 2013. "An Early Christian Reliquary in the Shape of a Sarcophagus in the University of Wisconsin-Milwaukee Art Collection." PhD diss. *Theses and Dissertations* 300. https://dc.uwm.edu/etd/300.

O'Reilly, A. 2019. "Matricentric Feminism: A Feminism for Mothers," *Journal of the Motherhood Initiative* 10 (1/2): 13–26.

Powell, A. ed. 1990. *Euripides, Women and Sexuality*. London: Routledge.

Reinhartz, A. 1998. *Why Ask My Name? Anonymity and Identity in Biblical Narrative*. Oxford: Oxford University Press.

Rostovtzeff, M.I. 1932. *Caravan Cities*. Oxford: Clarendon Press.

Rowan, C. 2011. "The Public Image of the Severan Women," *Papers of the British School at Rome* 79: 241–273.

Rowell, H.T. 1930. "Inscriptions grecques de Doura-Europos 1929–1930," *Comptes rendus des séances de l'Académie des inscriptions et belles-lettres* 74 (3): 265–274.

Schellenberg, A. 2016. "The Sensuality of the Song of Songs," in A. Schellenberg, and L. Schwienhorst-Schönberger (eds) *Interpreting the Song of Songs: Literal or Allegorical?* Biblical Tools and Studies 26. Leuven: Peeters, 103–129.

———. 2018. "'May Her Breasts Satisfy You at All Times' (Prov 5:19): On the Erotic Passages in Proverbs and Sirach and the Question of How They Relate to the Song of Songs," *Vetus Testamentum* 68: 252–271.

Sommer, M. 2016. "Acculturation, Hybridity, Créolité: Mapping Cultural Diversity in Dura-Europos," in T. Kaizer (ed.) *Religion, Society and Culture at Dura-Europos*. Cambridge: Cambridge University Press, 57–67.

Steinberg, F. 2006. "Women and the Dura-Europos Synagogue Paintings," *Religion and the Arts* 10 (4): 461–496.

Strong, A.K. 2016. *Prostitutes and Matrons in the Roman World*. New York: Cambridge University Press.

Tervanotko, H. 2013. "Speaking in Dreams: the Figure of Miriam and Prophecy," in J. Stökl, and C.L. Carvalho (eds) *Prophets Male and Female: Gender and Prophecy in the Hebrew Bible, the Eastern Mediterranean, and the Ancient Near East*. Atlanta: Society of Biblical Literature, 147–168.

———. 2015. "Members of Levite Family and Ideal Marriages in Aramaic Levi Document, Visions of Amram, and Jubilees," *Revue de Qumrân* 27 (2): 155–176.

Tsoucalas, G., M. Karamanou, and M. Sgantzos. 2014. "Midwifery in Ancient Greece, Midwife or Gynaecologist-Obstetrician?" *Journal of Obstetrics and Gynaecology* 34 (6): 547.

Weitzmann, K., and H.L. Kessler. 1990. *The Frescoes of the Dura Synagogue and Christian Art*. Washington, DC: Dumbarton Oaks.

Welles, C.B., R.O. Fink, and J.F. Gilliam. 1959. *The Excavations at Dura-Europos Conducted by Yale University and the French Academy of Inscriptions and Letters: Final Report V, Part I: The Parchments and Papyri*. New Haven: Yale University Press.

Wharton, A.J. 1994. "Good and Bad Images from the Synagogue of Dura Europos: Contexts, Subtexts, Intertexts," *Art History* 17 (1): 1–25.

Williamson, H.G.M. 2010. "Prophetesses in the Hebrew Bible," in J. Day (ed.) *Prophets and Prophecy: Proceedings of the Oxford Old Testament Seminar*. London: T&T Clark, 65–80.

Xeravits, G.G. 2017a. "Goddesses in the Synagogue?" *Journal for the Study of Judaism in the Persian, Hellenistic, and Roman Period* 48 (2): 266–276.

———. 2017b. "The Message of the West Wall of the Dura Synagogue," *Zeitschrift der Deutschen Morgenländischen Gesellschaft* 167 (1): 111–125.

Yon, J.-B. 2016. "Women and the Religious Life of Dura-Europos," in T. Kaizer (ed.) *Religion, Society and Culture at Dura-Europos*. Cambridge: Cambridge University Press, 99–113.

Zamfir, K. 2020. "Reading Motherhood in the Pastoral Epistles in the Light of Ancient Discourses on Mothers and Maternity," in U.E. Eisen, and H.E. Mader (eds) *Talking God in Society: Multidisciplinary (Re)constructions of Ancient (Con)texts. Festschrift Peter Lampe*, vol. 2: *Hermeneuein in Global Contexts: Past and Present*. Göttingen: Vandenhoeck & Ruprecht, 185–202.

9 Roman Charity

Nonnos of Panopolis, Support for Parents, and Questions of Gender

Tim Parkin

Introduction

> I had before dinner repeated a ridiculous story told me by an old man who had been a passenger with me in the stage-coach to-day. Mrs. Thrale, having taken occasion to allude to it in talking to me, called it "The story told you by the old *woman*." – "Now, Madam, (said I,) give me leave to catch you in the fact; it was not an old *woman*, but an old *man*, whom I mentioned as having told me this." (Boswell 1791, 2.188–189)

The story of Pero and Cimon, a father in captivity breastfed by his daughter, was a relatively popular one in antiquity (as the walls of Pompeii for one attest, as we shall see) with a long reception history, but it had until very recent times become forgotten. Most recently, however, the theme has become the focus of considerable renewed interest, especially among scholars both of Renaissance art history and of gender studies. Its popularity is perhaps also signposted by the fact that at a conference on motherhood and breastfeeding taking place at the University of Cyprus in 2021, three papers, by Sarah Shread, Sarah Beckmann, and me, all discussed aspects of the topic in antiquity. My own focus here is primarily on the textual evidence and on a single element – seemingly trivial – which, to be honest, has intermittently obsessed me for the past two decades, namely that the breastfed parent in the episode, Teiresias-like, appears to change gender.[1]

I begin, chronologically, late in antiquity, with the longest epic from antiquity, the over 20,000-line, 48-book epic by Nonnos of Panopolis, the *Dionysiaka* (*Dion.*). Dating almost certainly to the fifth century AD, the lengthy poem, in Homeric Greek and dactylic hexameters, has become not only much more accessible but also much better appreciated thanks to the 19 Budé volumes (1976–2006), edited by a team led

---

1 This chapter takes up a question I first discussed in Parkin 2003; I remain both entranced and mystified by the topic. The best modern discussion of the ancient tale of Pero and Cimon/Micon remains, in my opinion, that by Deonna 1956 and 1954, even if I am not fully persuaded of the idea that the breastfeeding here is symbolic of rejuvenation or transition to the next life (see also Köllner 1997). On the theme of *caritas Romana* note also Mulder 2017 and Knauer 1964.

DOI: 10.4324/9781003265658-12

by Francis Vian, and it has thus become the focus of much recent scholarship.[2] Its primary subject is the tale of Dionysos' triumphant campaign in India. In the course of that campaign, there feature a lot of breasts and a great deal of milk in Nonnos' work, as a search for the appropriate terms in the excellent lexicon by Werner Peek makes evident, and as Ron Newbold eloquently illustrated over two decades ago in his article "Breasts and Milk in Nonnus' *Dionysiaca*" (one of some 22 articles Newbold, based at the University of Adelaide in Australia, wrote over a period of 36 years).[3] Indeed, in many ways it is fitting that milk features widely in Nonnos, given the rivalry milk might have with wine as a thirst-quencher in antiquity – wine of course being the inevitable focus of so much of the Dionysiac work and milk having no one to champion it in quite the same way.

One episode, however, has been all but overlooked in the recent scholarship on Nonnos.[4] Yet it is a perfect illustration of the way that Nonnos draws on so many Hellenistic literary predecessors, particularly the Alexandrian authors.[5] I refer to the tale of Tektaphos (Τέκταφος), the Indian leader of the Bolinges. Tektaphos, we are told, would have previously perished in incarceration, if it had not been for his daughter Eerie (Ἠερίη), who saved her father's life with her breastmilk (*Dion.* 26.101–142). The story is introduced as part of Nonnos' narration – reminiscent of Homer's catalogue of the Trojan forces in *Iliad* Book 2 – of the build-up of the Indian forces under King Deriades. They are amassing to face Dionysos in battle (Zeus has ordered Dionysos to punish the Indians for their impious behaviour, as well as to civilize them, teaching them the properties of wine among other rites), a battle, of course, that Dionysos will ultimately win.[6]

Nonnos' description of the father breastfed in captivity by his daughter is the longest literary depiction from antiquity (and in fact the only one extant in Greek) of what is not an uncommon folk motif in various cultures.[7] "Far-shooter Tektaphos" ("Τέκταφος ... ἐκηβόλος," *Dion.* 26.101, ed. Vian 1990)[8] is introduced to the reader as one of the Indian leaders amassing his troops to support the Indian king Deriades in his upcoming campaign against Dionysos. We are immediately given more information about Tektaphos, namely that "once he had been saved

2 Scholarship is steadily growing, since the important collection of essays edited by Hopkinson (1994), still perhaps the best place to start. Nonnos can now boast his own handbook: Accorinti 2016. Further bibliography may also be found online at https://sites.google.com/site/hellenisticbibliography/empire/nonnus (accessed 17 September 2022), along with the three volumes in the series entitled *Nonnus of Panopolis in Context* (Doroszewski and Jażdżewska 2020; Bannert and Kröll 2017; Spanoudakis 2014).
3 Newbold 2000; cf. already Winkler 1974. In his 2016 paper, Newbold strikingly notes (p. 197), "Nonnus' exuberant fantasy projects a multi-nippled cosmos, where breasts and imbibers of breastmilk abound and where unexpected forms of suckling and nurturance occur."
4 Note, however, Mainoldi 1997.
5 On which general topic, see especially Hollis 1994; Chuvin 1991.
6 For the *Indiad*, see especially Vian 1994.
7 See e.g. Thompson 1955–1958, R 81, with H 807 and T 215.2. See also the rich entry on "Säugen" in the *Enzyklopädie des Marchens*, by Kawan 2004.
8 Translations of quoted *Dion.* passages are mine, as adapted from Rouse 1940.

from fate by sucking with starving lips the milk from a daughter's breast – she devised this trick to nourish her father" ("ὅς ποτε κούρης | χείλεσι πειναλέοισιν ἀλεξητήρια πότμου | πατροκόμου δολόεντος ἀμέλγετο χεύματα μαζοῦ," *Dion.* 26.101–103). Nonnos then describes in considerable detail the desperate physical straits to which the father had been reduced at the hands of Deriades (for reasons unknown): "parched, with crumbling skin, a living corpse" ("Τέκταφος, αὐαλέος ψαφαρῷ χροΐ, νεκρὸς ἐχέφρων," *Dion.* 26.104), Deriades has had him bound and imprisoned, filthy and starving, in a dark and mouldy pit. He is scarcely alive: "ugly whiffs came from his dry flesh as if he were a corpse" ("οἷα δὲ νεκροῦ | ἐκ χροὸς ἀζαλέοιο δυσώδεες ἔπνεον αὖραι," *Dion.* 26.115–116).

Enter the daughter, who addresses the guards (*Dion.* 26.121–134), assuring them that she brings nothing but her tears – they may search her if they so desire! – and urging them to allow her to die with her father. Thus, daughter is reunited with father in the pit and brings him back to life not with her tears but with her own milk.[9] Deriades is mightily impressed by this act of *pietas* (*Dion.* 26.138–139: "Ἡρίης δὲ θεουδέος ἔργον ἀκούων | Δηριάδης θάμβησε") – it is only now we learn her name. The father is set free, and the daughter's courage is celebrated throughout the land: "the Indian people praised the girl's breast which had saved a life by its cunning" ("στρατὸς Ἰνδῶν | μαζὸν ἀλεξικάκοιο δολοπλόκον ἤνεσε νύμφης," *Dion.* 26.141–142).

But ultimately the tale does not end happily: subsequently, in a scene as detailed as the breastfeeding episode (*Dion.* 30.127–186), Tektaphos is slain in battle by Eurymedon; Nonnos remarks that he could not escape his fate a second time, and no daughter's trick came to the rescue now. Tektaphos laments that his daughter can offer no help, no life-giving drink (*Dion.* 30.153), and the daughter herself, watching his dying agonies from the city wall, laments that she cannot save him this time; the father who had become her son in prison (*Dion.* 30.167) cannot now be saved by her breast or her milk, and she prays to be slain alongside her father.

Whether Nonnos created the tale himself or found a version of it in one of his literary sources, perhaps the *Bassarika* of a certain Dionysios,[10] we cannot say (as I have already mentioned, Nonnos' version is the only one that comes down to us in Greek), but what is clear, as I shall seek to elucidate here, is the tradition that Nonnos drew on from the classical world: the story of the daughter nourishing her parent in prison has both Hellenistic and Roman roots, many features of which (though not the happy ending) are drawn upon by Nonnos – not just the breast-feeding but also the prison, the guards, and the celebration of the deed – and all of which would go on beyond Nonnos to be immortalized in myriad works of art during the Renaissance, and especially in the Baroque period, such as Caravaggio's *Seven Works of Mercy* (ca. AD 1607, to be found in Pio Monte della Misericordia in Naples) and Rubens' several depictions entitled *Roman Charity* or *Cimon and*

9   It is strange that John Winkler (1974, 109) classifies her as a virgin.
10 See Vian 1994, 92–93; Chuvin 1991, 301.

Pero.[11] In almost all such depictions, before and after Nonnos, the parent is the father, but it is not always so, as we shall see.

The earliest traceable written account of the tale dates to the late first century BC or early first century AD, preserved in Festus' second-century AD *On the Meaning of Words*, an epitome of the *On the Significance of Words* of Verrius Flaccus, himself an antiquarian scholar in the employ of Augustus. It is brief:

> They say that a temple to *Pietas* was consecrated by Acilius at the spot where once upon a time there lived a woman whose father was shut up in prison. This woman secretly fed her father with her own breasts. Because of this deed he was granted impunity.
>
> Pietati aedem consecratam ab Acilio aiunt eo loco quo quondam mulier habitaverit, quae patrem suum inclusum carcere mammis suis clam aluerit: ob hoc factum, impunitas ei concessa est. (Festus, *On the Meaning of Words* 228, ed. Lindsay 1913)[12]

There is little detail here, but basic features stand out: we have the nameless father and daughter, the prison (though no guards), and the happy ending, including not just the release of the father but also the founding of a temple to that most Roman of virtues, *Pietas*.

Chronologically speaking, our next extant account comes from Valerius Maximus:

> Forgive me, most ancient hearth, give me your pardon, eternal fire, if the scheme of my work advance from your most sacred temple to a place in the city more necessary than splendid. For by no harshness of Fortune, no squalor, is the prize of dear *pietas* cheapened; on the contrary, the more unhappy in the trial, the more certain. A praetor had handed over a woman of free birth, found guilty at his tribunal of a capital crime, to the triumvir to be executed in prison. Received there, the head warder had pity on her and did not strangle her immediately. He even allowed her daughter to visit her, but only after she had been thoroughly searched to make sure she was not bringing in any food; for the warder expected that the prisoner would die of starvation. But after a number of days had passed, he asked himself what could be sustaining her so long. Watching the daughter more closely, he noticed her putting out her breast and relieving her mother's hunger with the succour of her own milk. This novel and remarkable spectacle was reported by him to the triumvir, by the triumvir to the praetor, and by the praetor to the board of judges. As a result, the woman's sentence was remitted. Whither does *Pietas* not penetrate, what does she not devise? In prison she found a new way to

---

11 On the later history of the theme, see the classic work by Steensberg 1976, and now especially Sperling 2016.

12 The translations of texts, unless otherwise indicated, are my own.

save a mother. For what is so extraordinary, so unheard of, as for a mother to be nourished by her daughter's breasts? This might be thought to be against nature, if to love parents were not nature's first law.

Ignoscite, vetustissimi foci, veniamque aeterni date ignes, si a vestro sacratissimo templo ad necessarium magis quam speciosum urbis locum contextus operis nostri progressus fuerit: nulla enim acerbitate Fortunae, nullis sordibus pretium carae pietatis evilescit; quin etiam eo certius quo miserius experimentum habet. Sanguinis ingenui mulierem praetor apud tribunal suum capitali crimine damnatam triumviro in carcere necandam tradidit. quo receptam is qui custodiae praeerat, misericordia motus, non protinus strangulavit: aditum quoque ad eam filiae, sed diligenter excussae, ne quid cibi inferret, dedit, existimans futurum ut inedia consumeretur. cum autem plures iam dies intercederent, secum ipse quaerens quidnam esset quo tam diu sustentaretur, curiosius observata filia animadvertit illam exerto ubere famem matris lactis sui subsidio lenientem. quae tam admirabilis spectaculi novitas ab ipso ad triumvirum, a triumviro ad praetorem, a praetore ad consilium iudicum perlata, remissionem poenae mulieri impetravit. quo non penetrat aut quid non excogitat Pietas, quae in carcere servandae genetricis novam rationem invenit? quid enim tam inusitatum, quid tam inauditum quam matrem uberibus natae alitam? putarit aliquis hoc contra rerum naturam factum, nisi diligere parentes prima Naturae lex esset. (Val. Max. *Memorable Doings and Sayings* 5.4.7, ed. and trans. Shackleton Bailey 2000, 498–501)

Once again, we have the prison, this time with a guard, and the release of the prisoner. Yet, other features are different: the nameless parent is described only as freeborn, the nameless daughter visits and breastfeeds the parent a number of times, not just once; there is no mention of a temple being set up, but instead a general moral lesson is expressed regarding how natural *pietas* is (as compared to a daughter breastfeeding a parent). And, of course, the father has become the mother.

Pliny the Elder, later in the first century AD, provides further details but is clearly following the same tradition[13]:

Of *pietas* there have, it is true, been unlimited examples all over the world, but one at Rome with which the whole of the rest could not compare. A plebeian woman of low position and therefore unknown, who had just given birth to a child, had permission to visit her mother who had been shut up in prison to be punished, and was always searched in advance by the doorkeeper to prevent her carrying in any food; she was caught feeding her mother with her own breasts. In consequence of this marvel the daughter's *pietas* was rewarded by the mother's release and both were awarded maintenance for life; and the place where it occurred was consecrated to the goddess concerned, a temple dedicated to *Pietas* being built on the site of the prison, where the Theatre

---

13 Cf. Beagon 2005, 314; Pavón 1997.

of Marcellus now stands, in the consulship of C. [*sic*, for Titus] Quinctius [Flamininus] and Manius Acilius [Balbus] [150 BC].

Pietatis exempla infinita quidem toto orbe extitere, sed Romae unum, cui comparari cuncta non possint. humilis in plebe et ideo ignobilis puerpera, supplicii causa carcere inclusa matre cum impetrasset aditum, a ianitore semper excussa ante, ne quid inferret cibi, deprehensa est uberibus suis alens eam. quo miraculo matris salus donata pietati est, ambaeque perpetuis alimentis, et locus ille eidem consecratus deae, C. Quinctio M'. Acilio cos. templo Pietatis extructo in illius carceris sede, ubi nunc Marcelli theatrum est. (Pliny the Elder, *Natural History* (*NH*) 7.36.121, ed. Rackham 1942; trans. with modifications Rackham 1942, 587)

We learn that the mother and daughter are lowly plebeians; there is again the mention of a guard and of the searching of the daughter, as well as of the visit happening on more than one occasion; the mother is released, both mother and daughter are rewarded (a new feature), and a temple to *Pietas* is later built on the site. Pliny has the wrong date because he (or a later copyist) has the wrong Acilius. The temple, in the Forum Holitorium, was in fact vowed in 191 BC by Manius Acilius Glabrio, one of the consuls of that year, on the eve of the Battle of Thermopylae against Antiochos, and while the construction was begun by him, the temple was dedicated by his son, also called Manius Acilius Glabrio, as duovir in 181 BC. In the temple, there was a gilded equestrian statue of his father. The temple was destroyed (or perhaps relocated?) in 44 BC by Julius Caesar, in order to build a theatre, later named the Theatre of Marcellus.[14]

In his *Collection of Memorable Matters* (*Coll. Rerum Mem.*), Solinus, probably writing in the third or early fourth century AD, follows Pliny very closely, as so often, but not in every detail. The parent and daughter are of humble origins, there are guards who search the daughter and there are repeated visits, the parent is released, and the site is thenceforth honoured as sacred to *Pietas*. But the mother has become the father again:

Of *pietas* evidence shone out quite nobly, it is true, in the house of the Metelli, but the most outstanding example is to be found in a plebeian woman who had just given birth to a child. This woman, of humble origin and therefore quite unknown, with difficulty gained entry to visit her father, who was being held in prison to be punished. She was regularly searched by the doormen in case she was trying to smuggle in some food to her parent. She was caught feeding her father with her own breasts. This act made both the place and the deed sacred. For the man who had been sentenced to death was handed over

---

14 Livy 40.34.5–6, ed. Yardley 2018; Val. Max. 2.5.1; Cassius Dio 43.49.2–3, ed. Cary 1916. It is worth remarking that in Paulus' epitome of Festus (105L), it is recorded that there was also in the Forum Holitorium a column (*lactaria columna*) to which infants were taken to be given milk; cf. Mulder 2017, 238–239.

to his daughter and his salvation became a memorial to the great event. The spot was dedicated to its *numen*, and a shrine to *Pietas* was set up there.

> pietatis documentum nobilius quidem in Metellorum domo effulsit, sed eminentissimum in plebeia puerpera reperitur. humilis haec atque ideo famae obscurioris cum ad patrem, qui supplicii causa claustris poenalibus continebatur, aegre obtinuisset ingressum, exquisita saepius a ianitoribus ne forte parenti cibum administraret, alere cum uberibus suis deprehensa est: quae res et locum et factum consecravit: nam qui morti destinabatur, donatus filiae in memoriam tanti praeconii reservatus est: locus dicatus suo numini Pietatis sacellum est. (Solin. *Coll. Rerum Mem.* 1.124–125, ed. Mommsen 1895)

The gender difference from the first-century version is all the more striking when one considers how closely Solinus has otherwise followed Pliny, not just in the other details but also in the very language used (examples highlighted here in bold):

Pliny the Elder, *Natural History* 7.36.121:	Solinus, *Collection of Memorable Matters* 1.124–125:
pietatis exempla infinita quidem toto orbe extitere, **sed** Romae unum, cui comparari cuncta non possint. **humilis in plebe et ideo ignobilis puerpera, supplicii causa** carcere inclusa matre cum **impetrasset aditum, a ianitore semper excussa** ante, **ne** quid inferret **cibi, deprehensa est uberibus suis alens eam.** quo miraculo matris salus **donata** pietati est, ambaeque perpetuis alimentis, et locus ille eidem **consecratus** deae, C. Quinctio M'. Acilio cos. templo Pietatis extructo in illius carceris sede, ubi nunc Marcelli theatrum est.	**pietatis** documentum nobilius quidem in Metellorum domo effulsit, **sed** eminentissimum in **plebeia puerpera** reperitur. **humilis haec atque ideo famae obscurioris** cum ad patrem, qui **supplicii causa** claustris poenalibus continebatur, aegre **obtinuisset ingressum, exquisita saepius a ianitoribus ne** forte parenti **cibum** administraret, **alere cum uberibus suis deprehensa est**: quae res et locum et factum **consecravit**: nam qui morti destinabatur, **donatus** filiae in memoriam tanti praeconii reservatus est: locus dicatus suo numini Pietatis sacellum est.

The gender shifting of the adult nursling in the story is fascinating and intriguing. In fact, of course, the father dominates most versions of the story and of the folk tale motif throughout history; the mother makes few appearances.

My focus in this chapter is on literary accounts, but at this point, the iconographic evidence is also worthy of mention. From the Bay of Naples, we have several instances – two identical statuettes and two (plus two now lost) wall paintings – of a father and daughter; from Southern Gaul, fragments of *terra sigillata*, also to be dated to the first century AD, which likewise depict the father and daughter.[15] In

---

15 Wall paintings (see also following item): Pompeii, casa IX, 2, 5, triclinium C, now in the Museo Nazionale Archeologico de Napoli, inv. 115398; Pompeii, casa VII, 4, 10, now lost; and from Pompeii or Herculaneum, Museo Nazionale Archeologico de Napoli, inv. 9040, now lost, but a drawing survives (*LIMC* 7.1.738, Pero II a 2–3, in fact the same item). Terracotta figurines from casa VI,

one particular Pompeian wall painting, in the house of Marcus Lucretius Fronto, the couple is also named – Pero and Micon – and a poetic text accompanies[16]:

> The nourishment which a mother was preparing for her small children was turned into sustenance for her father by cruel fortune. This creation merits eternity; see, the old man's veins in his wizened neck now [swell?] with milk, and at the same time, with … countenance, Pero herself massages [? reading *fricat*] Micon; sad modesty together with *pietas* is present here.
>
> > quae parvis mater natis alimenta parabat,
> >> fortuna in patrios vertit iniqua cibos.
> > aevo dignum opus est: tenui cervice seniles
> >> as[pice, ia]m venae lacte …
> > …]q(ue) simul voltu fri<c>at ipsa Miconem
> >> Pero; tristis inest cum pietate pudor (Pompeii, casa V, 4, 2 and 11; *CIL* 4.6635 = *CLE* 2048)

As in the other accounts, the decrepitude of the aged father is emphasized. What is novel here, of course, is that we have the couple named, with very Greek names at that.[17] Here from Pompeii, we are seeing a version of the tale based on a Greek tradition – a tradition also preserved, in fact, by Valerius Maximus, alongside the Roman version which we quoted above. Here is Valerius Maximus' account of the Greek version, with the same protagonists as at Pompeii (although variants of the names have survived on manuscripts):

> Let the same be considered as predicated concerning the piety of Pero, whose father Cimon/Mycon was in a like sorry plight and equally under prison guard. A man in extreme old age, she put him like a baby to her breast and fed him. People's eyes are riveted in amazement when they see the painting of this act and renew the features of the long bygone incident in astonishment at the spectacle now before them, believing that in those silent outlines of limbs they see living and breathing bodies. This must happen to the mind also, admonished to remember things long past as though they were recent by painting, which is considerably more effective than literary memorials.
>
> Idem praedicatum de pietate Perus existimetur, quae patrem suum Cimona [AL; Mycona Muncker] consimili fortuna adfectum parique custodiae traditum, iam ultimae senectutis velut infantem pectori suo admotum aluit. haerent ac stupent hominum oculi, cum huius facti pictam imaginem vident, casusque antiqui condicionem praesentis spectaculi admiratione renovant, in illis mutis membrorum liniamentis viva ac spirantia corpora intueri

---

13, 19: Museo Nazionale Archeologico de Napoli, inv. 22580, 124846. *Terra sigillata*: Staatliche Museen zu Berlin, Bode-Museum, inv. 31737; cf. *LIMC* 7.1.328–329; Gricourt 1969; Renard 1955.

16 Cf. Valladares 2011; Köllner 1997, 72–73; Tontini 1997.

17 Chuvin 1991, 57, 301, 317–319.

credentes. quod necesse est animo quoque evenire, aliquanto efficaciore pictura litterarum <monumentis> [add. SB] vetera pro recentibus admonito [Lipsius: -tos AL] recordari. (Val. Max. 5.4.ext.1.; trans. with modifications Shackleton Bailey 2000, 500–503)

Aside from the names, Valerius Maximus here provides little detail of the scene (much less than in his description of the Roman version), except to make it clear that it is very much a visual depiction, such as that which survives from Pompeii, that he has in mind as he writes. And it is this Greek tradition that Nonnos clearly has also in mind, replacing names – but still very Greek names, despite the Indian context! – in his own version. The Greek version is also extant in the writings of Hyginus (also probably dating to the 1st c. AD), again with some name changes: "Xanthippe offered her own milk to her father Mycon, who was locked up in prison, as a means of sustenance" (*Xanthippe Myconi patri incluso carcere lacte suo alimentum vitae praestitit*, Hyg. *Fables* 254.3, ed. Marshall 2002).

That the parent was the father is also recorded much later than Nonnos, in a twelfth-century Greek manuscript account; it is the solution to the riddle: "How could my father, the husband of my mother, become my son and then my father again?" (cod. Paris. 2991A, *ad* Tzetzes, *Allegoriae Iliadis* 24.331, ed. Boissonade 1851). One thinks again of Nonnos' daughter calling her father her son. The riddle features widely in later centuries, often with the father named Cimon, the daughter nameless, and the *topos* also appears in other folktales (Irish, Spanish, and Jewish, for example), typically of a daughter feeding a father (sometimes a husband) through a crack in the prison wall.[18] Again, the beneficiary adult nursling is always male. The mother never reappears.

To sum up where our exploration has taken us: the Greek version of the tale presents us with a named father and daughter: Pero and an extremely old Cimon/ Mycon in Valerius Maximus, Pero and an aged Micon on the walls of Pompeii, Xanthippe and Mycon in Hyginus, Eerie and a very decrepit Tektaphos in Nonnos, and a nameless daughter and her aged father Cimon in subsequent riddles. On the Roman side, however, we have a nameless daughter and father in Verrius Flaccus (*apud* Festus), a nameless daughter and *ingenua* mother in Valerius Maximus, a *humilis plebeia* daughter and mother in Pliny the Elder, and a *humilis plebeia* daughter and father in Solinus. The Greek version emphasizes the age and decrepitude of the father, with the protagonists identified by name, whereas on the Roman side we see no names but more on the status of the protagonists. And, of course, the father briefly becomes the mother before reverting back, Teiresias-like, to being male.

So, what is going on regarding this metamorphosis in gender? Several people have suggested to me that it might be because Romans of the early principate underwent a sense of prudery, temporarily, at the thought of a father being suckled by his daughter. But we should hardly think of Romans of the time as prudish.[19]

18 See n. 7 above; cf. Bronzini 1999; Taylor 1948; Ohlert 1897.
19 Although note the perceptive comments of Seiringer 2011, 129–133.

A number of scholars have remarked on the transformation, and a few have also tried to account for it. Franz Kuntze in 1904 thought the explanation obvious: Romans did not like to see men of *virtus* in an inferior or degraded position; I do not find that idea persuasive, not least given the heroic *pietas* involved in all versions of the story. More recently, Richard Saller, quoting (in passing) the version of Valerius Maximus and Pliny with the mother, refers in a footnote to the gender shift in Festus' version with the father. The reference is mistakenly assumed to be to Glabrio's father, and the change of gender likewise wrongly justified as predicated on the need to account for the dedication of the temple.[20] Not at all: "patrem suum" in Festus (quoted above) refers to the woman, not to Acilius – otherwise it would be Acilius' breasts ("mammis suis") as well! Indeed, Lord Byron's friend Sir John Hobhouse (Lord Broughton), in his *Italy: Remarks Made in Several Visits from the Year 1816 to 1854*, briefly mentions the tale and the different versions and suggests "the change of sex was, perhaps, occasioned by some confusion of the father of Glabrio with the mother of the pious matron."[21]

I do not think there is any real confusion, but clearly something has happened in the intervening period, between Verrius Flaccus and Solinus. Perhaps in the early principate more direct reciprocity was seen as more pleasing: the mother had fed the daughter as a child, now the daughter feeds the mother. What we might also be seeing is something symptomatic of tensions within a patriarchal society concerned about gender roles in terms of the raising of infants – the sort of concerns one can see also in Favorinus' well-known chauvinistic diatribe about maternal breastfeeding in Aulus Gellius.[22] I still believe that the change of gender may also in part be explained by considering the debate that was going on at the time of the late Republic and the early Empire about the role of *cognati*. In the context of that debate, the question was raised, as I suggest, about the reciprocal duties owed by relatives in the maternal as well as in the paternal lines, and the degree to which *pietas* operates beyond agnatic lines or between individuals not affected by *patria potestas*.

Ulpian, in his work *On the Duties of a Consul*, written probably in AD 215, discusses specific circumstances where the consul or *iudex* may need to intervene to require a son to maintain a father: for example, a son may have an obligation towards his *pater familias*, but what if the son had been emancipated before the age of puberty? He is no longer under the paternal *potestas* and therefore, technically, under no obligation to his father. Ulpian states that in such a case a son may be compelled (by the *iudex*) to support his father, if the former is financially able and the latter is in need (*patrem inopem alere cogetur*, Justinian, *Digest* (*Dig.*) 25.3.5.13, ed. Mommsen 1870). The duty is seen again as a moral or natural one, rather than one strictly required by the letter of the law.

Ulpian then goes on to consider other situations. Since one was not legally under the *potestas* of one's ascendants on the maternal side (such as the *avus maternus*,

20 Saller 1994, 106–108.
21 Broughton 1859, 121–124.
22 Aulus Gellius, *Attic Nights* 12.1, ed. Marshall 1968. For Aulus Gellius, see also Chapter 5 in this volume.

but also one's mother), the question is raised as to whether *pietas* should extend to the maintenance of such older people as well as to those in the paternal line:[23]

> Must we support only our father, our paternal grandfather, paternal great-grandfather, and other relatives of the male sex, or are we compelled also to support our mother and other relatives in the maternal line?
>
> Utrum autem tantum patrem avumve paternum proavumve paterni avi patrem ceterosque virilis sexus parentes alere cogamur, an vero etiam matrem ceterosque parentes et per illum sexum contingentes cogamur alere, videndum. (*Dig.* 25.3.5.2)

Ulpian states that the *iudex* should also consider these relatives' physical and financial position:

> It is better to say that in each case the judge should intervene, so as to give relief to the necessities of some of them and the infirmity of others. Since this obligation is based on justice and affection between blood relations, the judge should balance the claims of each person involved. The same is true in the maintenance of children by their parents.
>
> et magis est, ut utrubique se iudex interponat, quorundam necessitatibus facilius succursurus, quorundam aegritudini: et cum ex aequitate haec res descendat caritateque sanguinis, singulorum desideria perpendere iudicem oportet. Idem in liberis quoque exhibendis a parentibus dicendum est. (*Dig.* 25.3.5.2–3)

Ulpian goes on to cite a rescript of Antoninus Pius regarding the link between grandchildren and maternal grandparents:[24] "The deified Pius also says that a maternal grandfather is compelled to support his grandchildren" (*Item Divus Pius significat, quasi avus quoque maternus alere compellatur, Dig.* 25.3.2.5).

In other words, despite the strict letter of the law regarding legal duties related to *patria potestas*, *pietas* should require care between cognates also. Of related legal interest at the time was the benefit grandchildren might bring to the grandfather in relation to the *ius liberorum*. By the letter of the law, only grandchildren by a son counted. Ulpian here is explicit that that rule holds, and he goes on to cite a related *oratio* of Marcus Aurelius.

Such questions are indicative not only of the significant issue of the role of cognates as opposed to agnates alone and the role of the family as opposed to the *familia*, but also, I think, of the tension between the force of law and the force of morals, the tension between civil law and natural law. Indeed, one declamatory exercise preserved by Seneca the Elder makes the point rather well, and it is with this that I would like to finish this chapter. When, in an exercise from the declamatory

---

23 Interestingly, there is no mention of female relatives on the paternal side.
24 Compare this with *Dig.* 25.3.8 (Marcellus) and Ulpian, *Frag. Vat.* 195, ed. Mommsen 1890.

school, two brothers die in the home of their father and stepmother, a maternal grandfather steps in and takes away the third brother, who is already ailing:

> A man lost two sons, who had a stepmother. The attendant symptoms suggested either indigestion or poison. The maternal grandfather snatched away the man's third son, who had not been allowed in to visit his ailing brothers. When the father started making enquiries through a crier, the grandfather said he was at his house. He is accused of violence.
>
> Quidam duos filios sub noverca amisit: dubia cruditatis et veneni signa insecuta sunt. Tertium filium eius maternus avus rapuit, qui ad visendos aegros non fuerat admissus. Quaerenti patri per praeconem dixit apud se esse. Accusatur de vi. (Sen. Elder, *Controversies* (*Controv.*) 9.5, preface, ed. Winterbottom 1974)

In the debate over this hypothetical situation (and I am fully aware that in Roman declamatory exercises we are not talking about Roman law per se), every kind of possibility and innuendo is considered, in particular the role of the stepmother in all this. However, it is *never* suggested that the grandfather, though described as a *violentus et inpotens senex* (*Controv.* 9.5.1), should mind his own business or should not have the welfare of a maternal grandson at heart. That, I think, is reflective of a wider reality in, and general attitude of, Roman society. Legal definitions of responsibility for support might be outweighed by feelings of, and moral obligations entailed by, *pietas*. With similar logic, Seneca goes on to report, sometimes a grandfather may chastise and punish a grandchild. The ties felt between a maternal grandfather and his grandchildren are a result of nature rather than of laws: "Certain rights are given to us not by law but by nature" (*quaedam iura non lege sed natura nobis attributa, Controv.* 9.5.7). One thinks again of the words of Valerius Maximus quoted above in regard to the Roman version of our tale, namely that to love parents is nature's first law.

Nor need it be assumed that a legal obligation held more force than a moral one or an unwritten law. The opposite could in fact be true, especially if a law is imposed to mend a breakdown in social sanctions. It is of course a literary and general *topos*, common to most (if not all) societies and periods of history, that people nowadays are so degenerate that they need laws to enforce what in the good old days human nature ensured. So, Sallust in his *War of Catiline* (*Cat.* 9.1, ed. Reynolds 1991) observes that in archaic Rome the city was marked by good morals, everyone was happy, and justice and goodness prevailed as a result not so much of laws as of nature (*non legibus magis quam natura*). In like fashion, Tacitus noted of the Germans: "among them good morals have more effect than good laws do elsewhere" (*plusque ibi boni mores valent quam alibi bonae leges, Germania* 19.2, ed. Köstermann 1970). On the other hand, it is also worth adding that, if we apply the realities of Roman law to this declamatory case, it is never suggested – though it would suit the defence's case – that this grandfather (not, of course, the *pater familias*) had an automatic right to take the grandson. The nuclear family and agnatic lines were the *primary* legal focus of obligations.

Conclusions

The care of older members of the Roman family was felt to lie naturally with one's children. The institution of *patria potestas* in theory meant that the *pater familias* could expect total and immediate support from his dependants for as long as he lived and continued to control the purse strings.[25] The position of other ageing relatives, such as the mother and the maternal grandparents, who did not carry such sway in legal terms but some of whom might well be expected to outlive the *pater familias*, is less straightforward, and the expectation that they would receive support rested on general feelings of *pietas*, at times enforced by the decision of a *iudex*. That a daughter should support a needy mother, as opposed to a father, may not have stood up so easily in a court of law, but it was seen as fitting to natural *pietas*.

It is the support of ageing kin by younger generations that I think underlies our tale of a parent nourished and saved by a daughter, and it is a story which, with a variety of features and names, has had a long history, one which Nonnos drew on and expanded. What is very remarkable to me remains the fact that over two millennia, until very recent times, the *topos* with its very long history in art and fable almost universally portrays a daughter with her father rather than with her mother. A few depictions of daughter and mother do survive,[26] but they are few and far between, aside from several striking literary *exempla* from Roman times, as we have seen here. Clearly the Romans, for their own reasons, saw fit to change the sex of the parent, albeit only for a limited time. I have made here a few suggestions about its significance and possible motivations. Ultimately, of course, it may be a trivial detail or a slip – but I doubt it.

References

Texts: Editions and Translations
Beagon, M. ed. and trans. 2005. *The Elder Pliny on the Human Animal: Natural History Book 7*. Oxford: Oxford University Press.
Boissonade, J.F. ed. 1851. *Tzetzae Allegoriae Iliadis*. Paris: Dumont.
Cary, E. ed. and trans. 1916. *Dio Cassius: Roman History*, vol. 4: *Books 41–45*. Loeb Classical Library 66. Cambridge, MA: Harvard University Press.
Köstermann, E. ed. 1970. *P. Cornelii Taciti libri qui supersunt*, vol. 2.2: *Germania*. Leipzig: Teubner.
Lindsay, W.L. ed. 1913. *Sexti Pompeii Festi De verborum significatu quae supersunt cum Pauli Epitome*. Leipzig: Teubner.

---

25 For the patriarchal structure and mindset of these societies, see also Chapters 1 and 2 in this volume.
26 A striking example is the printer's device employed by Sébastien Cramoisy in the seventeenth century (see Winger 1976, although he misidentifies the relevant scenes): with two storks – ancient symbols of *pietas* – central, in each corner are relevant scenes: *pius* Aeneas; Tobias curing his father's blindness; and a daughter breastfeeding in turn her father and her mother. Note also Sperling 2016, 41, and Bellhouse 1999, for discussion of Etienne-Barthélémy Garnier's (1759–1849) painting *Roman Charity*, where the aged parent is the mother.

Marshall, P.K. ed. 1968. *A. Gellii Noctes Atticae*. Oxford: Oxford University Press.
———. 2002. *Hyginus: Fabulae*. Leipzig: Saur.
Mommsen, T. ed. 1870. *Digesta Iustiniani Augusti*. Vol. 1. Berlin: Weidmann.
———. 1890. "Iuris Anteiustiniani fragmenta quae dicuntur Vaticana," in P. Krüger (ed.) *Collectio librorum Iuris Anteiustiniani in usum scholarum*. Berlin: Weidmann, 1–106.
———. 1895. *C. Iulii Solini Collectanea rerum memorabilium*. Berlin: Weidmann.
Rackham, H. ed. and trans. 1942. *Pliny: Natural History*, vol. 2: *Books 3–7*. Loeb Classical Library 352. Cambridge, MA: Harvard University Press.
Reynolds, L.D. ed. 1991. *C. Sallusti Crispi Catilina*. Oxford: Oxford University Press.
Rouse, W.H.D. ed. and trans. 1940. *Nonnos: Dionysiaca*, vol. 2: *Books 16–35*. Loeb Classical Library 354. Cambridge, MA: Harvard University Press.
Shackleton Bailey, D.R. ed. and trans. 2000. *Valerius Maximus: Memorable Doings and Sayings*, vol. 1: *Books 1–5*. Loeb Classical Library 492. Cambridge, MA: Harvard University Press.
Vian, F. ed. 1990. *Nonnos de Panopolis: Les Dionysiaques*, vol. 9: *Chants XXV–XXIX*. Paris: Les Belles Lettres.
Winterbottom, M. ed and trans. 1974. *Seneca the Elder: Declamations*, vol. 1: *Controversiae, Books 1–6*. Loeb Classical Library 463. Cambridge, MA: Harvard University Press.
Yardley, J.C. ed. and trans. 2018. *Livy: History of Rome*, vol. 11: *Books 38–40*. Loeb Classical Library 313. Cambridge, MA: Harvard University Press.

Secondary Works

Accorinti, D. ed. 2016. *Brill's Companion to Nonnus of Panopolis*. Leiden: Brill.
Bannert, H., and N. Kröll. 2017. *Nonnus of Panopolis in Context II: Poetry, Religion, and Society. Proceedings of the International Conference on Nonnus of Panopolis, 26th–29th September 2013, University of Vienna, Austria*. Mnemosyne Supplement 408. Leiden and Boston: Brill.
Bellhouse, M.L. 1999. "Crimes and Pardons: Bourgeois Justice, Gendered Virtue, and the Criminalized Other in Eighteenth-Century France," *Signs: Journal of Women in Culture and Society* 24: 959–1010.
Boswell, J. 1791. *The Life of Samuel Johnson LLD*. 2 vols. London: Henry Baldwin.
Bronzini, G.B. 1999. "La giglia che allatta il padre: Analisi morfologico-strutturale del motivo incestuoso nella letteratura popolare," *Lares* 65: 187–208.
Broughton, Lord, G.C.B. 1859. *Italy: Remarks Made in Several Visits from the Year 1816 to 1854*. 2 vols. London: Murray.
Chuvin, P. 1991. *Mythologie et géographie dionysiaques: Recherches sur l'oeuvre de Nonnos de Panopolis*. Clermont-Ferrand: Adosa.
Deonna, W. 1954. "La légende de Pero et de Micon et l'allaitement symbolique," *Latomus* 13: 140–166, 356–375.
———. 1956. "Les thèmes symboliques de la légende de Pero et de Micon," *Latomus* 15: 489–511.
Doroszewski, F., and K. Jażdżewska. 2020. *Nonnus of Panopolis in Context III: Old Questions and New Perspectives*. Mnemosyne Supplement 438. Leiden and Boston: Brill.
Gricourt, J. 1969. "La légende de Pero et de Micon sur un 'nouveau' vase de la Graufesenque: Examen de quelques poinçons associés," in J. Bibauw, and M. Renard (eds) *Hommages à Marcel Renard*. Vol. 3. Collection *Latomus* 103. Brussels: Latomus, 272–287.
Hollis, A. 1994. "Nonnus and Hellenistic Poetry," in Hopkinson 1994, 43–62.

242   *Tim Parkin*

Hopkinson, N. ed. 1994. *Studies in the Dionysiaca of Nonnus*. Cambridge: Cambridge Philological Society.

Kawan, C.S. 2004. "Säugen," in R.W. Brednich, H. Alzheimer, H. Bausinger, W. Brückner, D. Drascek, H. Gerndt, I. Köhler-Zülch, K. Roth, and H.-J. Uther (eds) *Enzyklopädie des Märchens: Handwörterbuch zur historischen und vergleichenden Erzählforschung*. Vol. 11. Berlin: De Gruyter, 1156–1163.

Knauer, E.R. 1964. "Caritas Romana," *Jahrbuch der Berliner Museen* 6: 9–23.

Köllner, L. 1997. *Die töchterliche Liebe: Ein Mysteriumgeheimnis. Die sogenannte Caritas Romana*. Frankfurt am Main: Peter Lang.

Kuntze, F. 1904. "Die legende von der guten Tochter in Wort und Bild," *Neue Jahrbücher für das klassische Altertum* 13: 280–300.

Mainoldi, C. 1997. "Eria e Tectafo nelle Dionisiache di Nonno," in Raffaelli, Danese, and Lanciotti 1997, 161–170.

Mulder, T. 2017. "Adult Breastfeeding in Ancient Rome," *Illinois Classical Studies* 42: 227–243.

Newbold, R.F. 2000. "Breasts and Milk in Nonnus' *Dionysiaca*," *Classical World* 94: 11–24.

———. 2016. "The Psychology in the *Dionysiaca*," in Accorinti 2016, 193–212.

Ohlert, K. 1897. "Zur antiken Räthseldichtung," *Philologus* 56: 612–615.

Parkin, T. 2003. "Honour Thy Father – and Thy Mother? An Act of *pietas*," in J. Davidson, and A. Pomeroy (eds) *Theatres of Action: Papers for Chris Dearden*. Prudentia Supplement. Auckland: Polygraphia, 194–210.

Pavón, P. 1997. "La *pietas* e il carcere del foro olitorio: Plinio, *NH*, VII, 121, 36," *Mélanges de l'École française de Rome, Antiquité* 109: 633–657.

Peek, W. 1968–1975. *Lexicon zu den Dionysiaka des Nonnos*. 4 Vols. Berlin: Akademie Verlag.

Raffaelli, R., R.M. Danese, and S. Lanciotti. eds. 1997. *Pietas e allattamento filiale: La vicenda, l'exemplum, l'iconografia. Colloquio di Urbino, 2–3 maggio 1996*. Urbino: QuattroVenti.

Renard, M. 1955. "La légende de Pero et de Micon sur les vases de la Graufesenque," *Latomus* 14: 285–289.

Saller, R.P. 1994. *Patriarchy, Property and Death*. Cambridge: Cambridge University Press.

Seiringer, I. 2011. "*Sedula me nutrix ducit* (Ov. *epist.* 21,95): Die Amme in der römischen Literatur – eine Mittlerin zwischen den Generationen und Geschlechtern?" in H. Brandt, A.M. Auer, J. Brehm, D. de Brasi, and L.K. Hörl (eds) *Genus & generatio: Rollenerwartungen und Rollenerfüllungen im Spannungsfeld der Geschlechter und Generationen in Antike und Mittelalter*. Bamberg: University of Bamberg Press, 119–136.

Spanoudakis, K. 2014. *Nonnus of Panopolis in Context I: Poetry and Cultural Milieu in Late Antiquity with a Section on Nonnus and the Modern World. Trends in Classics* Supplementary Volume 24. Berlin: De Gruyter.

Sperling, J.G. 2016. *Roman Charity: Queer Lactations in Early Modern Visual Culture*. Bielefeld: Transcript.

Steensberg, A. 1976. *Caritas Romana: The Concept of Culture*. Copenhagen: National Museum of Denmark.

Taylor, A. 1948. "Straparola's Riddle of Pero and Cimon and Its Parallels," *Romance Philology* 1: 297–303.

Thompson, S. 1955–1958. *Motif-Index of Folk-Literature: A Classification of Narrative Elements in Folk-Tales, Ballads, Myths, Fables, Mediaeval Romances, Exempla, Fabliaux, Jest-Books, and Local Legends*. Copenhagen: Rosenkilde and Bagger.

Tontini, A. 1997. "L'epigramma *CIL* IV 6635 (= *CLE* 2048)," in Raffaelli, Danese, and Lanciotti 1997, 141–160.

Valladares, H. 2011. "*Fallax imago*: Ovid's Narcissus and the Seduction of Mimesis in Roman Wall Painting," *Word and Image* 27: 378–395.

Vian, F. 1994. "Dionysus in the Indian War: A Contribution to a Study of the Structure of the *Dionysiaca*," in Hopkinson 1994, 86–98.

Winger, H.W. 1976. "The Cover Design," *The Library Quarterly: Information, Community, Policy* 46: 62–63.

Winkler, J.J. 1974. "In Pursuit of Nymphs: Comedy and Sex in Nonnos' Tales of Dionysos." PhD diss. Austin: The University of Texas at Austin.

10 Children in Distress

Agonizing Mothers as Intercessors in Early Byzantine Miracle Collections*

Andria Andreou

Introduction

Healing miracles – tales recounting cures performed by Christian saints – topped the list of popularity in Byzantine Greek miracle collections, which also include punishments, salvations, the finding of lost objects, and the thwarting of hostile attacks.[1] A precondition for healing miracles is the occurrence of a physical illness (for example a hernia), a mental illness (for example demonic possession), or an accident (for example a fall). In turn, such events are unavoidably joined with the patients' intense suffering and agony that is usually voiced by the hagiographers. When, however, the patients involved in the healing process are children, certain differences arise in the organization of the miracle tale as a short narrative.[2] By focusing on early Byzantine miracle collections, this chapter investigates the twists that appear in the narrative plot and structure of healing tales in cases where the suffering patient is a child. The discussion will draw on five miracle collections that present cases of child patients: the fifth-century *Miracles of Thekla* (*MT*),[3] the sixth-century *Miracles of Kosmas and Damianos* (*MKD*),[4] and three seventh-century collections: the *Miracles of Kyros and John* (*MKJ*) penned by Sophronios

* The research for this chapter was co-funded by the European Regional Development Fund and the Re-public of Cyprus through the Foundation of Research and Innovation (Project: Post-Doc/0718/0021). Furthermore, some of the ideas that inform the chapter's arguments were developed in the framework of the project "Network for Medieval Arts and Rituals" (NetMAR), which received funding from the European Union's Horizon 2020 research and innovation programme under grant agreement nr 951875. The opinions expressed in this document reflect only the author's view and in no way reflect the European Commission's opinions. The European Commission is not responsible for any use that may be made of the information it contains.

1 For miracle collections, see Efthymiadis 2014 and 1999; Johnson 2006. For healing miracles, see Constantinou 2014, 2013, and 2010.
2 For the characteristics of early Byzantine tales, including miracles, see Constantinou and Andreou 2022.
3 *MT*, ed. Dagron 1978. For this collection, see especially Narro 2010 (language and style); Johnson 2006, 172–220 (comparison with paradoxography); Dagron 1978, 13–30 (dates, authorship).
4 *MKD*, ed. Rupprecht 1935; ed. Deubner 1907. For the saints' cult, see Booth 2011, 115–128.

DOI: 10.4324/9781003265658-13

of Jerusalem,[5] the *Miracles of Artemios* (*MA*),[6] and the *Miracles of Anastasios the Persian* (*MAP*).[7]

Tales involving children in miracle collections are few in number. Specifically, in miracle collections of the early Byzantine period, children appear only in the aforementioned five texts, and in a total of 24 tales. Another issue that needs to be addressed before the undertaken investigation is the fact that what is understood by the term "child" and, in turn, the child's relation to its kin might not directly respond to contemporary understandings of such terms. In cultures where the average lifespan was much shorter, the age at which an individual "ceased" being a child and became an adult differed considerably from our own Western notion of adulthood (beginning at the age of 16 or 18 years). Actually, despite the fact that, legally, people were considered minors until the age of 25, women could get married at the age of 12 or 13 years (with betrothal taking place considerably earlier),[8] and men at 15 years of age.[9] The age span of a family member considered to be a child was thus much shorter than the contemporary conception, while a person might pass from childhood to adulthood abruptly following an arranged marriage.

The terminology depicting the understanding on the part of miracle tales' authors of a character being a child is extremely rich. Specifically, the collections in question might indicate the age of a child vaguely, with terms such as "τέκνον" ("child"), "παιδίον" ("child") "παῖς" ("child," "son"), "βρέφος" ("newborn," "infant," or "toddler"), "κόριον" ("female child"), "υἱός" ("son"), "θυγάτριον" ("little daughter," "girl"), and "μειράκιον" ("child," usually in puberty, between 6 and 14 years).[10] In other cases, hagiographers might opt to be more specific, using epithets to narrow down the age of the child, such as "υἱὸν νήπιον" ("boy toddler"), "βρέφος παραμάσθιον" ("nursling"), and "παιδὶ μικρὸν" ("small child"). Additionally, in a number of tales the age and gender of the child are referred to with concise accuracy, as for instance with terms such as "υἱὸν ὡς ἐτῶν ἐννέα" ("son of about 9 years old"). To complicate matters, some of these terms, such as "παῖς," "παιδίον," and "υἱός," are also employed in tales in which the "child" is in fact understood as an adult, as, for example, in the case of a father protagonist who is said to have a "son of about 16 years of age" ("υἱὸν ἔσχεν ὡς ἐτῶν δεκαὲξ," *MAP* p. 137, line 2).[11]

---

5 Sophronios of Jerusalem, *MKJ*, ed. Marcos 1975. For the saints' cult and the miracle collection, see Gascou 2007 and 2006.

6 *MA*, ed. Papadopoulos-Kerameus 1909. For the saint's cult and the miracle collection, see Alwis 2012; Efthymiadis 2004; Crisafulli and Nesbitt 1997, 8–19; Lieu 1996.

7 *MAP*, ed. Flusin 1992. For the text, see Kažhdan 1996; Flusin 1992, 2.329–352.

8 For marriage and consent in Byzantium, see e.g. Laiou 2011; Ritzer 1970.

9 Moffatt 1986, 706; Antoniadis-Bibicou 1973. For childhood in Byzantium, see Cojocaru 2022; Ariantzi 2018 and 2012; Papaconstantinou and Talbot 2009; Hennessy 2008.

10 See also Prinzing 2009, 16–23 on the terminology of describing the child's various stages of life. However, the terminology employed in miracle collections to describe a child seems to disregard the exact stages of life, with terms more generally and/or figuratively employed. See especially pp.17–18 for terms employed in an overlapping manner to describe various stages.

11 Translations, unless otherwise indicated, are mine.

As regards the relations of a child to its kin, scholars such as Leslie Brubaker and Ruth Macrides have already pointed out the discrepancy between the modern model of a closed family unit formed by parents and children and the usually more extended Byzantine family that included slaves,[12] adoptive children, nurses, and godparents.[13] Despite the lack of concise specificity in the terminology referring to children in the investigated corpus, and setting aside the aforementioned discrepancy between the Byzantine and modern understanding of family bonds, it seems that miracle tales portraying what is understood in the context of the narrative as a child patient (that is, a dependent family member who has not yet reached the age of adulthood) present certain structural and content differences from tales portraying adult patients. These differences are directly related to the bond developed between the child and the mother, or in some cases the child and the nurse, or the father. It is to these differences that this chapter turns in an effort to unravel the narrative workings behind the portrayal of child patients. The analysis turns to the two axes on which the differences between tales presenting children in relation to adult patients are made manifest: structure and plot.

Narrative Structure

Most frequently, healing miracles follow a rather ritualistic structure, with repetitive elements that run through each collection in question.[14] Healing miracles are usually presented in the following narrative structure: the protagonist's profile is sketched through information pertaining to his/her gender, name, nationality, and profession. Following the biographical information, details of the patient's illness are usually presented: the nature of the illness, symptoms, and period of suffering. The saint's appearance and the healing process are then described, followed by the patient's and bystanders' gratitude toward the saint and the patient's departure from the church or the locus of cure.

When a child enters the narrative, on the other hand, a different structural organization is in place. Specifically, in addition to the child's biographical details, which would constitute the first section of the ritualistic structure of healing miracles described above, biographical information concerning the parents is also offered. Moreover, there are cases in which nothing is said about the child except that it is ill, but information about the parent(s) is still provided. This structural modification, which is found in all miracles with child patients, differentiates healings of children from those of adults. In fact, the information pertaining to children is almost as a rule less than the information concerning their parents. Details

---

12 In e.g. Miracle 53 of the *MKJ* (53.§3–5), narrating the healing of a certain man named Prokopios, there is added an episode concerning his so-called "young" slave named Theodoros, who was playing in the sea and was dragged into the sea by a big fish. Theodoros prays for salvation, but Prokopios is not implicated in the process.

13 Brubaker 2013; Macrides 1999.

14 See Constantinou 2014.

often mentioned as regards children are their gender and age (vaguely or with more specificity). This information is usually followed by the description of the child's illness. Indicatively for the purposes of this analysis, of the 24 tales with child patients, only nine mention their name, while five are found in the Kyros and John collection, whose author tends to name all protagonists. The tendency not to name children is in contrast with the hagiographers' inclination to provide the parent(s)' name and other detailed information, such as their gender, origin, and occupation. This form of narrative organization points to the child being considered an additional aspect of the parent(s)' assets.

A characteristic example of this difference between miracle tales involving children (and their parents) and tales devoted to adult patients is the miracle collection of Artemios, who specializes in healing afflictions affecting the male genital area. The typical beginning of the miracles in Artemios' collection is portrayed in the following sentence: "A certain man by the name of Euporos, a Chian by birth, a merchant had a hernia for very many years" ("Ἀνήρ τις τοὔνομα Εὔπορος, τῷ γένει Χῖος, πραγματευτής, ἐκ πλείστων χρόνων καταβαρὴς ὢν," *MA* 1.1; trans. Crisafulli and Nesbitt 1997, 85). The protagonist is introduced by a reference to his gender, name, origin, and occupation, followed by his health problem and its duration. When a child enters the storyline, the structural order is modified as follows: "A certain silver dealer, Akakios by name, had a son of about seven years who fell victim to the same disease" ("Ἀκακίῳ τοὔνομά τινι ἀργυροπράτῃ ὑπῆρχεν υἱὸς ὡς ἐτῶν ἑπτά, ὃς ... τῇ αὐτῇ περιέπεσεν νόσῳ," *MA* 10.7–8; trans. Crisafulli and Nesbitt 1997, 95). Here the father's name and occupation are still mentioned, but there is an addition to his attributes or possessions, which is his ill child. This structural twist eventually suggests that children are introduced in the narratives as paired with their parents. They are not treated as independent characters. Thence, the typical structure of the miracle tale is modified to accommodate the parent–child pair, by introducing first the father or mother (or, rarely, another relative or the nurse), followed by the dependent child.

In addition to the narrative being expanded to accommodate the child as the parent(s)' possession, the structure might acquire further parameters guided by the choice of a child patient in relation to the parent who escorts the child. A usual addition to this information concerns, for example, the difficulties parents face while taking the child to the saint's shrine, or the parents' effort to have their child cured through visits to doctors. A case in point is Miracle 36 from Artemios' collection. In this tale, the repeated effort of a mother to bring her son to doctors is followed by the doctors' absurd financial demand. This demand is then succeeded by the mother's repeated withdrawal of effort, due to her poverty. The solution to this cycle of persistence and withdrawal is offered when the mother decides to visit the miraculous saint's shrine (*MA* 36). This repetitive structural pattern serves the narrative development and the narrative's goal of offering praise to Artemios. In particular, as the mother's repeated failure prolongs the child's suffering, the persistence of the suffering underlines the incapability of doctors compared to Artemios' subsequent instantaneous cure.

In certain cases, the interdependence of child and parent might become more explicit as it is manifested on a macrostructural level – that is, extending to more than one tale. For example, Miracle 10 of the Kyros and John collection, which concerns the healing of a little girl, comes after Miracle 8, which concerns the saving of the girl's father from an accident, and Miracle 9, which reports the healing of the girl's mother. The author comments in the short prologue of Miracle 10 that, since he has related miracles involving the parents, he will "add" one involving the daughter: "let us add the daughter to the parents" ("καὶ τοῖς τεκοῦσιν προσθήσωμεν τὸ θυγάτριον," *MKJ* 10.§1.1–2). The tale concerning the girl thus completes the series of miracles concerning firstly the father and secondly the mother. What is more, in this last miracle of the series, devoted to the child, the girl appears as a co-protagonist of the plot with her mother, which is not the case with the miracles devoted to the father and the mother respectively.

Another feature of the macrostructure which points to the special treatment of miracles concerning children is manifested in at least two of the examined collections. This relates to a tendency for miracles involving children to be grouped close together or to reappear in small units of two in the *Miracles of Artemios* and in the Kyros and John collection (*MA* 4, 10, 11, 12, 28, 31, 33, 34, 36, 38, 42, 43, 45; *MKJ* 10, 11, 34, 41, 44, 54). The Kosmas and Damianos collection and the Thekla collection include only two miracles involving children (*MKD* 22 Rupprecht, 36 Deubner; *MT* 11, 24), while the Anastasios the Persian collection contains only one such miracle (*MAP* 11). Thus, an accurate argument as to the grouping of miracles involving children on the part of the hagiographers cannot be made. However, the tendency observed in the *Miracles of Artemios* and the *Miracles of Kyros and John* might testify to an awareness on the part of the hagiographers that miracles involving mothers (or fathers, or nurses) and children constitute a special subcategory and should be grouped together, as is the case with other categories of miracles.[15]

Narrative Content

When a child patient acquires a central role in a miracle tale, certain thematic parameters emerge or are altered compared to tales concerning adult patients. First, mothers seem to acquire a prominent role, and to act as the link between the child and the saint.[16] The relationship between the mother and the child is dealt with in detail and acquires narrative importance; namely, it becomes the kernel around which the plot unfolds. Second, the body of the child seems to receive a different treatment from the saint compared to the treatment an adult in need of a cure receives.

---

15 A case in point is the *MT*, in which Thekla's defeat of the pagan gods is succeeded by healings of priests, then healings of individuals with their own subgroups (i.e. healings at sea, over land, of women, etc.).

16 On different ways in which the maternal identity of biblical maternal prophetic figures is again defined via their bond with and care for their offspring, see Chapter 8 in this volume.

Mothers as Intercessors

As already mentioned, children enter a miraculous shrine escorted by a guardian; even if the cure takes place in another setting (for example the child's home), the child's guardian is still present in the narrative. In most cases, the child's mother appears, while in rarer cases it is the nurse, the grandmother, or the father that escorts the child. Notably, mothers appear as active participants in miracles that involve their children, since in almost every case the cures are administered following their intercession. Since small children cannot voice their request or go on their own to the place of healing, mothers take action. They carry their infants to the saint's shrine, they perform customary rites, they pray for the children's well-being, they care for their needs,[17] and they suffer for them.[18] This range of actions, supplemented by emotional engagement, unveils the fact that a child's illness is shared in a metaphorical way by the mother. The strong bond between a mother and her child can be witnessed in Miracle 10 of Artemios' collection, which concerns a herniated boy:

> His parents brought him to the all-holy and honoured martyr of Christ. They had spent some time in the church of St. John when they … departed … But the mother did not desist from coming with him, tearfully exhorting the holy martyr since she was especially afflicted in her soul. Now it is worthwhile as well to lend an ear to her child's inarticulate speech and lisping since, although these things occasion much laughter for the present, they would reveal much pity for those who reflect. For as though entreating his own father face to face, he confidently begged the holy martyr thus: "St. Artemios, take away my hernia." After the child and mother had acted in this way …, the saint appeared to the wife in a dream, while they were passing time at home and he said to her: "Bring me your son." She, seeming to lift him up, gladly leaned the boy's head against the martyr's feet. Artemios, after he took hold of him by the chin, straightened up from a stooped position and said to him: "Do you want me to take away your hernia?" The child replied: "Yes, sir, take away my hernia." Then making the sign of the precious cross all over his body, the saint said: "Behold, from now on you do not have a hernia." These things the woman saw in her dream, and after awakening she found the child, just as she had seen, restored to health.

---

17 A noteworthy example of the mother caring for her child's needs is Mary, the mother of the child protagonist of Miracle 41 in the Kyros and John collection. Menas, her son, has his tongue hanging out of his mouth and cannot eat properly. Therefore, the mother is said to come up with a novel way to administer food, bypassing the tongue and spilling the food directly into the mouth. The author refers to this as "a certain device" ("μηχανῇ τινι," *MKJ* 41.§4).

18 Perpetua's maternal thinking for her biological and spiritual children in the *Passion of Perpetua and Felicity* (*PPF*) is likewise an exemplar (through her prayers, suffering, and other intercessions for their salvation); see Chapters 1 and 5 in this volume.

Τοῦτον ἄγουσιν οἱ γονεῖς πρὸς τὸν πάνσεπτον καὶ τίμιον μάρτυρα τοῦ Χριστοῦ. Τινὰ δὲ αὐτῶν χρόνον διαγόντων ἐν τῷ τοῦ ἁγίου Ἰωάννου ναῷ ... ἀπαναχωροῦσιν. ἡ δὲ μήτηρ οὐ διέλειπεν σὺν αὐτῷ ἐρχομένη, μετὰ δακρύων παρακαλοῦσα τὸν ἅγιον μάρτυρα, μάλιστα κατώδυνος τῇ ψυχῇ τυγχάνουσα. ἄξιον δὲ καὶ αὐτοῦ τοῦ παιδὸς τῶν ψελλισμάτων καὶ τραυλισμῶν ἀκοῦσαι, ἅπερ γέλωτα πολὺν πρὸς τὸ παρὸν ἐμποιοῦντα οἶκτον πολὺν τοῖς λογιζομένοις ἐνέφαινον· οἷα γὰρ οἰκεῖον πατέρα ὄψιν πρὸς ὄψιν δεόμενος ἐξῄτει πεπαρρησιασμένως τὸν ἅγιον μάρτυρα, φάσκων· "Ἅγιε Ἀρτέμιε, ἔπαρον τὴν κήλην μου." Τούτων δὲ οὕτως παρὰ τοῦ παιδὸς καὶ τῆς μητρὸς αὐτοῦ πραττομένων ..., φαίνεται κατ' ὄναρ τῇ γυναικὶ ὁ ἅγιος, ἐν τῷ οἴκῳ διαγόντων αὐτῶν, καὶ λέγει αὐτῇ· "Φέρε μοι τὸν υἱόν σου." ἡ δὲ δόξασα βαστάζειν αὐτόν, χαίρουσα ἔκλινεν τὴν κεφαλὴν αὐτοῦ πρὸς τοὺς πόδας τοῦ μάρτυρος· ὁ δὲ τοῦ πώγονος αὐτοῦ λαβόμενος ἀνώρθωσεν αὐτὸν κεκυφότα, καὶ φησι πρὸς αὐτόν· "Θέλεις ἐπάρω τὴν κήλην σου;" Τὸ δὲ παιδίον ἀπεκρίνατο· "Ναι, κῦρι, ἔπαρον τὴν κήλην μου." Τότε ὁ ἅγιος σφραγίσας αὐτὸ κατὰ παντὸς τοῦ σώματος τῷ τιμίῳ σταυρῷ ἔφη· "Ἴδε ἀπὸ τοῦ νῦν κήλην οὐκ ἔχεις." Ταῦτα ἑώρα ἡ γυνὴ καθ' ὕπνους, καὶ διυπνισθεῖσα ηὗρεν τὸν παῖδα, καθὼς ἐθεάσατο, ὑγιῆ καθεστῶτα. (*MA* 10; trans. Crisafulli and Nesbitt 1997, 95–97)

Here the child is carried to the saint's church by his parents, but the family is obliged to leave after a while. At this point, we are offered a glimpse into the mother's emotional world. In particular, the mother hesitates to leave with her still-suffering child, and, as the author points out, she exhorts the martyr in tears, deeply afflicted in her heart. In fact, such explicit statements on the part of the hagiographer pertaining to a character's strong emotions in the face of a patient's suffering are unusual not only in this collection but in the other collections as well. Generally, in miracle collections, hagiographers offer no information concerning other relatives' emotions in the face of their adult loved ones' suffering, even though relatives of-ten act as patients' escorts;[19] nevertheless, these relationships of escort relatives to adult patients acquire no narrative importance, since they do not significantly con-tribute to the unravelling of the plot. In the case of child patients, on the other hand, the mothers' emotions are voiced and, as the above passage shows, the mother often becomes the central emotional focus of the miracle. Moreover, the healing of the child also takes place in the mother's dream after she begs, prays, and presents the child to the martyr.[20]

A variety of terms is employed to showcase the mothers' acute grief and reac-tion in the face of their child's suffering. For example, mothers are said to lament

19 An indicative example is Miracle 1 of the Artemios collection, in which a certain man named Anthi-mos brings his 20-year-old son to the saint's church and, despite the information that the young man did not even have the strength to go to the latrines by himself, the father, we are told, just performs the ordinary rites (*MA* 1.14). No emotional involvement on the part of the father is encountered.

20 Cf. Dinokrates' case in the *PPF*, where healing again takes place within the context of a dream (Chapter 1 in this volume).

("ὠλοφύρετο," *MKD* 36.10 Deubner), to experience pain in their gut ("τὰ σπλάγχνα πλέον ἐδάπτετο"; "ὀδυνωμένης τὰ σπλάγχνα," *MKJ* 36.§5; *MA* 42.14), to yell or wail ("μετὰ κραυγῶν"), to shed tears ("[μετὰ] δακρύων"; "σὺν δάκρυσιν," *MKJ* 36.§5; *MA* 28.25). In a number of healing miracles, the mother's grief follows an emotional climax which is resolved with the saint's appearance and the child's cure. A telling example is Miracle 34 of the collection of Kyros and John. In this tale, Dorothea's son has accidentally swallowed a snake's egg, with the result that the egg has hatched in his stomach and the snake is eating up the child's intestines. Dorothea is said first to be "pierced in her gut," then to "wail" and "shed tears," an emotional stance that climaxes in a mourning prayer formed of rhetorical questions addressed to the saints. The monologue takes up more than half a printed page (of a miracle extending to about two printed pages) and concludes with the mother begging that if her son is being punished for a fault of hers, that *she* be punished instead of him; or that *she* die so that she does not have to face the loss of her child; or, alternatively, that her child be spared and returned to her (*MKJ* 34). Her reaction hints first at a view of illness as a punishment that might extend to the little child because of her, that is, as a punishment that was intended for her. This possibility for a mother's punishment to befall the child hints at the mother being considered a unit with the child, not only according to her own view but also in the view of the saints and God, who decide upon her punishment. Moreover, this view is shared by the hagiographer who communicates the mother's monologue to the audience of the collection and by the members of the audience, who are offered no further explanation, so that it is received as "natural" truth.

Besides being involved in the healing process and in their children's suffering, mothers also function as the launchpad that triggers the saints' cures. Such is the role of the mother of Marou. Marou is the little girl who is the protagonist of the above-mentioned Miracle 10 in the collection of Kyros and John. Marou develops an abscess on her teeth which eventually leads to a nest of worms that causes her deafness. The following passage neatly describes the resolution of the child's condition:

> The one who had given birth to the girl, upon watching her, and as she could not bear it, was planning … to bring the child to the doctors to treat it … For she was, at the time, at the saints' church. And that night …, falling asleep she saw an empty doctor's room. And there was a monk sitting in the room. The seated man was Kyros … The saint, who was supposedly sitting on a throne, said to the woman: "Lady, why did you come here?" She replied that she sought a doctor's office. "And I thought this small house would be one …" And he replied in this way: "Search, and whatever you find, put in the in-fected ears and your daughter will be healed." She, examining the whole house closely, saw a small opening and within it a glass of honey … She … did as instructed and she poured a bit of honey in the ears of the infant, and she drew out a nest of worms four fingers long and equally wide. And the little girl was immediately relieved from the cause of her suffering and the great trouble that could arise from it.

Ἅπερ ἡ τὴν παῖδα γεννήσασα βλέπουσα, καὶ φέρειν ἐπὶ πολὺ μὴ ἰσχύσασα
… ἐβουλεύσατο … τὸ παιδίον ἰατροῖς προσενέγκασθαι, ἰαθησόμενον …·
εἰς τὸ τῶν ἁγίων γὰρ τότε διέτριβεν τέμενος. Καὶ κατ' ἐκείνην τὴν νύκτα …,
ἔρημον ὁρᾷ καθευδήσασα ἰατροῦ τὸ δωμάτιον· εὕρισκεν καὶ μοναστὴν ἐν
αὐτῷ καθεζόμενον. Κῦρος ἦν οὗτος ὁ φανεὶς καθεζόμενος … Πρὸς ἣν ὁ ἅγιος
ὁ δῆθεν ἐπὶ θρόνου καθήμενος ἔλεξεν· Ἐνθάδε, ὦ γύναι, τί παραγέγονας; Ἡ
δέ, Ἰατρεῖον ζητοῦσα, πρὸς αὐτὸν ἀπεκρίνατο· καὶ τοιοῦτον μὲν ἐγὼ τόνδε τὸν
οἰκίσκον νενόμικα … Ὁ δὲ πρὸς αὐτὴν ἀκριβῶς ἀπεκρίνατο· Ἐρεύνησον, καὶ
ὅπερ ἂν εὕροις, ὠσὶ τοῖς πάσχουσιν ἔμβαλε, καὶ ἰαθήσεταί σου τὸ θυγάτριον. Ἡ
δὲ τὸν οἶκον ἅπαντα περινοστήσασα, θυρίδα μικρὰν ἐθεάσατο, καὶ μέλιτος ἐν
αὐτῇ ποτήριον κείμενον … τὸ λεχθὲν αὐτῇ διεπράξατο, καὶ βραχὺ τοῦ μέλιτος
τοῖς ὠσὶ τοῦ βρέφους ἐγχέασα, σκωληκόμεστον ἀνήγαγεν θύλακα, δακτύλων
τὸ μῆκος τεττάρων, καὶ πλάτος ἀνάλογον ἔχοντα· καὶ τούτου λυτρωθεῖσα
παραχρῆμα τὸ κόριον οὗπερ αὐτῇ τῶν ἀλγηδόνων ταμεῖον ἐγένετο, καὶ τῶν
ἀπλέτων τικτομένων δεινῶν ἐλυτροῦτο κολάσεων. (*MKJ* 10.§57)

As with the previous examples, the mother is in charge and undertakes action.
Here, however, she plans to take the child to a doctor after spending some time in
the saints' shrine and losing her hope for a miraculous cure. It is the mother's plan
to leave that triggers the saints' intervention. She thus becomes the narrative occasion for the child's imminent cure. What is more, the mother acts as the saint's instrument through which the therapy is executed. Part of the cure takes place within
the dream, as she is instructed what to do to effect the cure and she initiates a search
within the dream, while the actual practical process is also performed by her, as she
applies the ingredient she finds to the child's ear.

In some of the examined tales, the mother's emotional involvement constitutes
a sufficient reason to cause the intervention of the supernatural. Such an example
is Miracle 36 from the collection of Kosmas and Damianos. This story concerns a
child who loses his eyesight. It reads as follows:

A woman had a four-year-old child who, as a result of devil's machinations,
immediately became totally blind, and she lamented in the face of her child's
suffering. The saints, feeling pity for her, appeared in a dream and told her: "If
you want your child to regain his eyesight, go to the church of Saints Kosmas
and Damian and ask the priests … to apply some of this blessed medicine on
the eyes of your child …" She, filled with joy, hastened over, and gave the
light to the blinded child, and, as usual, God was glorified through his saints.

Γυνή τις ἔχουσα παιδίον ὡς ἐτῶν τεσσάρων, ὅπερ ἀθρόον ἐκ διαβολικῆς
ἐνεργείας ἐν παντελεῖ ἀβλεψίᾳ κατέστη, ὠλοφύρετο ἐπὶ τῇ συμβάσῃ τοῦ
τέκνου αὐτῆς συμφορᾷ. Ταύτῃ συμπαθήσαντες οἱ ἅγιοι κατ' ὄναρ φανέντες
λέγουσιν αὐτῇ· "εἰ βούλει ἀναβλέψαι τὸ τέκνον σου, ἄπελθε ἐν τῷ ναῷ
τῶν ἁγίων Κοσμᾶ καὶ Δαμιανοῦ καὶ διαίτησαι παρὰ τῶν κληρικῶν … ἵνα
ἐπιχρίσωσιν τοὺς ὀφθαλμοὺς τοῦ τέκνου σου τοῦ εὐλογημένου ἐκείνου
φαρμάκου …" Τῆς δὲ μετὰ πάσης χαρᾶς προσδραμούσης παραχρῆμα
περιποιήθη τὸ φῶς τῷ τυφλωθέντι παιδίῳ, καὶ συνήθως ἐδοξάσθη ὁ θεὸς ἐν
τοῖς ἁγίοις αὐτοῦ. (*MKD* 36.18–30 Rupprecht)

The mother has an emotional attitude to her child's suffering, which is communicated through the use of a strong verb, "ὠλοφύρετο" ("lamented"). In this case, the child is not reported to feel pain, as the problem it encounters is blindness. However, the mother is in pain. It is precisely the mother's intense suffering that initiates the saints' intervention since, strictly speaking, she does not undertake any action (such as taking the child to the saints' church, or praying). Instead, in this case, the mother is in a state of emotional breakdown. As the narrator notes, the saints appeared because they felt pity for her. As in the previous example, the mother eventually becomes the saints' instrument in order for the child to achieve a cure. This time the instrument of the cure, the saints' ointment, is not applied by the mother herself. Nevertheless, her intercession is needed, as it is *she* who shoulders the responsibility of begging the priests to administer the medicine. Once again, the mother intercedes, this time between the child and the saints and between the priests and the child.

Mothers thus seem to assume a protagonistic role in the examined tales. They create the context for the cure to take place (carrying their ill children to the shrine, praying, and performing the customary rites). They also enable the practical aspects of the cure (following the saints' instructions, administering the cure), but they are also the characters who voice the praise toward the saints when the cure is finally performed. Their central role, therefore, might also be related to the fact that small children could not accurately narrate the process of their healing, and thus the miraculous saint(s) would not be properly praised. Hence, hagiographers exploit the emotional bond between mother and child to provide a character who can narrate what exactly happened during the supernatural healing process and properly praise the saints. Consequently, mothers acquire importance as extensions of and intercessors for their children.

The Child's Body

In early Byzantine miracle collections, most healings are performed either in a patient's dream, or in waking reality. The saint might touch the infected bodily part or direct a patient to do something in order for favourable circumstances to arise and for a cure to take place. The saint might also instruct another character, or even another saintly figure, on how to perform the healing. In the case of children, as already inferred from the previous discussion, the mother is the character who functions as the saint's instrument. Children are hardly implicated in the healing process despite the fact that their bodies are the locus on which the cure is performed.

Compared to the suffering adult's body, that of the child receives a different miraculous treatment. The child's body is not treated in the violent ways in which an adult's body is approached by the miraculous saint(s). If a child's body has to be touched in the framework of the miraculous healing, this bodily contact is usually performed by the mother. More specifically, in our tales, the following methods of treatment are encountered: honey administered as ointment (for example *MKJ* 10); making the sign of the cross (for example *MA* 10, 31, 38); shaking the child upside down (for example *MA* 28); play (for example *MKJ* 41; *MT* 24); administering drink or food (for example *MKJ* 44; *MA* 43); application of pork meat (for example *MKJ* 54); anointing with the ashes of burnt wool (for example *MT* 11); touch (for example *MA* 12, 36); application of an ointment (for example *MKD* 36 Deubner; *MA* 33).

Artemios' miracles allow an illustrative comparison between healing methods deemed suitable for adults and those that are proper for children. Artemios not only touches his adult patients' genitals, but he often becomes extremely violent in his choice of healing methods. The saint squeezes or pricks his patients' genitals (for example *MA* 2, 13), he performs forced incisions on their body (for example *MA* 44), and he steps on their stomach (for example *MA* 7). Artemios even devises strange methods to bring about treatment with the help of other characters, such as the hitting of a patient's testicles with a blacksmith's hammer (*MA* 26). Revealingly, when children are the protagonists of a story, Artemios' healing ritual is as simple as possible and as painless as possible. Anointing the child's forehead, offering edible medicine, and instructing the mother to take simple steps are some of Artemios' most common healing methods when patients are children. It seems, therefore, that cruel cures and generally touching a child's body, especially on sexually charged bodily members, are avoided.

What is more, children's cures seem to be tailored to their needs. In a number of miracles involving adults in the collections under examination, the saint(s) order patients to consume things that are inedible (such as sheep's pubic hair, *MKD* 3 Deubner, 6 Rupprecht); or to consume things which have an unpleasant taste (such as cedar, *MKD* 11 Deubner, 13 Rupprecht). When a child is involved, by contrast, it is offered food which is pleasant in taste (for example a piece of cake or jujube berries, *MA* 43, 45). Moreover, when the child's guardian is not involved in the cure, the cure itself assumes the form of a happening in the course of the child's daily activities, such as play. An illustrative example is the following miracle from Thekla's collection:

> A little boy … was in danger of losing one of his eyes … This boy's wet nurse took him and … presented the child to the martyr with incessant lamentations, prayers, and tears … and praying that the martyr not disregard a child … The miracle was accomplished more through childish play than through a serious endeavour. This is what happened in the forecourt of the church … One day this child was playing here and having fun, sometimes chasing a bird with peals of laughter and the next moment, being chased by one of the birds, which resulted in great entertainment for the onlookers and gave them cause for laughter. One of the cranes, apparently because it was being hindered by the boy from its feeding … jumped at the boy and pecked with its beak that eye which was already afflicted and had now lost its sight. The child started wailing at the attack, and all the women who were there also cried out, as if something terrible had happened. The elderly wet nurse … all but gave up the ghost because his malady had taken a turn for the worse and any hope for the future had been extinguished. In reality, this event was the remedy and the cure of his suffering.
>
> Παιδίον τὸν ἕτερον τῶν ὀφθαλμῶν ἐκινδύνευσεν. Τοῦτο ἡ τίτθη λαβοῦσα …, διέτριβεν ἀεὶ μετ' ὀδυρμῶν καὶ λιτῶν καὶ δακρύων προκομίζουσα τὸ

παιδίον τῇ μάρτυρι ... καὶ δεομένη μὴ παριδεῖν τὸ παιδίον ... παιδιᾶς δὲ
... ποιεῖται τὸ θαῦμα. Καὶ γάρ τι συμβαίνει τοιοῦτο κατὰ τὴν αὐλὴν αὐτοῦ
τοῦ νεώ ... Ἐνταῦθα καὶ τὸ παιδίον τοῦτό ποτε ἀθύρον καὶ τερπόμενον ἦν,
ποτὲ μὲν διῶκον ὄρνιν μετὰ γέλωτος, ποτὲ δὲ καὶ διωκόμενον ὑπό τινος τῶν
ὀρνίθων, ὡς καὶ τέρψιν εἶναι τοῦτο τοῖς θεωμένοις καὶ γέλωτος ἀφορμήν.
Καὶ δὴ μία τῶν γεράνων, ὡς ἅτε δὴ παρὰ τοῦ παιδίου κωλυομένη φαγεῖν
... ἐμπηδᾷ τῷ παιδίῳ, καὶ τῷ ῥάμφει τὸν ὀφθαλμὸν ἐκεῖνον ἐγκολάπτει
τὸν καὶ ἤδη πεπονθότα καὶ ἀποσβεσθέντα λοιπόν. Καὶ ἀνωλόλυξε μὲν τὸ
παιδίον ὑπὸ τῆς πληγῆς, συνεξεβόησαν δὲ καὶ αἱ παροῦσαι γυναῖκες, ὡς ἂν
καὶ ἀτόπου μεγάλου τινὸς γεγονότος. Ἡ δὲ πρεσβῦτις ἡ τίτθη ... μικροῦ καὶ
ἀφῆκε τὴν ψυχήν, ὡς καὶ πρὸς τὸ χεῖρον ἔτι τοῦ πάθους ἐλάσαντος καὶ τὸ
λεῖπον ἐκκόψαντος τῆς ἐλπίδος. Τόδε ἄρα θεραπεία ἦν τοῦ πάθους καὶ ἄκος.
(*MT* 24; trans. Johnson 2012, 97–99)

This story presents the only case in which a wet nurse is involved. The wet nurse takes the same emotional and practical stance as that observed with regard to mothers.[21] She laments, prays, cries, and presents the child to the saint asking for a cure. The cure is carefully orchestrated and effected in the form of play to meet the needs of the child patient. Neither the saint nor the wet nurse is practically involved in the cure. Instead, a crane pierces the child's eye in an instantaneous manner. Besides being tailored to a child's routine, the choice of play as a method of cure in this case creates suspense: a happy everyday scene turns into a nightmare witnessed by all the bystanders. This creates the framework through which the miracle can cause a strong impression: the bystanders realize that instead of worsening, the child's health had in this unorthodox manner been restored.

Even though this chapter mainly concerns mothers and their ill children, it would be worthwhile to compare the mother–child bond with the father–child relationship. As already pointed out, fathers are rarely encountered in cases of (small) child patients. Specifically, of the 24 tales involving child patients from infancy to puberty, only four involve fathers, and all concern boy patients, with one of them eventually centring on the mother, while the father is sidelined. One case involves an infant (*MAP* 11), one a boy of speaking age (*MKJ* 54), and two boys of unspecified age (*MA* 4, 33). In addition to the difference in the number of tales concerning fathers as compared to mothers, the treatment of this relationship seems also to differ in respect to the fathers' reaction to their children's condition but also in respect to the fathers' practical engagement in the situation. A case in point is Miracle 33 of Artemios' collection. This tale presents a father whose son suffers from hernia. The father brings his son to Saint John's Church in Oxia.

A certain man named Theodore had a son who suffered from hernia and who was in acute pain. Hearing about the miracles of St. Artemios, he said to his beloved friend named Theognios ...: "Lead me to St. Artemios because my

21 For the figure of the wet nurse, see Chapters 1–3 and 7 in this volume.

child is in great distress, being afflicted in his testicles." ... Both waited – the father of the child with the child, as well as the aforesaid Theognios ... Theognios ... fell asleep and saw the one who is quick to help – the glorious servant of Christ Artemios speaking to him: "Get up, and take some of the prepared wax-salve and anoint your chest and eat some of it. Also anoint the testicles of the child reclining with you and both of you will be well." ... The man recounted how: ... "I rose immediately ... I also roused those reclining with me and ... I anointed my own chest and I ate some of it in accordance with the saint's command. But, as bidden, I also anointed the child's testicles and both of us were restored to health."

Τὶς ὀνόματι Θεόδωρος, ἔχων υἱὸν καταβαρῆ καὶ ὀδυνώμενον πικρῶς, ἀκούσας περὶ τῶν τοῦ ἁγίου Ἀρτεμίου θαυμάτων λέγει τῷ ἀγαπητῷ αὐτοῦ ὀνόματι Θεογνίῳ ...· "Ἄγαγέ με εἰς τὸν ἅγιον Ἀρτέμιον, ὅτι δεινοπαθεῖ τὸ παιδίον μου ἐκ τῶν διδύμων αὐτοῦ ἀσθενοῦν." ... Παραμένουσιν ἀμφότεροι, ὅ τε πατὴρ τοῦ παιδίου μετὰ τοῦ τέκνου καὶ ὁ ῥηθεὶς Θεόγνιος ... καὶ ἐτράπη εἰς ὕπνον καὶ ὁρᾷ τὸν σύντομον πρὸς βοήθειαν, τὸν ἔνδοξον τοῦ Χριστοῦ θεράποντα Ἀρτέμιον λέγοντα αὐτῷ· "Ἀνάστηθι, καὶ ἐκ τῆς γενομένης κηρωτῆς λαβὼν ἄλειψαί σου τὸ στῆθος καὶ φάγε ἐξ αὐτῆς· ἄλειψον δὲ καὶ τοὺς διδύμους τοῦ σὺν σοὶ ἀνακειμένου παιδίου, καὶ καλῶς ἔξετε." Διηγεῖτο τοίνυν ... ὁ ἀνήρ, ὅτι ... "ἠγέρθην οὖν εὐθέως ... ἐξήγειρα δὲ καὶ τοὺς μετ' ἐμοῦ ἀνακειμένους, καὶ ... λαβόντες ἀμφότεροι τῆς ἁγίας κηρωτῆς ἤλειψα τὸ ἴδιόν μου στῆθος καὶ ἔφαγον ἐξ αὐτῆς κατὰ τὴν κέλευσιν τοῦ ἁγίου· ἤλειψα δε, ὡς ἐπετράπην, καὶ τοὺς διδύμους τοῦ παιδὸς καὶ ἀμφότεροι ὑγιεῖς ἀπεκατέστημεν." (*MA* 33; trans. Crisafulli and Nesbitt 1997, 174–176)

Like the mothers discussed previously, the father takes his child to the miraculous shrine. A small divergence from the scheme, however, is that the father asks a friend of his, named Theognios, to lead him to the location, this introducing another character into the father–child team. Eventually, Theognios acquires the status of a protagonist, as he is also suffering – from a chest disease – and the tale concentrates on the treatment of his disease. In fact, the child's cure seems to be almost an afterthought in the general plotline, since Theognios prays just for himself. As an answer to his prayer, the saint appears and instructs him how to cure himself, adding the child's cure as part of Theognios' cure ("also anoint"). Moreover, the father is completely overshadowed, as he seems to perform no other action besides asking Theognios to lead him to the church. He is neither actively nor emotionally involved.[22] What is more, it is not he who acts as the conduit for the cure, but

---

22 The only case in which a father is said to "shed tears" is in a tale from the *MKD* (20 Deubner; in the Rupprecht edition, there is no mention of the shedding of tears). However, this tale obviously concerns an older child compared to the cases discussed here, who is able to address complicated arguments and requests to the doctor left there for his care. Moreover, the father sheds tears not on account of the pain he feels for his son's illness, but to supplicate the saint. And even if we do not take these details into account, this father departs from the church, leaving the child in the care of a doctor. Hence, he does not display any profound emotional engagement.

Theognios. Furthermore, in mother–child cases, the indication that the child is in pain is usually joined to an indication that the mother suffers. In this case, the child is said to be "in acute pain" ("ὀδυνώμενον πικρῶς") but no respective reaction on the part of the father is given. This absence of emotions and active engagement might be related to the general Byzantine ideology of the woman being considered more prone to emotional crises and more tied to worldly affairs (her relation to her children included); the man was instead traditionally thought to be more spiritual and uninvolved with worldly affairs.[23]

A similar treatment may be observed in the other cases involving father–son relationships: Miracle 11 of the *Miracles of Anastasios the Persian*, Miracle 4 of the *Miracles of Artemios*, and Miracle 54 of the *Miracles of Kyros and John*. In all these cases, the father is introduced first, followed by the indication that the boy is the only male child and is thus the only one to continue the family line. These statements introduce a different parameter of importance; it is vital for the fathers to save their only male heir, while mothers behave in the same way independently of the child's gender.

Another notable difference between the treatment of mother–child and father–son pairings in healing miracles concerns the dynamics of paternal faith and saintly intervention. In the collection of Anastasios the Persian, the tale is presented as a power play between the father and the saint: the father doubts the ability of Anastasios' relic to cure his son – a doubt which is explicitly voiced by the father. Anastasios asserts his power by curing the boy in an unspecified manner. A difference in the dynamics of the mother's faith related to saintly intervention is observable in these terms, since the doubting of the mother, when present, is silent. One such example is the healing of Marou already discussed above. The intention of Marou's mother to depart from the saints' church and take the girl to conventional doctors in search for a cure shows a lack of fervent belief in the power of the saints to heal her daughter, which is, however, silenced. In the case of the father, it is instead flagged. In the third case that concerns the healing of a son in which the father is present, Miracle 4 of the Artemios collection, the cure is again unspecified, as the father goes alone to the shrine and lights a votive lamp. We have no case of a mother leaving her child behind.

In the fourth tale in which a father appears, a boy is attacked by a demon while in the bath. It is noteworthy that whereas the tale begins by introducing the father, after the child becomes ill both parents take the child to doctors, and thus the mother enters the tale, too. In fact, the father eventually withdraws from the narrative, as he disappears after sending the mother along with the child to the saints' shrine. The child's treatment is undertaken by the mother, who in a dream is directed what to do. Moreover, in this case the main thematic strand of the tale is the fact that the

---

23 See e.g. the hagiographer's comment in the *Life of Andronikos and Athanasia* (*BHG* 123a) p. 250.§4, ed. Alwis 2011, when the couple's children die; Athanasia has a strong emotional reaction, while Andronikos remains calm and distant. The hagiographer reports that despite Athanasia's piety, she was still tortured by her maternal love and the rules of nature.

cure (the covering of the child's body with pork meat) contradicts the mother's belief against eating pork. The mother is a pagan, and the narrator informs us that, through their choice of healing method, the saints aimed to attack the mother's pagan disposition: "they devised to attack Julia's faith, for that was the name of the mother, who was led astray to the pagan fallacy, and because of this [she] ... refrained from eating pork" ("βεβλάφθαι γὰρ τὴν Ἰουλίαν, τοῦτο γὰρ αὐτῆς ὑπῆρχε τὸ ὄνομα, περὶ τὴν πίστιν ἐφήμιζον, πρὸς πλάνην Ἑλληνικὴν ἀποκλίνουσαν καὶ ταύτῃ ... τὰ κρέα παραιτεῖσθαι τὰ ὕεια," *MKJ* 54.§6). Hence, the whole healing ritual centres around the mother.[24] In these terms, one could infer that even in cases in which the father enters the scene, when actual action is involved and when the method of cure is mentioned, it is to the mother that the plot turns. Despite our lack of further evidence, one could suggest that a gender-based difference is at work, whereby the child and the mother are treated as one unit, whereas the father–child bond is not considered as strong.

That the treatment of child patients discussed here seems to be consciously engineered by the hagiographers is illustrated by a case in which the scheme followed so far, namely of parents (especially mothers) acting as a constituent part of the child's healing process, is reversed. Specifically, it seems that parents, as the child's guardians, can act the other way round and cause their child's distress as well. In Chapter 38 of Artemios' Miracles, a child becomes ill because his parents are impious. Their lack of virtue is premised on their profession of bartering.

> A certain child named George with the nickname Koutales about nine years old became a reader in the often-mentioned church of the holy Forerunner and Baptist John of the Oxeia. He had parents who pursued a living through the business of bartering and exchanging gold. George was being trained by them to master such a business ... He ... withdrew quietly from his parents' spiritually deleterious education ... Then after a great commotion was made by the parents, they succeeded, virtually by force, in bringing him back home. And after a few days this same George succumbed to a sickness ... His parents brought him to the church of St. John ... and after they accomplished the customary rites, they let go of him and withdrew ... [A]s he lay sleeping ... in his sleep he saw St. Artemios ... And stretching out his hand and starting from the patient's head all the way down to his toenails, the saint made the precious sign of the cross ... The ailing George, after waking up and remembering the dream, touched himself and found himself healthy in his whole body. So it was possible to see the child who could not move leaping up and running off and giving thanks to Christ our Saviour and to His saints since he had been deemed worthy of such a great gift and of a divine visit.

---

24 A similar treatment of the child's cure centring on the ill disposition of the mother may also be observed in *MA* 34. The salvation of a girl in this miracle is equated with the mother's spiritual correction.

Παῖς τις ὡς ἐτῶν ἐννέα ἀναγνώστης γεγονὼς τοῦ πολλάκις εἰρημένου ναοῦ τοῦ ἁγίου προδρόμου καὶ βαπτιστοῦ Ἰωάννου τῆς Ὀξείας, ὀνόματι Γεώργιος, τὸ ἐπίκλην Κουτάλης, ἔχων γονεῖς διὰ τοῦ χρυσοκαταλλακτικοῦ καὶ σημαδαρικοῦ πόρου, μετερχομένους, ἐξεπαιδεύετο παρ' αὐτῶν τὴν τοιαύτην πραγματείαν καταμαθεῖν ... Οὗτος ... ὑπεχώρησεν ἡσύχως ἐκ τῆς τῶν γονέων ψυχοβλαβοῦς παιδαγωγίας ... Πολλῆς οὖν κινήσεως γενομένης ἐκ τῶν γονέων, ἴσχυσαν βίᾳ σχεδὸν ἀπαγάγαι αὐτὸν εἰς τὰ ἴδια· καὶ μετ' ὀλίγας ἡμέρας περιπίπτει εἰς ἀσθένειαν ὁ αὐτὸς Γεώργιος ... ἄγουσιν αὐτὸν οἱ γονεῖς ἐν τῷ ναῷ τοῦ Προδρόμου ... καὶ ποιήσαντες τὰ ἐν ἔθει ἀφέντες αὐτὸν ἀνεχώρησαν ... κοιμωμένου αὐτοῦ ... ὁρᾷ ἐν τῷ ὕπνῳ αὐτοῦ ... τὸν ἅγιον Ἀρτέμιον ... καὶ ἐκτεῖνας ὁ ἅγιος τὴν χεῖρα αὐτοῦ καὶ ἀρξάμενος ἀπὸ τῆς κεφαλῆς αὐτοῦ τοῦ νοσοῦντος μέχρι τῶν ὀνύχων τῶν ποδῶν αὐτοῦ ἐποίησεν τὸν τίμιον σταυρὸν ... ἔξυπνος δὲ γενόμενος ὁ νοσῶν Γεώργιος καὶ πρὸς τὸν ὄνειρον ἐν ἑαυτῷ γενόμενος ψηλαφᾷ ἑαυτὸν καὶ ηὗρεν ὅλον τῷ σῶμα αὐτοῦ ὑγιῆ ὄντα· ἦν δὲ ἰδεῖν τὸν ἀκίνητον ἐξαλλόμενον καὶ ἀποτρέχοντα καὶ τῷ σωτῆρι Χριστῷ εὐχαριστοῦντα καὶ τοῖς αὐτοῦ ἁγίοις, ὡς τοιαύτης καὶ τοσαύτης καὶ θείας ἐπισκέψεως ἠξιωμένος. (*MA* 38; trans. Crisafulli and Nesbitt 1997, 197–200)

Compared to the previous examples, this miracle has several differences. In this tale, the child is introduced before the parent(s) in the manner an adult protagonist would be introduced. Specifically, his name (and nickname) is offered, followed by his age and vocation (a reader in the church of the Forerunner). Moreover, in contrast to the observations made so far with regard to miracles concerning children, this time it is the parents' biographical profile that is lacking. They remain anonymous, with only their occupation mentioned (bartering and exchanging gold). This mention of their profession, as it seems, occurs only because it becomes relevant to the plot (the child despises the parents' occupation). Furthermore, a difference from other healings of children discussed so far is also observed in regard to the mother's actions. As discussed, mothers maintain an active stance, bringing their child to the saint's shrine and praying, executing saintly directions, and assisting the process of the cure. In this case, however, though the parents do take the child to the church of the Forerunner to be healed, surprisingly enough, after they perform the customary rites, they "dump" the child there and leave. The cure is performed in the child's dream, with the child acquiring an active role.

It would, therefore, seem that in this miracle the parents are almost an afterthought in the whole process, a development which severely compromises the hermeneutic path followed in this investigation. Nevertheless, a more careful glance changes this picture, as it seems that it is because the hagiographer intentionally subverts some well-known conventions that the impression of reversal arises. In particular, the meaning of this miracle tale is contained in the fact that this child is not an ordinary child, and this is implied by the hagiographer from the very beginning, in the phrase "even though he was a child" ("εἰ καὶ παῖς ἐτύγχανεν"), through the use of which the hagiographer mentions that the child did not approve of his parents' business although he was trained to follow it. Hence, this child protagonist is invested with attributes and wisdom not ordinary for his age. In turn, since he is not an ordinary child, he is not silent like other child protagonists of healing miracles. Instead, George acquires a voice after his cure, and after he wakes up, he runs about glorifying God. In this respect, he also acts as the implied first storyteller of his cure since no other character besides George witnessed the dream. Hence, the hagiographer, exploiting the conventions that arise when the child is the subject of the miracle tale, reverses them to highlight the case of a spiritually advanced child. The treatment of George as a special and not an ordinary child is further exploited in the next tale of the collection (Miracle 39), which serves as the continuation of the story of George. This chapter relates that George decided to become a monk. After he is pursued and confronted by his impious parents, who wanted to prevent him from becoming a monk, he is finally allowed to follow his spiritual vocation. Thus, the different treatment of the child (compared to that of other children) in the first tale becomes the launching pad for the author to narrate the child's spiritual career in the second tale.

Conclusions

In sum, it seems that Byzantine hagiographers realized that when the protagonist of their miracle tale was a child, both typical structure and plot needed to be adjusted. Depending on the escort of the child, a mother or – rarely – a father, a grandmother or a wet nurse, other characters might also enter the scene of the miracle, adding more strands to the common elements of form and content. These adjustments resulted in a healing process which was premised on the mother–child relationship. The child seems to be treated as a unit along with the mother, who shares the child's pain and acts as the cause of the cure and the link between the child and the saint. This bond is treated as essential in narrative terms since it constitutes a force that drives the plot forward. Moreover, certain gender-based differences between the relationship of mothers and children and that of fathers and children have been unveiled, since fathers seem to be more emotionally distant and less practically engaged with the child's situation. Another important aspect that is made manifest in healing tales about children are the restrictions as regards the method of cure on the part of the saint. The child's body seems to be treated with respect, and cures come to be tailored to its needs and daily routine instead of assuming an extravagant or ambiguous form. It would thus seem that Byzantine authors were alert in their choice of the suffering patient and extremely methodical in the manner in which structure and plot needed to be manipulated in order to accommodate that choice.

References

Texts: Editions and Translations

Alwis, A. ed. 2011. *Celibate Marriages in Late Antique and Byzantine Hagiography: The Lives of Saints Julian and Basilissa, Andronikos and Athanasia, and Galaktion and Episteme*. London: Bloomsbury Academic, 250–268.

Crisafulli, V.S., and. J.W. Nesbitt. trans. 1997. *The Miracles of St. Artemios: A Collection of Miracle Stories by an Anonymous Author of Seventh-Century Byzantium*. Leiden, New York and Cologne: Brill.

Dagron, G. ed. 1978. *Vie et miracles de sainte Thècle: Texte grec, traduction et commentaire*. Subsidia Hagiographica 62. Paris: Société des Bollandistes, 285–412.

Deubner, L. ed. 1907. *Kosmas und Damian: Texte und Einleitung*. Leipzig and Berlin: Teubner.

Flusin, B. ed. 1992. *Saint Anastase le Perse et l'histoire de la Palestine au début du VIIe siècle*. Vol. 1. Paris: CNRS Editions, 108–153.

Gascou, J. ed. 2006. *Miracles des saints Cyr et Jean (BHG 477–79)*. Paris: De Boccard.

Johnson, S.F. trans. 2012. "Miracles of Saint Thekla," in A.-M. Talbot, and S.F. Johnson (eds) *Miracle Tales from Byzantium*. Dumbarton Oaks Medieval Library 12. Cambridge, MA and London: Harvard University Press, 2–183.

Papadopoulos-Kerameus, A. ed. 1909. *Varia graeca sacra*. St Petersburg: Kirschbaum, 1–75.

Rupprecht, E. ed. 1935. *Cosmae et Damiani sanctorum medicorum vita(m) et miracula e codice Londinensi*. Berlin: Junker und Dünnhaupt.

Marcos, N.F. ed. 1975. *Los Thaumata di Sofronio: Contribucion al estudio de la 'incubatio' cristiana*. Madrid: Instituto Antonio de Nebrija.

Secondary Works

Alwis, A. 2012. "Men in Pain: Masculinity, Medicine and the *Miracles* of St. Artemios," *Byzantine and Modern Greek Studies* 36 (1): 1–19.

Antoniadis-Bibicou, H. 1973. "Quelques notes sur l'enfant de la moyenne époque byzantine (du VIe au XIe siècle)," *Annales de démographie historique: Enfant et sociétés*, 77–84.

Ariantzi, D. 2012. *Kindheit in Byzanz: Emotionale, geistige und materielle Entwicklung im familiären Umfeld vom 6. bis zum 11. Jahrhundert*. Millennium-Studien 36. Berlin and Boston: De Gruyter.

———. 2018. *Coming of Age in Byzantium: Adolescence and Society*. Millennium-Studien 69. Berlin and Boston: De Gruyter.

Booth, AP. 2011. "Orthodox and Heretic in the Early Byzantine Cult(s) of Saints Cosmas and Damian," in P. Sarris, M. Dal Santo, and P. Booth (eds) *An Age of Saints? Power, Conflict and Dissent in Early Medieval Christianity*. Leiden and Boston: Brill, 114–128.

Brubaker, L. 2013. "Preface," in L. Brubaker, and S. Tougher (eds) *Approaches to the Byzantine Family*. Birmingham Byzantine and Ottoman Studies 14. Farnham: Ashgate, xix–xxv.

Cojocaru, O.-M. 2022. *Byzantine Childhood: Representations and Experiences of Children in Middle Byzantine Society*. London: Routledge.

Constantinou, S. 2010. "Grotesque Bodies in Hagiographical Tales: The Monstrous and the Uncanny in Byzantine Collections of Miracle Stories," *Dumbarton Oaks Papers* 64: 43–54.

———. 2013. "Healing Dreams in Early Byzantine Miracle Collections," in S. Oberhelman (ed.) *Dreams, Healing, and Medicine in Greece: From Antiquity to the Present*. Farnham: Ashgate, 189–198.

———. 2014. "The Morphology of Healing Dreams: Dream and Therapy in Byzantine Collections of Miracle Stories," in C. Angelidi, and D. Calofonos (eds) *Dreaming in Byzantium and Beyond*. Farnham: Ashgate, 21–34.

Constantinou, S., and A. Andreou. 2022. "The Voices of the Tale: The Storyteller in Early Byzantine Collective Biographies, Miracle Collections, and Collections of Edifying Tales," *Byzantine and Modern Greek Studies* 46 (1): 24–40.

Efthymiadis, S. 1999. "Greek Byzantine Collections of Miracles: A Chronological and Bibliographical Survey," *Symbolae Osloenses* 74 (1): 195–211.

———. 2004. "A Day and Ten Months in the Life of a Lonely Bachelor: The *Other Byzantium* in *Miracula S. Artemii* 18 and 22," *Dumbarton Oaks Papers* 58: 1–26.

———. 2014. "Collections of Miracles (Fifth–Fifteenth Centuries)," in S. Efthymiadis (ed.) *The Ashgate Research Companion to Byzantine Hagiography*, vol. 2: *Genres and Contexts*. Farnham: Ashgate, 103–142.

Gascou, J. 2007. "Les origines du culte des saints Cyr et Jean," *Analecta Bollandiana* 125: 241–281.

Hennessy, C. 2008. *Images of Children in Byzantium*. Aldershot: Ashgate.

Johnson, S.F. 2006. *The Life and Miracles of Thekla: A Literary Study*. Hellenic Studies 13. Cambridge, MA: Harvard University Press.

Kažhdan, A. 1996. "Two Notes on the *Vita of Anastasios the Persian*," in C.N. Constantinides, N.M. Panagiotakes, E. Jeffreys, and A.D. Angelou (eds) *ΦΙΛΕΛΛΗΝ: Studies in Honour of Robert Browning*. Venice: Istituto Ellenico di Studi Bizantini e Postbizantini di Venezia, 151–157.

Laiou, A.E. 2011. *Women, Family and Society in Byzantium*. Edited by C. Morrisson, and R. Dorin. Ashgate: Variorum.

Lieu, S. 1996. "From Villain to Saint and Martyr: The Life and After-Life of Flavius Artemius, *dux Aegypti*," *Byzantine and Modern Greek Studies* 20: 56–76.

Macrides, R. 1999. "Substitute Parents and Their Children in Byzantium," in M. Corbier (ed.) *Adoption et fosterage*. Paris: Editions de Boccard, 307–319.

Moffatt, A. 1986. "The Byzantine Child," *Social Research* 53 (4): 705–723.

Narro, Á. 2010. "Lo scontro tra formazione classica e pensiero cristiano: La vita e miracoli di santa Tecla," *Greco-Latina Brunensia* 15: 127–138.

Papaconstantinou, A., and A.-M. Talbot. eds. 2009. *Becoming Byzantine: Children and Childhood in Byzantium*. Washington, DC: Dumbarton Oaks. Research Library and Collection

Prinzing, G. 2009. "Observations on the Legal Status of Children and the Stages of Childhood in Byzantium," in Papaconstantinou and Talbot 2009, 15–34.

Ritzer, K. 1970. *Le mariage dans les églises chrétiennes du Iᵉʳ au XIᵉ siècle*. Paris: Editions du Cerf.

Index

Note: **Bold** page numbers refer to tables; *italic* page numbers refer to figures and page numbers followed by "n" denote endnotes.

Elisha, Hebrew prophet 219, 220
emotions 17, 21, 34, 38, 39, 41–43, 74,
    78, 86, 132, 139, 146, 202, 210,
    215, 223, 249–253, 255–257, 260;
    gendered 4
Empiricism 163; *see also* Galen
Enkomion on Andrew of Crete 13n50
Enkomion on Kirikos and Ioulitta 13n50
epilepsy 72, 73n13, 111, 118–119, 126, 161
Erasistratus of Ceos, physician, 3ʳᵈ c. BC,
    171n47
ethnography 152, 153, 155n9, 156n11,
    164–169, 165n33, 165n35, 176, 177
Eucharist 199
Euchologion 97
Eunice, mother of Timothy the Apostle 217
Euripides, Greek tragedian, 5ᵗʰ c. BC, 215
Euryphon of Knidos, physician, 460–440
    BC 108
Eusebios (Eus.), bishop and Church
    Historian, AD ca. 264–ca. 340, 38,
    39; *Ecclesiastical History* (*EH*)
    38n125
Eve, biblical figure 185n10
Exodus (*Ex*) 206, 211–216, 224n100
eye disease 35, 109–113, 120, 124, 125
Ezekiel the Tragedian, Jewish dramatist,
    ca. 3ʳᵈ c. BC 46, 214–216; *Exagoge*
    (Ezek.) 214, 224, 224n100

father 7, 7n23, 7n24, 14–18, 20, 30, 39–41,
    43–46, 131, 215, 216, 219, 222,
    223, 228–240, 240n26, 245–250,
    255, 256–258, 256n22, 260
Fausta, empress, AD 290–326, 183,
    187–189, *188, 190,* 191
Favorinus, sophist philosopher, AD ca.
    85–ca. 155, 14, 145n42, 237
Fecunditas, personification 188, 189
Felicitas, personification 17, 26, *188,* 189
Felicity, Christian martyr, 2ⁿᵈ–3ʳᵈ c. AD,
    6–9, 7n23–24, 17, 18, 22–30, 37,
    45, 130–132, 147
Feriale Duranum, military calendar of
    feast days dating from the rule of
    Severus Alexander 223
fertility 45, 196, 199, 200, 207–209; *see
    also Fecunditas,* personification
Festus Pompeius Sextus, scholar, late
    2ⁿᵈ c. AD 231; *On the Meaning of
    Words* 231
fever 29, 31, 110, 111, 113, 119, 131, 143
figurine 46, 185n10, 189, *190,* 234n15
Fine, S.(teven) 218, 218n72

foetus 11n41, 15, 23, 23n82, 24, 26, 145,
    153n3, 156, 173
food: consumption 75–81; semi-solid
    food/solid food 34n110, 132, 134,
    135; *see also* infant, nutrition of;
    weaning
Formisano, M.(arco) 6n22, 7n23, 8n26,
    9n32, 17, 17n64, 36, 36n117, 130n1
Forum Holitorium 233, 233n14
Frankfurter, D.(avid) 94, 94n13, 96, 96n23,
    96n26–30, 130n2

galaktology 152–155; elite authorship of
    184–185, 164n32; ethnocentrism
    of 153n3, 156n11, 164–169;
    vocabulary of milk in 31, 137
Galenism 116, 155, 160, 162; *see also*
    Galen
Galen (Gal.), physician, AD 129–ca.
    216/217, 14, 73n11, 109, 111,
    113–114, 117, 125, **140**, 153–154,
    157–158, 162–163, 168–169,
    169n42, 176–177; *Affected Parts*
    (*Loc. Aff.*) 156, 157, 157n12, 170;
    On the Anatomy of the Uterus
    108n22; *Bloodletting* (*[Ven.
    Sect.]*) 171n47; *Bloodletting
    against Erasistratus* (*Ven. Sect.
    Er.*) 171, 171n47–48, 172,
    174n52; *Bloodletting against
    the Erasistrateans at Rome* (*Ven.
    Sect. Er. Rom.*) 171n47; *On the
    Capacities of Foodstuffs* (*Alim.
    Fac.*) 114n63, 115n66; *On the
    Capacities of Simple Drugs*
    (*SMT*) 114n63, 115, 115n65, **143**,
    162n22; *On the Composition of
    Drugs According to Places* (*Comp.
    Med. Loc.*) 113n55–56, 115n67;
    *On the Function of the Parts of
    the Body* (*UP*) 14n60, 115n66,
    171n49; *On Good and Bad Humour*
    108n19; *Hygiene* (*San. Tu.*) 28n95,
    34n110, 83, 115n68, 133, 133n13,
    134, 153n3, 158, 159, 159n16,
    161, 165n34, 166, 173, 174,
    174n50–51; *Therapeutic Method*
    (*MM*) 106, 108, 120, 124, 155,
    168; *On Withering* 108n19; *see
    also* Empiricism; Galenism; Galen
    pseudo-
Galen pseudo- (Ps.-Gal.): *Medical
    Definitions* (*[Def. Med.]*) 81n28;
    On Procurable Drugs 118n88;

For Product Safety Concerns and Information please contact our EU
representative GPSR@taylorandfrancis.com
Taylor & Francis Verlag GmbH, Kaufingerstraße 24, 80331 München, Germany

www.ingramcontent.com/pod-product-compliance
Lightning Source LLC
Chambersburg PA
CBHW060447240326
41598CB00088B/3944

*9 7 8 1 0 3 2 2 0 8 7 6 3 *